Social Stigma and Drug Use

Telmo Mota Ronzani
Editor

Social Stigma and Drug Use

Gender Perspectives, Family Contexts and Intersections

Springer

Editor
Telmo Mota Ronzani
Department of Psychology
Universidade Federal Juiz de Fora
Juiz de Fora, Minas Gerais, Brazil

ISBN 978-3-031-94812-1 ISBN 978-3-031-94813-8 (eBook)
https://doi.org/10.1007/978-3-031-94813-8

The original submitted manuscript has been translated into English. The translation was done using artificial intelligence. A subsequent revision was performed by the author(s) to further refine the work and to ensure that the translation is appropriate concerning content and scientific correctness. It may, however, read stylistically different from a conventional translation.

This Springer imprint is published by the registered company Springer Nature Switzerland AG
The registered company address is: Gewerbestrasse 11, 6330 Cham, Switzerland

Preface

Social Stigma has been widely discussed in various sectors, especially in the field of health. From the work of Goffman, several authors from different areas of knowledge have been deepening conceptually the theme and producing derived concepts, which in turn have allowed for the production of some theoretical reflections, understandings of contexts, formulation of hypotheses, and empirical investigations. In particular, attention is drawn to the fact that Social Stigma and all its conceptual derivations have a significant impact at different levels, from individual and daily life to public policies that affect people with certain characteristics.

For more than 20 years, our research group has been investigating the theme, especially in relation to the area of alcohol, tobacco, and other drugs, and other health conditions. Over these decades, our research has also been improving and seeking to understand more complex and dynamic processes about the impacts that stigma has on the life of certain groups. Our initial studies focused on a more interactionist base and on the stigmatized/stigmatizer relationship, from a specific frame that characterized the interaction between the groups and how theoretically we could understand such a relationship.

Our research pointed to a high degree of stigmatization of people who use drugs or experience some type of mental suffering, especially among professionals in Primary Health Care or even Mental Health professionals. In addition, we sought to evaluate the impacts of stigma from the perspective of stigmatized groups (self-stigma). From such data, we sought to develop or adapt interventions to reduce stigma among people who use drugs, whether from self-stigma or stigmatization by professionals. From such work, we closed a cycle of our research, focusing on different social actors involved in the process of stigmatization. However, from field observations, theoretical deepening, and qualitative research, we discussed that there was a very important contextual and social substrate to understand such processes. Especially, we understand that the discrimination of specific groups and the issue of drug use in general occur from a specific social reality and not directly due to a given behavior or certain health condition, but in relation to the social context.

In this sense, we published the book entitled "*Drugs and Social Context. Social Perspectives on the Use of Alcohol and Other Drugs,*" where we sought to address how the social context influences the social perception of consumption, prevention, treatment and policies on drugs, mainly from specific social categories. In the same direction, we expanded our discussion that social stigma plays an important role in the formulations and implementations of drug policies, especially in the definition of repressive and excluding strategies of care for people who use drugs and their relationship with the violation of Human Rights.

Thus, we emphasize the importance of considering the Social Determinations in Health, which fundamentally influence access to care, the quality of prevention actions, treatment and social reintegration, and public policies. That is, from social categories like race/ethnicity, gender, territory, and social class, among others, the impacts of alcohol and other drug use and social stigma are better qualified.

Therefore, in this work we advance in the direction of understanding, in a contextual and intersectional way, how social stigma impacts the lives of people, drawing special attention to the issue of gender and family contexts, important topics but often neglected or even discussed in a decontextualized way and based on moralizing discourses. In this book we discuss, from a gender perspective, how such crossings impact the lives of people who use drugs in different conditions or even, indirectly, through the concept of Courtesy Stigma, aimed at people who do not present certain characteristics or are the direct target of stigmatization, but who are part of their daily lives, like the relatives of people who use drugs. Here, we draw attention mainly to women, especially mothers and partners of users who, due to the expectation of the social role of "caregiver," are often blamed for the condition or worsening of the family member's situation and, as a consequence, face prejudice, discrimination, increased mental care load, social isolation, etc.

Thus, this book is the result of the research and studies of the Research, Intervention and Evaluation Center on Alcohol and Other Drugs (CREPEIA), from the Federal University of Juiz de Fora (UFJF)—Brazil, which has been coordinating the Ibero-Latin American Network on Stigma and Drug Use for years. This book is funded by the National Council for Scientific and Technological Development (CNPq), through the Call CNPq/MCTI N° 10/2023, process 402075/2023-4. The authors are from different nationalities such as Brazil, Chile, Colombia, Spain, Mexico, and Uruguay and are also characterized by interdisciplinarity, from areas such as Biology, Social Sciences, Nursing, Medicine, Dentistry, Psychology, and Social Work.

The book is a collection composed of two parts and 17 chapters. The first part, called "Social Stigma and the Use of Psychoactive Substances Among Different Groups," begins with the chapter "Stigma in Problematic Uses and Public Health in Latin America and Spain," by Rodrigo Goycolea Martinic, Aldo Gabriel Tomassini Urti, Laura Pérez-Martorell de Vicente, and Víctor José Villanueva-Blasco, who provide a general conceptualization of the different types and levels of stigma and discuss their impacts in the context of alcohol and other drug use. In the second chapter "Stigma, Morality and Intersectionality in Drug Use," by Andrés Felipe Tirado-Otálvaro, Sandra Milena Velásquez-Vergara, and Edgar Orlando Arroyave-Álvarez, the authors present a critical perspective on how the topic is intersected by intersectionality, especially by gender, ethnicity, and social class categories and how it perpetuates situations of discrimination against specific groups. The chapter "Poverty, Gender, Drug Use and Stigma: An Intersectional Discussion from the Perspective of Homeless Women" by Weverton Corrêa Netto, Gabriel Martins Silva, Aldo Tomassini, Alexandre Aranha Arbia, Marina Fernandes Toledo Lourenço, Viviane Souza Pereira, and Telmo Mota Ronzani presents a discussion on the intersection of gender, social class, and race, from the scenario of homeless women, users of alcohol and other drugs. The chapter "Stigma in Vulnerable Drug-Using Populations: Migrants, Incarcerated Individuals, and Women," by Bárbara González Amado, Carolina Gorlero, Raquel Gallego and Víctor José Villanueva-Blasco, goes in the same direction, with a focus on people in refugee, immigration, and deprivation of liberty situations, and how such situations affect women who use drugs.

In the chapter "Stigma and Diagnostic Overshadowing in People with Mental Disorder and Substance Addiction," Concepción Martínez-Martínez, Leticia Olave, Vicente Gea-Caballero, and Víctor José Villanueva-Blasco bring a discussion on how the wrong ways of making and treating the diagnosis of mental disorders and problems with drug use are often loaded with stigma and bring direct consequences to the treatment and life of these people. The chapter "Stigma and Behavioral Addictions: Problematic Gambling and Video Game Addiction" by Víctor José Villanueva-Blasco, Dalila Eslava Pérez, and Antonio Rial-Boubeta discusses a growing topic which is game and internet dependencies, especially among young people, which are also loaded with stigma, and explores what are the consequences for these people. The chapter "Evaluation of an Online Intervention to Reduce Stigma Among Healthcare Workers in Latin America" by Jazmín Mora Ríos, Hugo Noel Valdivia Ramos, Jimena Kalawski Isla, and José Luis Vázquez Martínez is an empirical research where the effectiveness of an online intervention aimed at health professionals was evaluated with the aim of promoting changes in attitudes about drug use. The results suggest that such an intervention was promising in relation to the objectives.

In the chapter by Mario J. Domínguez García and Hugo César Moreno, "Extreme Experiences: Social Exclusion of Young Users of Inhalants, Crack, and Heroin in Mexico," through qualitative research among young Mexican drug users, accounts are presented and discussed regarding how the stigmatizing view turns into discrimination, especially with some cuts based on ethnicity and social class. The last chapter of the part by Jazmín Mora Rios, Marcela Tiburcio Sainz, and Adán Emir Aranda Reynoso "Stigma, Discrimination, and Substance Use. An Intersectionality-Based Approach" precisely highlights the importance of analysis through intersectionality, highlighting gender, race/ethnicity, and social class for a more contextualized understanding of the stigmatization processes affecting certain groups that consume alcohol and other drugs.

Part II, "Social Stigma, Gender, Family Contexts and Drug Use" begins with the chapter "Stigma, Prejudice and Media: Impacts on the Care of Relatives of People Who Use Drugs" by Joanna Gonçalves de Andrade Tostes-Bianchetti, Telmo Mota

Ronzani, Rodrigo Goycolea Martinic, and Pollyanna Santos da Silveira, where it is discussed how the media in general are a source of dissemination and reinforcement of stigmas, especially about gender role expectations and at the same time an important means of disseminating knowledge and awareness for the reduction of stigma. In the following chapter "An Analysis of Bibliographic Productions About the Use of Substances by LGBTQIA+ Youth in Brazil: Debating Stigma and Prejudice" by Juliana Perucchi, Caroline Nazar Machado Cândido, Fernanda Zeloschi, Arthur de Paula Ribeiro, and Thamiris Ribeiro, the authors present a systematic review that analyzes scientific productions in Brazil that investigate drug use among sexual minorities, more specifically among the LGBTQIA+ population, pointing to the consequences, not only of use, but also of prejudice toward these people. In the same direction, Rafael Ballester-Arnal, Maria Dolores Gil-Llario, Cristina Giménez-García, and Estefanía Ruiz-Palomino, in the chapter "When Drug Addiction Coexists with HIV Infection: The Interaction of Two Powerful Stigmas" make an important discussion between the intersections between stigma about drug use and people with HIV/AIDS, relating to prejudices about sexuality and gender.

In the chapter "Intrafamily Violence, Substance Use and Gender," Marianne Ramos Feijó, Eroy Aparecida da Silva, and Richard Alecsander Reichert draw attention to the contexts of intrafamily violence, mainly focused on gender issues and alcohol and other drug use and the importance of implementing actions and reinforcing public policies in the area. Antonio Vidal Infer, Juan Carlos Valderrama-Zurián, and Andrea Sixto Costoya in the chapter "Accessibility Barriers to Treatment from a Gender Perspective" discuss the main barriers to care in relation to alcohol and other drug use due to still hegemonic models that disregard the perspective of gender and sexuality as a way to improve access and quality of treatments. The same authors present another chapter entitled "The Role of the Caregiver in the Addiction Treatment Process" in which they draw attention to the need for support and support for caregivers and family members of people who use drugs, emphasizing that they are subjects fundamental in care processes and bear a significant burden of care, and are also stigmatized due to the health condition of their relatives. In the chapter "Stigmatization of Women Who Consume Alcohol in a Rural Indigenous Community in Central Mexico" by Marcela Tiburcio Sainz, Jazmín Mora Ríos, and Pilar Bernal Pérez, who also focus on the issue of gender in relation to the categories of territory and ethnicity with a study among indigenous women living in rural Mexico, where accounts of these women are presented, highlighting the difficulties of access to care, prejudice, and discrimination due to these social categories. The book concludes with the chapter "Addictive behaviors, gender and stigma: contributions to the understanding of the Portuguese case", authors Sandra Mendes, Sara Melo and Idalina Machado make a relationship between stigma, substance use and gender, using drug policies in Portugal as a backdrop.

As can be seen, this is a book with varied themes, which has as its backdrop the stigma in its different characterizations in relation to the consumption of psychoactive substances and the understanding of such phenomenon from the perspective of intersectionality, mainly with the categories of gender, sexuality, race/ethnicity, territory, and social class. As already mentioned, this is an interdisciplinary work with a rich discussion on the topic and precisely for this reason the work is of interest to various areas of knowledge, with different audiences such as academics and researchers, health professionals, managers and policy makers, activists, among others. We hope that with this work made by many hands and many perspectives we can contribute to the advancement and mainly to the change of the conditions of care and access to people who use drugs, as a form of basic human right.

Juiz de Fora, Brazil
December 2024

Telmo Mota Ronzani

Contents

Part I Social Stigma and the Use of Psychoactive Substances Among Different Groups

1 **Stigma in Problematic Uses and Public Health in Latin America and Spain** . . . 3
Rodrigo Goycolea Martinic, Aldo Gabriel Tomassini Urti, Laura Pérez-Martorell de Vicente, and Víctor José Villanueva-Blasco

2 **Stigma, Morality, and Intersectionality in Drug Use** . . . 15
Andrés Felipe Tirado-Otálvaro, Sandra Milena Velásquez-Vergara, and Edgar Orlando Arroyave-Álvarez

3 **Poverty, Gender, Drug Use, and Stigma: An Intersectional Discussion from the Perspective of Homeless Women** . . . 29
Weverton Corrêa Netto, Gabriel Martins Silva, Aldo Tomassini, Alexandre Aranha Arbia, Marina Fernandes Toledo Lourenço, Viviane Souza Pereira, and Telmo Mota Ronzani

4 **Stigma in Vulnerable Drug-Using Populations: Migrants, Incarcerated Individuals, and Women** . . . 45
Bárbara González Amado, Carolina Gorlero, Raquel Gallego, and Víctor José Villanueva-Blasco

5 **Stigma and Diagnostic Overshadowing in People with Mental Disorder and Substance Addiction** . . . 59
Concepción Martínez-Martínez, Leticia Olave, Vicente Gea-Caballero, and Víctor José Villanueva-Blasco

6 **Stigma and Behavioral Addictions: Problematic Gambling and Video Game Addiction** . . . 71
Víctor José Villanueva-Blasco, Dalila Eslava Pérez, and Antonio Rial-Boubeta

7 **Evaluation of an Online Intervention to Reduce Stigma Among Healthcare Workers in Latin America** 85
Jazmín Mora-Rios, Hugo Noel Valdivia Ramos, Jimena Kalawaski, and José Luis Vázquez

8 **Extreme Experiences: Social Exclusion of Young Users of Inhalants, Crack, and Heroin in Mexico** 97
Mario Joaquín Domínguez and Hugo César Moreno

9 **Stigma, Discrimination, and Substance Use: An Intersectionality-Based Approach** 113
Jazmín Mora-Rios, Marcela Tiburcio, and Adán Aranda

Part II Social Stigma, Gender, Family Contexts and Drug Use

10 **Stigma, Prejudice, and Media: Impact on the Care of Relatives of People Who Use Drugs** 125
Joanna Gonçalves de Andrade Tostes-Bianchetti, Telmo Mota Ronzani, Rodrigo Goycolea Martinic, and Pollyanna Santos da Silveira

11 **An Analysis of Bibliographic Productions About the Use of Substances by LGBTQIA+ Youth in Brazil: Debating Stigma and Prejudice** 137
Juliana Perucchi, Caroline Nazar Machado Cândido, Fernanda Zeloschi, Arthur de Paula Ribeiro, and Thamiris Ribeiro

12 **When Drug Addiction Coexists with HIV Infection: The Interaction of Two Powerful Stigmas** 153
Rafael Ballester-Arnal, Maria Dolores Gil-Llario, Cristina Giménez-García, and Estefanía Ruiz-Palomino

13 **Intrafamily Violence, Substance Use, and Gender** 167
Marianne Ramos Feijó, Eroy Aparecida da Silva, and Richard Alecsander Reichert

14 **Accessibility Barriers to Treatment from a Gender Perspective** 189
Antonio Vidal Infer, Juan Carlos Valderrama-Zurián, and Andrea Sixto-Costoya

15 **The Role of the Caregiver in the Addiction Treatment Process** 205
Antonio Vidal Infer, Juan Carlos Valderrama-Zurián, and Andrea Sixto-Costoya

16 **Stigmatization of Women Who Consume Alcohol in a Rural Indigenous Community in Central Mexico** 219
Marcela Tiburcio Sainz, Jazmín Mora Ríos, and Pilar Bernal Pérez

17 Addictive Behaviors, Gender, and Stigma: Contributions to the Understanding of the Portuguese Case 231
Sandra Mendes, Sara Melo, and Idalina Machado

Index 249

About the Editor and Contributors

About the Editor

Telmo Mota Ronzani Psychologist, Master in Social Psychology, Doctor in Health Sciences. Postdoctoral training in Mental Health, Public Health and Psychology. Full Professor of the Department of Psychology at the Federal University of Juiz de Fora (UFJF). Researcher at the Research and Intervention Center on Alcohol and Other Drugs (CREPEIA). Research Productivity Fellow 1C CNPq. Email: telmo.ronzani@ufjf.br

About the Contributors

Bárbara González Amado Doctor Cum Laude in Psychology with a doctoral award from the University of Santiago de Compostela (USC). Expert Psychologist in Forensic Psychology and Criminologist. Member of the Research Group on Health and Psycho-Social Adjustment (GI-SAPS) and Director of the Master's Degree in Legal Psychology at the Valencian International University (VIU). Email: barbara.gonzaleza@professor.universidadviu.com

Adán Emir Aranda Doctoral student of the Doctorate Program in Psychology. Faculty of Psychology, National Autonomous University of Mexico. UNAM. Lines of interest: Stereotypes, prejudices and discrimination, mental health, and its social determinants. Email: adan.arandar@gmail.com

Alexandre Aranha Arbia Social Worker. Doctor in Social Service from the Federal University of Rio de Janeiro (UFRJ). Professor of the permanent staff of the Postgraduate Program in Social Service at the Federal University of Juiz de Fora (UFJF). Brazil. Main areas of study: social theory, ideology, poverty and homeless population. Email: alexandre.arbia@ufjf.br

Edgar Orlando Arroyave-Álvarez Psychologist, Master in Philosophy, PhD. in Social and Human Sciences. Professor of the Faculty of Social and Human Sciences of the Universidad de Antioquia, Medellín, Colombia. Research Group: Psychology, Society and Subjectivity. Areas of study: Gender, psychology, psychology and politics of exclusion, contemporary sexualities. Email: edgar.arroyave@udea.edu.co

Rafael Ballester-Arnal PhD in Psychology. Full Professor at the University Jaume I of Castelló (Spain) in the Department of Basic Psychology, Clinical and Psychobiology. Director of the Castellón Salusex team. He works on promoting sexual health and psychological treatments for sexual problems in areas such as HIV infection, risky sexual behaviors, male sex workers, LGTBQIA+ population, sexual compulsivity, cybersex, sexuality and ICTs, paraphilias and minors in conflict with the law. Email: rballest@uji.es

Antonio Rial Boubeta Doctor in Social Psychology and Full Professor at the University of Santiago de Compostela. Author of more than 150 articles in international impact scientific journals and director of 21 doctoral theses. Member of the UNESCO High Commissioner for the fight against school bullying and cyberbullying. Collaborates with reference research centers such as the Center for Adolescent Behavioral Health Research (Harvard University), the Cognitive and Affective Regulation Laboratory (University of Lausanne) or the National Anti-Bullying Centre (Dublin City University). Email: antonio.rial.boubeta@usc.es

Caroline Nazar Machado Cândido Psychologist, doctoral student in Psychology in the line of Psychosocial Processes in Health, at the Federal University of Juiz de Fora (UFJF) and is part of the Research and Practice Center in Social Psychology, Public Policies and Health (PPS). She has a master's degree in psychology from the same university. She works in the areas of Social Psychology, Community Psychology, gender and sexualities and public policies. Email: nazarcarol@gmail.com

Andrea Sixto Costoya Graduate in Social Work and Doctor from the University of Valencia. Assistant Doctor Professor in the Department of Social Work, Faculty of Social Sciences, University of Valencia (Spain). Research line: Drug addiction, Gender and Health, Science Evaluation and Bibliometrics, Open Science and Open Data. Email: Andrea.Sixto@uv.es

Mario J. Domínguez García Department of Social Sciences in Health, Ramón de la Fuente Muñiz National Institute of Psychiatry, Mexico City, Mexico. Co-researcher at the University of Southern California. Collaborating Professor of the Research Line Youth and Contemporary Societies of the Graduate Program in Social Anthropology of the National School of Anthropology and History. Professor of the Psychology of Addictions Residency at the National Autonomous University of Mexico and INPRFM. Member of the National Hispanic Science Network (NHSN). Email: mariodom@inprf.gob.mx

Marianne Ramos Feijó Graduated in Psychology from Universidade Paulista; holds a Master's degree and PhD in Clinical Psychology from Pontifícia Universidade Católica de São Paulo (PUC-SP), with postdoctoral research at the Department of Psychobiology at Escola Paulista de Medicina—Universidade Federal de São Paulo (EPM-UNIFESP). She serves as an Assistant Professor and Supervisor in the Department of Psychology at Universidade Estadual Paulista (UNESP). Email: marianne.r.feijo@unesp.br

Raquel Gallego Cum Laude Doctor in Psychology from USC and expert in Forensic Psychology and Family Mediation, combines her work as a psychologist at the Women's Information Center attending to victims with her research career. Author of several scientific publications and speaker at conferences, she was awarded the Professor Mariano Yela Award for her contribution in the legal-forensic field. Member of the Health and Psycho-Social Adjustment Research Group (GI-SAPS). Email: raquel.gallego.gonzalez@gmail.com

Vicente Gea-Caballero Dean of the Faculty of Health Sciences of the Valencian International University (VIU). Nurse, Doctor in Health Sciences. Principal Researcher SALCOM Research Group. Main research lines: Community health, health literacy, chemsex, wastewater analysis, health services, healthcare in diversity. Member of Asociación de Enfermería Comunitaria (AEC) and Sociedad Española de Salud Pública y Administración Sanitaria (SESPAS). Editor in chief of the Revista Iberoamericana de Enfermería Comunitaria (RIdEC). Email: vagea@universidadviu.com

María Dolores Gil-Llario PhD in Psychology. Full Professor at the University of Valencia (Spain) in the Department of Developmental and Educational Psychology. Director of the Valencia Salusex team. Her work focuses on sexting, affective-sexual education in adolescents and young people who are in the protection system, and in people with intellectual development disorder. Email: dolores.gil@uv.es

Cristina Giménez-García Doctor in Psychology. Associate Professor of the Department of Basic Psychology, Clinical and Psychobiology at the Faculty of Health Sciences of the University Jaume I de Castelló (Spain). Her scientific-technical career, as part of the Salusex team, has sought to deepen the understanding and promotion of health behaviors, as well as the prevention of risk behaviors, in particular, those linked to online and offline sexuality. Email: gimenezc@uji.es

Carolina Gorlero Degree in Psychology and Master in Community Mental Health from the Universitá Degli Studi di Cagliari. She has more than 15 years of clinical experience in substance use disorders. Author of publications and research on SUD and its intersection with gender, human rights, migration and deprivation of liberty. Consultant for OAS-CICAD, IOM-UN Migration and PAHO. Member of the Argentine Chapter of ISSUP; and of the ITTC, Argentina. Coordinator of the Latin America subgroup on Stigma and Women with SUD for the OAS-CICAD; and part of the Board of Directors of ISSSUP Global since 2024. Email: gorlecaro@gmail.com

Antonio Vidal Infer Bachelor in Psychology and Doctor from the University of Valencia. Full Professor at the Department of History of Science and Documentation, Faculty of Medicine and Dentistry, University of Valencia (Spain). Co-director of the ITTC Spain. Research line: Drug addiction, Science Evaluation and Bibliometrics, Open Data. Email: Antonio.Vidal-Infer.@uv.es

Jimena Kalawski Head of the Demand Reduction Unit. Organization of American States. United States of America. Lines of interest: Demand reduction policies that include as essential elements, universal, selective and indicated prevention, environmental prevention, health promotion, early intervention, treatment, care, rehabilitation, social integration, recovery, reduction of adverse consequences and related support services. Chile. Email: kalawski@oas.org

Marina Fernandes Toledo Lourenço Psychologist from the Federal University of Juiz de Fora (UFJF). Master's in Social Service from UFJF. Currently a doctoral student in Social Psychology at the University of São Paulo (USP). Brazil. Main areas of study: Social psychology, female work; public policies. Email: marinaftoledo@gmail.com

Idalina Machado Sociologist, Master and Doctor in Sociology from the Faculty of Letters of the University of Porto. Assistant Professor at the Higher Institute of Social Service of Porto. Invited Assistant Professor at the Faculty of Letters of the University of Porto. Integrated Researcher at the Institute of Sociology of the University of Porto. Her research interests focus on Gender, Poverty, Social Exclusion, as well as the Right to the City and Housing. Email: idalina.machado@isssp.pt

Concepción Martínez Martínez Biologist and Specialist Nurse in Mental Health Care. Doctor in Health Sciences from the University of Alicante. Professor at the Universitat de València (Spain). The research lines in which I work are stigma and human rights in people with mental disorders. Collaborator with the ASIEM Mental Health Association in carrying out various activities with the associates. Email: concepcion.martinez-martinez@uv.es

Rodrigo Goycolea Martinic Research professor at the University of San Sebastián. Occupational Therapist from the University of Playa Ancha and Master in Drug Addiction from the University of Barcelona. Student of the Doctorate in Community Mental Health at the National University of Lanús. Young researcher of the millennium core for the evaluation and analysis of public drug policies. Specialist in evidence-based practices in the areas of prevention and treatment of drugs in adolescent and adult population with and without law infringement. Research line of instrument validation and stigma in people with mental health conditions. Email: rodrigo.goycolea@uss.cl

Sara Melo Bachelor in Sociology (2002) from FLUP, Master in Development and Social Insertion (2007) by FEP-UP and PhD in Sociology (2015) by FLUP. She is an Assistant Professor at the Higher Institute of Social Service of Porto and an Integrated Researcher at the Institute of Sociology of the University of Porto (ISUP).

Her current research interests focus, among others, on Social Intervention Projects through Art, Gender and Sexualities, and Sociology of Deviant Behavior. Email: sara.melo@isssp.pt

Sandra Mendes PhD (2020) in Social Service from ISCTE-IUL, Master's (2014) in Sociology from FLUP and Bachelor's (2012) in Social from ISSSP. Assistant Professor at the Higher Institute of Social Service of Porto; Integrated Researcher of the Lusíada Center for Research in Social Service and Social Intervention at the Lusíada University of Lisbon. Her current research interests focus on Addictive Behaviors and Dependencies with Psychoactive Substances, as well as Gender studies. Email: sandra.mendes@isssp.pt

Jazmín Mora-Ríos PhD in Psychology. Directorate of Epidemiological and Social Research, Mexico, Interventions to reduce stigma and discrimination in mental health and substance use. Mexico. Email: morarj@inprf.org.mx

Hugo César Moreno Member of the National System of Researchers CONHACyT Level 2. Collaborating Professor of the Line Youth and Contemporary Societies of the Graduate Program in Social Anthropology of the National School of Anthropology and History. Full time professor at the Institute of Social Sciences and Humanities "Alfonso Vélez Pliego" of the Benemérita Universidad Autónoma de Puebla. Email: hcmor@hotmail.com

Weverton Corrêa Netto Psychologist and master's student in Collective Health at the Federal University of Juiz de Fora (UFJF). Researcher at the Research, Evaluation and Intervention Center on Alcohol and other Drugs (CREPEIA/UFJF), Brazil. Main areas of study: Homeless Population, Prevention and Promotion in Mental Health and Alcohol, Tobacco and other Drugs. Email: weverton.correa@estudante.ufjf.br

Viviane Souza Pereira Social Worker. Associate Professor of the Faculty of Social Service of the Federal University of Juiz de Fora (UFJF). PhD in Social Service from the Federal University of Rio de Janeiro (UFRJ), Brazil. Main areas of study: Social issue, homeless population, management and public policies. Email: vivianesouza.pereira@ufjf.br

Dalila Eslava Pérez Doctor in Health Sciences. She has experience in school prevention and in addiction care in the prison population. She has worked as a researcher in the Research Network in Primary Care of Addictions (RIAPAd) and as an associate professor at the University of Zaragoza. She is currently a teacher at the Valencian International University (VIU) and a member of the Health and Psycho-Social Adjustment Research Group (GI-SAPS). Email: dalila.eslava@universidadviu.com

Juliana Perucchi Psychologist. Associate Professor IV of the Department of Psychology at the Federal University of Juiz de Fora (UFJF). Master and Doctor in psychology from the Federal University of Santa Catarina (UFSC). She leads the Research and Practice Center in Social Psychology, Public Policies and Health (PPS), linked to the

Postgraduate Program in Psychology at UFJF. She works in the areas of health, education, youth, public policies, sexual rights and sexualities, gender and feminisms, community psychology, and research-intervention. Email: juliana.perucchi@ufjf.br

Leticia Olave Porrúa Doctor in Psychology from the Complutense University of Madrid. Health and Forensic Psychologist. Research lines in substance addictions (alcohol, cannabis, cocaine, etc.), behavioral addictions (physical exercise, shopping, sex addiction, social networks, etc.), attachment, self-esteem, cognitive schemas, impulsivity, emotional dependence, violence in relationships. Email: leticiaolave@ucm.es

Richard Alecsander Reichert Graduated in Psychology from Universidade do Vale do Itajaí (UNIVALI); Postgraduate specialization in Neuropsychology, Psychopathology and Mental Health from Universidade do Extremo Sul Catarinense (UNESC); and PhD in Sciences at the Department of Psychobiology at Escola Paulista de Medicina—Universidade Federal de São Paulo (EPM-UNIFESP), with specialization in Medicine and Sociology of Drug Abuse. He works as a Researcher affiliated with the Drug Dependence Unit (UDED-UNIFESP); Researcher at the Interdisciplinary Center for Studies in Neuroscience, Health and Education in Adolescence (CIENCIA-UNIFESP); Collaborator at the Laboratory of Basic and Applied Cognitive Psychology at Universidade Federal de Santa Catarina (LPCOG-UFSC); and member of the Brazilian Association of Behavioral Psychology and Medicine (ABPMC), the Brazilian Multidisciplinary Association for Drug Studies (ABRAMD), the International Network on Brief Interventions for Alcohol and Other Drugs (INEBRIA), and the Confederación de Adolescencia y Juventud de Iberoamérica, Italia y Caribe (CODAJIC). Email: reichert@unifesp.br

Arthur de Paula Ribeiro Psychologist, master's student in Psychology from the Federal University of Juiz de Fora (UFJF), in the line of Psychosocial Processes in Health. He is part of the Research and Practice Center in Social Psychology, Public Policies and Health (PPS). Postgraduate (lato sensu) in Public Health from Paulista University (UNIP). He works in the areas of gender and sexuality studies in intersection with Critical Social Psychology and also Community Psychology, in addition to the constant dialogue with public health and mental health. Email: arthurribeiropsi@gmail.com

Thamiris Ribeiro Psychologist, master in Psychology from the Federal University of Juiz de Fora (UFJF). She is part of the Core of Research and Practices in Social Psychology, Public Policies and Health (PPS). Activist of the social movement Levante Popular da Juventude. She works in the areas of public policies, alcohol and other drugs, Community Social Psychology, decoloniality, and black feminism. Email: ribeirothamiris97@gmail.com

Estefanía Ruíz-Palomino Associate Professor of the Department of Basic Psychology, Clinical and Psychobiology in the Faculty of Health Sciences at University Jaume I of Castelló (Spain). Doctorate in Psychology, her research has focused on the modeling of risky sexual behavior in young people and the design and validation of a preventive intervention. As part of the Salusex team, she has participated in projects on promoting health behaviors, cybersex addiction, and psychosocial aspects related to AIDS. Email: eruiz@uji.es

Eroy Aparecida da Silva Graduated in Psychology from Organização Paulista de Educação e Cultura da Faculdade Paulistana; Specialist in Social Psychology from Instituto Sedes Sapientiae; Specialist in Family and Couple Therapy from Pontifícia Universidade Católica de São Paulo (PUC-SP); and PhD in Sciences at the Department of Psychobiology at Escola Paulista de Medicina—Universidade Federal de São Paulo (EPM-UNIFESP), with specialization in Medicine and Sociology of Drug Abuse. She works as a Psychologist and Coordinator of the School Clinic at the Drug Dependence Unit (UDED) in the Department of Psychobiology at UNIFESP; and is a member of the Brazilian Multidisciplinary Association for Drug Studies (ABRAMD) and the Brazilian Mental Health Association (ABRASME). Email: eroyntc@gmail.com

Gabriel Martins Silva Undergraduate in Psychology at the Federal University of Juiz de Fora (UFJF). Researcher at the Center for Research, Evaluation and Intervention in Alcohol and other Drugs (CREPEIA/UFJF), Brazil. Main areas of study: Social Psychology, Psychometrics and Community Psychology. Email: martinssilvagabriel@gmail.com

Pollyanna Santos da Silveira Psychologist, Master in Psychology and Doctor in Health Sciences. Professor of the Graduate Programs in Psychology at the Catholic University of Petrópolis (UCP) and Federal University of Juiz de Fora (UFJF). Researcher at the Center for Research, Intervention and Evaluation in Alcohol and Drugs (CREPEIA/UFJF). Email: pollyannassilveira@gmail.com

Andrés Felipe Tirado-Otálvaro Nurse, Master in Epidemiology, PhD. in Public Health. Professor at the Faculty of Nursing, Universidad Pontificia Bolivariana, Medellín, Colombia. Research Group in Care. Areas of study: stigma toward people who use drugs, public health, epidemiology, and care. Email: felipe.tirado@upb.edu.co

Aldo Tomassini Psychologist, PhD in Psychology from the University of the Republic (Udelar) and Master in Clinical Psychology, researcher at the Clinical Research Center in Psychology of the Faculty of Psychology of Udelar and Technical Secretary of the Departmental Board of Drugs of Montevideo in the Municipality of Montevideo. My studies focus on clinical interventions in psychology and the study of substance use in general. Email: Aldo.Tomassini@imm.gub.uy

Joanna Gonçalves de Andrade Tostes-Bianchetti Psychologist, Master and Doctor in Psychology. Federal University of Juiz de Fora, Institute of Human Sciences, Postgraduate Program in Psychology, Reference Center in Research, Intervention and Evaluation in Alcohol and Other Drugs (CREPEIA). Email: joanna@tostes.org

Juan Carlos Valderrama-Zurián Doctor of Medicine from the University of Valencia. University Professor in the Department of History of Science and Documentation, Faculty of Medicine and Dentistry, University of Valencia (Spain). Director of the UISYS group and co-director of the ITTC Spain. Research line: Drug addiction, Gender and Health, Science Evaluation and Bibliometrics, Open Data. Email: Juan.Valderrama@uv.es

Hugo Valdivia-Ramos PhD in Medical Sciences. Master's and Doctoral Program in Medical and Dental Sciences. National Autonomous University of Mexico (UNAM). Mexico. Interventions to reduce the stigma and discrimination of mental illnesses. Mexico. Email: hnvaldiviar@gmail.com

José Luis Vázquez Specialist in Demand Reduction. Organization of American States. United States of America. Lines of interest: Demand reduction policies that include as essential elements, universal, selective and indicated prevention, environmental prevention, health promotion, early intervention, treatment, care, rehabilitation, social integration, recovery, reduction of adverse consequences and related support services. Email: jvazquez@oas.org

Sandra Milena Velásquez-Vergara Nurse, Specialist in Quality Management and Audit of Health Services, PhD. in Nursing. Professor at the Faculty of Nursing, Universidad de Antioquia, Medellín, Colombia. Research Group: Social Policies and Health Services. Areas of study: Care, perioperative care, gender, contemporary sexualities, masculinity, stigma. Email: sandra.velasquez3@udea.edu.co

Laura Pérez-Martorell de Vicente General Health Psychologist and Educational Counselor. Expert in problematic uses, Personality Disorders and Eating Behavior Disorders. She works with child and adolescent population at Centro Puerta Abierta (Logroño, La Rioja). Email: lauraperezdevte@gmail.com

Víctor José Villanueva-Blasco Doctor in Psychology. Professor and Director of the Master's Degree in Prevention of Drug Addiction and other Addictive Behaviors at the Valencian International University (VIU). Member of the Research Network in Primary Care of Addictions (RIAPAd); of International Society of Substance Use Professionals (ISSUP), Spain; of the International Center for Technology Transfer in Addictions (ITTC), Spain. Associate Editor of International Journal of Mental Health and Addiction and Journal of Prevention. Email: vjvillanueva@universidadviu.com

Fernanda Zeloschi Psychologist, master's student in Psychology in the line of Psychosocial Processes in Health at the Federal University of Juiz de Fora (UFJF) and part of the Research and Practice Center in Social Psychology, Public Policies and Health (PPS). She has a lato sensu postgraduate degree (specialization) in Social Psychology and Communities from the Faculty of Governance Engineering and Education (FGE). She works in the areas of Social Psychology, Community Psychology, gender and sexualities, and public policies. Email: fernandazeloschi@gmail.com

Part I
Social Stigma and the Use of Psychoactive Substances Among Different Groups

Chapter 1
Stigma in Problematic Uses and Public Health in Latin America and Spain

Rodrigo Goycolea Martinic, Aldo Gabriel Tomassini Urti, Laura Pérez-Martorell de Vicente, and Víctor José Villanueva-Blasco

1.1 Introduction

Goffman (1963) defines stigma as a social process where an individual is negatively classified due to a specific attribute. Link and Phelan (2001) propose a multidimensional approach to stigma, describing it as a process that involves several interrelated components: the attribution of differences, labels between groups, the creation of negative stereotypes, and the separation between "them" and "us," which reinforces discrimination. This process of categorization is a feature of the functioning of social cognition, a cognitive mechanism that labels and classifies people based on the social and cultural construction forged from interpersonal relationships, and imposes a negative label on certain people (Michaels et al., 2012). The emotional reactions of the stigmatized group and the stigmatizer are key to identifying the stigmatizing dynamics (Jones et al., 1984; Link et al., 2004) and describe six dimensions of stigma: concealability, course, disruptiveness, aesthetics, origin, and

R. G. Martinic
Escuela de Terapia Ocupacional, Facultad de Odontología y Ciencias de la Rehabilitación, Universidad San Sebastián, Santiago, Chile
e-mail: rodrigo.goycolea@uss.cl

A. G. T. Urti
Centro de Investigación Clínico en Psicología, Facultad de Psicología, Universidad de la República, Montevideo, Uruguay

Departamento de Desarrollo Social, Intendencia de Montevideo, Montevideo, Uruguay
e-mail: aldo.tomassini@imm.gub.uy

L. P.-M. de Vicente
Centro Puerta Abierta, Logroño, Spain

V. J. Villanueva-Blasco (✉)
Valencian International University, Valencia, Spain
e-mail: vjvillanueva@universidadviu.com

T. Mota Ronzani (ed.), *Social Stigma and Drug Use*,
https://doi.org/10.1007/978-3-031-94813-8_1

dangerousness, each of which influences how stigma affects social interactions. The process of stigmatization is dependent on the culture, education, and morality of each society at a given historical moment (Pedersen, 2005).

Intersectional stigma, which particularly affects Black and Hispanic people, exacerbates the negative effects of drug dependence, creating persistent health inequalities and also people with multiple stigmatized identities face intensified stigma, which can hinder access to healthcare and support services (Walters et al., 2023). A global understanding of the stigma system can guide public health strategies (Friedman et al., 2021).

1.2 Concept and Impact of Stigma in Problematic Uses

People with problematic uses are often negatively labeled, and their problems are perceived as a lack of will or a "vice," rather than a health problem, which aggravates their situation (Mota et al., 2014). Likewise, substance use disorders (SUDs) are among the most stigmatized conditions (Ronzani et al., 2009; Van Boekel et al., 2013). This means that people who have a substance abuse disorder are treated at a legal and social level (Prado et al., 2015).

Stigma reinforces social and psychological barriers that make it difficult to seek help for fear of discrimination or legal problems (Cunningham et al., 1993; Link et al., 1997). Stigma affects during and after treatment, reducing adherence and increasing treatment abandonment (Mota et al., 2014). In addition, drug users are legally penalized, which reinforces stigma and hinders their inclusion (Cañarte-Quimis et al., 2023).

1.2.1 Types of Stigma and Their Consideration from Problematic Uses

The literature identifies several types of stigma:

1. Social or public stigma: This stigma occurs when society manifests prejudices and negative stereotypes toward people with problematic uses, resulting in discrimination (Vicario Cañas & De la Villa Moral Jiménez, 2016).
2. Structural/institutional stigma: Refers to systematic discrimination in organizations and policies that perpetuate stigma (Hatzenbuehler & Link, 2014).
3. Provider stigma: Is the prejudice exercised by health professionals that can affect patient care (Da Valle-Chervellera et al., 2024; Knaak et al., 2017). In addition, the stigma surrounding non-medical substance use leads to internalized shame and fear of professional repercussions among providers (McNeely et al., 2023).

4. Self-stigma: Occurs when individuals internalize the prejudices and see themselves as inferior or "guilty" of their condition, which can reduce self-esteem and hinder their recovery (Brohan et al., 2010).
5. Vicarious or courtesy stigma: This type of stigma affects people close to the person suffering from an addiction, such as family members or health professionals, who are also stigmatized and may suffer social and emotional isolation (El-Tantawy et al., 2010).

1.2.2 Stigma in Problematic Use and Public Health

Stigmatization and discrimination are intrinsically linked to inequalities (Breilh, 2010; Vázquez & Stolkiner, 2009). In this line, Hatzenbuehler et al. (2013) underline that stigma generates health inequalities, which poses a challenge to social justice. In the field of public health, this discrimination affects drug users, who, when labeled as patients with substance use disorders (SUD), face barriers in accessing fundamental rights such as health, education, and work (Link et al., 2006).

Conventional public health, from its functionalist approach, perceives the population as objects and addresses problems from an instrumental reason, which limits its ability to respond to complex phenomena such as drug use (Valencia Arredondo, 2011). Thus, solutions such as penalization and medicalization are proposed, which do not address the problem from its social roots but from a perspective that individualizes collective problems (Conrad, 1992; Vázquez & Stolkiner, 2009). Medicalization, driven by the dominant biomedical discourse, has negative implications for social justice, as it facilitates the adoption of medical solutions instead of economic or political approaches (Conrad, 1992). This approach is reinforced by the association between the use of illegal substances and crime, which legitimizes both penalization and medicalization (Conrad, 1992; Vázquez & Stolkiner, 2009). Likewise, discourses that equate the recreational use of illegal drugs with SUDs distort and magnify the phenomenon, associating it with crime and danger, which objectifies the problem and makes individuals invisible (Vázquez & Stolkiner, 2009). This invisibility is aggravated by the limitations of traditional public health, which tends to marginalize vulnerable sectors and ignore minorities (Valencia Arredondo, 2011).

Corrigan (2004) points out that this can result in unemployment, housing exclusion, and low quality of life. Hatzenbuehler and Link (2014) indicate that public health policies often marginalize people with problematic uses, especially in vulnerable populations, perpetuating health inequalities. In this sense, the World Health Organization (WHO) (2005) emphasized the importance of reducing stigma to improve the quality of health services and proposed policies that promote their inclusion.

On the other hand, health professionals perpetuate stigmas through discriminatory attitudes, which also contribute to treatment abandonment. Corrigan et al. (2017) and Mojtabai et al. (2011) underline that those patients who perceive these attitudes among health professionals are less likely to seek help. Provider stigma is manifested in the lack of trust in users and in decisions that are imposed without taking into account their opinions (Fernández, 2017). This causes users to avoid going to health services even in extreme situations due to shame and the stigmatizing treatment they perceive, which affects their confidence in the health system (Garpenhag & Dahlman, 2021; Van Boekel et al., 2015). On the other hand, this stigma generates incorrect diagnoses and prejudices, negatively affecting the therapeutic relationship and perpetuating the social exclusion of these patients (Lucas-Choez et al., 2021). This dynamic exacerbates the problems of self-esteem and self-efficacy of patients, which reduces adherence to treatment and worsens their health status (Rusch et al., 2005). Consequently, the insufficient training of health professionals on the stigma associated with SUDs remains a key barrier to improving care and the recovery of these people (Garpenhag & Dahlman, 2021). Interventions aimed at reducing stigma underline the need for comprehensive training and commitment to affected people (Cazalis et al., 2023; Guerrero et al., 2023; Magnan et al., 2023).

In Chile, the translation of the Opening Minds Scale for Healthcare Practitioners (OMS-HC) instrument has been adapted to Spanish and with an analysis of its content validation, for the evaluation of stigma toward people with mental illnesses in health professionals, enabling new studies that analyze its criterion validity, and the exploration of its utility at the local level (Gajardo et al., 2021). The results are consistent with previous literature referring to moderate-low levels of stigmatizing attitudes toward people with mental illnesses. The incipient differences between first- and fourth-year students make new studies with a larger sample size and in other contexts relevant (Gajardo et al., 2022).

Research addressing the intersection between stigma, public health, and drug prevention, treatment, and recovery policies highlight the widespread impact of stigma on health outcomes and recovery processes. Stigma, particularly within the criminal justice system, should also be considered to intervene and reduce stigma among criminal justice staff and clients (Moore et al., 2023). Addressing these stigma-related challenges is crucial to developing effective public health policies and interventions that promote better health outcomes and support recovery (Abu-Ba'are et al., 2024; Antin & Sanders, 2023).

Thus, the impact that stigma would have on the care of people with problematic uses within the Public Health system can be specified in:

(a) *Access to health care:* Stigma prevents many people from seeking treatment or continuing with therapies due to fear of being labeled or discriminated against.
(b) *Adherence to treatments:* People who perceive stigma will be less likely to adhere to the recommended treatments, which will worsen their prognosis.
(c) *Social exclusion:* Stigma leads to social isolation, job loss, and difficulties in interpersonal relationships, which increases the vulnerability of the affected individuals.

(d) *Impact on public policies:* Stigma undermines the effectiveness of public health policies, particularly those focused on the prevention and treatment of stigmatized diseases.

1.3 Stigma in Problematic Uses in Spain and Latin America

Public health stigma is a phenomenon that affects people with various diseases, mental disorders, and problematic uses, both in Spain and in Latin America, and has a negative impact on the quality of healthcare and the social integration of the affected individuals. Next, in Spain and Latin America, drug prevention, treatment, and recovery are discussed, focusing on evidence-based strategies that can reduce the incidence of drug use and minimize its negative impacts on health and society.

Evidence-based strategies to reduce stigma among people who use drugs (PWUD) include peer recovery interventions, educational programs, and harm reduction training. Peer recovery specialists can effectively change stigma-related barriers by providing support and promoting positive perceptions of treatment, especially in underserved populations (Kleinman et al., 2024).

Culturally sensitive strategies can address stigma in public treatment centers for problematic uses, improving engagement with health services (Khazaee-Pool et al., 2024). Training of health professionals in the principles of harm reduction has been shown to significantly improve attitudes toward PWUD, thus reducing stigma in clinical settings (Avra et al., 2024). Interventions such as Acceptance and Commitment Therapy can effectively reduce self-stigma among PWUD (Sibley et al., 2024). Tailored messages that incorporate personal recovery stories can be especially effective in rural areas, highlighting the need for contextualized approaches to stigma reduction (Ashworth et al., 2024).

1.3.1 Public Health Stigma in Spain

In Spain, stigma toward people with mental disorders, problematic uses, and infectious diseases such as HIV remains a significant challenge in the field of public health. Cazalis et al. (2023) analyze how the stigma associated with drug use in Spain causes delays in seeking treatment for addiction, as patients fear being labeled as "drug addicts" or criminals. In this same sense, a report from the National Plan on Drugs highlights that people with SUD are often stigmatized, which hinders their access to appropriate treatment and contributes to social isolation.

In Spain, there are other considerations of the public health system that must be taken into account, as they may be favoring structural stigma in the field of problematic uses. In Spain, care for problematic uses is not fully integrated within the public health system, which creates significant barriers for patients to receive appropriate treatment. The availability and type of treatment services vary significantly among the different autonomous communities, leading to inequalities in access to healthcare.

In addition, studies like that of Muñoz et al. (2009) underline that the stigma toward people with mental disorders has decreased with awareness campaigns, but significant barriers persist in areas such as employment and access to mental health services.

1.3.2 Public Health Stigma in Latin America

According to the Pan American Health Organization, stigma and discrimination are key barriers in the effective implementation of public health policies. In the context of substance use disorders, people with problematic uses are perceived as a "moral problem" rather than patients who require medical care. According to Hansen (2019b), stigma toward drug users in health settings translates into inadequate treatments, late care, and the perpetuation of prejudices in the general population.

1.4 Strategies and Public Policies for the Prevention and Reduction of Stigma in Problematic Uses from Public Health

1. Educational and contact-based interventions: Education and direct contact with people suffering from substance use disorders are effective in reducing stigma among medical students and professionals (Aronowitz & Meisel, 2022; Livingston et al., 2012). Contact-based training and education programs aimed at health professionals, such as visual campaigns and narrative vignettes, can reduce stigmatizing attitudes and increase empathy (Aronowitz & Meisel, 2022).
2. Positive empathy interventions: Positive empathy interventions, in which individuals are exposed to positive stories and imagined positive contact with people who inject drugs, significantly reduce maintained stigma (Clinton & Pollini, 2021).
3. Therapeutic interventions for self-stigma: Group-based acceptance and commitment therapy has shown promise to reduce self-stigma among people with substance use disorders (Livingston et al., 2012).
4. Structural and policy interventions: The integration of health services into community organizations frequented by injectable drug users can create non-stigmatizing environments and improve the use of healthcare (Biancarelli et al., 2019). Addressing the stigma of intervention toward medications for opioid use disorder (OUD) through provider training and policy changes can improve access and reduce patient barriers (Madden et al., 2021).

5. Reduction of public and social stigma: Motivational interviewing and the communication of positive stories about people with substance use disorders are effective strategies for reducing social stigma (Livingston et al., 2012).

Based on scientific studies, several strategies have been proposed:

(a) *Education and training of healthcare providers:* Educating health professionals about addiction as a chronic disease, rather than a moral defect, is crucial to reducing provider stigma. Corrigan et al. (2017) and Wakeman et al. (2016) highlight the importance of training programs that foster understanding and compassion toward people with SUD.
(b) *Public awareness campaigns:* Public health campaigns that destigmatize SUD and promote it as a treatable condition can change social attitudes. Studies like Livingston et al. (2012) show that media campaigns and community outreach initiatives can effectively challenge negative stereotypes, thus reducing public stigma and encouraging people to seek help.
(c) *Enhancing the autonomy of affected individuals:* Generating greater self-efficacy and fostering active involvement in the treatment process can favor the reduction of stigma (Mota et al., 2014).
(d) *Peer support:* It has been shown that involving people in recovery as peer support specialists reduces stigma and improves treatment outcomes. Knaak et al. (2017) suggest that peer-led programs provide a model of hope and success, which helps combat self-stigma among those seeking treatment.
(e) *Policy reform for inclusive care:* According to Hatzenbuehler and Link (2014), policies that decriminalize drug use and prioritize treatment over punishment can reduce the stigmatization of SUD. Programs like needle exchange and safe consumption spaces also align with this approach by reducing harm and promoting recovery.
(f) *Legislation against discrimination:* It is essential to enforce legal protections against discrimination in healthcare and employment for people with SUD. Link and Phelan (2001) advocate for stricter anti-discrimination laws that protect people in recovery from being denied work, housing, or healthcare services based on their addiction history.
(g) *Integrated care models:* Providing integrated care that combines SUD treatment with general medical care can reduce stigma. Saunders-Adams et al. (2020) found that the integration of mental health, SUD services, and primary care reduces the compartmentalization of SUD treatment, thus normalizing SUD care within the broader healthcare system.
(h) *Community-based participatory approaches:* Involving communities in the development and implementation of prevention and treatment programs is another way to address stigma. Mora-Ríos and Bautista (2014) highlight that community-based initiatives allow for culturally sensitive interventions that address both stigma and the social determinants of SUD.

Similarly, Hansen (2019a) proposes several recommendations for addressing stigma toward people with SUD specifically from public health care services:

Programs and services should be reviewed to ensure equity in access and retention, as well as the language used in documentation and in the interaction between professionals and users. The language should be inclusive, non-stigmatizing, and non-sexist.

Trainings should be experiential and led by experts, integrating the human rights (HR) perspective in the treatment of problematic uses, with the aim that these trainings are reflected in therapeutic interventions. It is recommended to hold supervision meetings where issues related to the vulnerability and discrimination of users are discussed, fostering the team's participation in networks and platforms that promote policies with an HR approach in the field of problematic uses.

It is essential to review the power relations between professionals and users, avoiding directive practices that infantilize or limit the autonomy of service users. Encourage an open attitude in work teams and volunteers to discuss stigma, promoting self-reflection on beliefs and attitudes. It is necessary to generate review spaces to agree on appropriate ways of relating to service users.

In therapeutic interventions, it is necessary to create and maintain therapeutic groups that address stigma and ensure that these activities are regularly imparted by professionals trained in human rights and drugs, avoiding perpetuating stereotypes. Coordination with primary care is vital to improve case detection and referral and to network with other devices to optimize the therapeutic response. The concept of intersectionality should be integrated as a framework for analysis, considering the impact of multiple stigma based on gender, race, social class, or sexual orientation. Import and reproduce good practices that have previously worked in reducing stigma in other contexts.

Work with the families of the users on how stigma influences recovery and family emotional burden. These recommendations underline the need for an inclusive and equitable approach that integrates the human rights perspective to improve care for substance users within public health services.

1.5 Final Considerations

The stigma in problematic uses is directly connected with the Sustainable Development Goals (SDGs), particularly with SDG 3: Health and Well-being, which seeks to ensure universal access to health and promote well-being. Stigma acts as a crucial barrier to achieving this goal, as it hinders people with problematic uses from accessing necessary health services. Likewise, SDG 10: Reduction of Inequalities is affected by criminalization and social rejection, which deepen inequalities by preventing affected people from enjoying a dignified life and accessing their social and economic rights.

To confront this problem, it is necessary to work on intersectional interventions that recognize different factors of vulnerability and discrimination. In addition, public health strategies should include the education of health professionals, awareness campaigns, and the integration of care. These evidence-based measures can significantly improve the treatment of problematic uses and ensure equitable access to health services, addressing both public and structural stigma.

The public health system's response to this stigma is multifaceted, aiming to reduce its impact on people seeking help. Public health efforts can inadvertently reinforce it by focusing too much on substance use and not on the affected people. This highlights the need for a balanced approach that fosters understanding and support. Reducing stigma among drug users is crucial to improving their health and social outcomes. Various strategies have been researched to address this problem, focusing on different target groups and employing various methods.

References

Abu-Ba'are, G. R., Hogarty, S., Shamrock, O. W., Russell, H., Manchisi, K., Smith, V., & Mericle, A. (2024). Investigating experiences of stigma and its impact on substance use recovery among residents of recovery residences in the United States: A scoping review protocol. *BSGH020*. https://doi.org/10.1101/2024.08.22.24312414

Antin, T. M., & Sanders, E. (2023). *Stigma and public health*. Edward Elgar Publishing. https://doi.org/10.4337/9781800885691.ch57

Aronowitz, S., & Meisel, Z. (2022). Addressing stigma to provide quality care to people who use drugs. *JAMA Network Open, 5*(2), e2146980. https://doi.org/10.1001/jamanetworkopen.2021.46980

Ashworth, M., Thunström, L., Clancy, G. L., Thompson, R. A., Johnson, D., & Fletcher, E. (2024). 5. Addressing rural and non-rural substance use disorder stigma: Evidence from a national randomized controlled trial. *Addictive Behaviors Reports, 19*, 100541. https://doi.org/10.1016/j.abrep.2024.100541

Avra, T., Cowan, A., Friedman, J., Fukushima, J., Nelson, A., Truman, K., Stevens, A., Bourgois, P., Hansen, H., Shover, C., & Goodman-Meza, D. (2024). Decreasing stigma toward people who inject drugs: Harm reduction training for first-year medical students. *Academic Medicine*, 10–97. https://doi.org/10.1097/acm.0000000000005675

Biancarelli, D., Biello, K., Biello, K., Childs, E., Drainoni, M., Salhaney, P., Edeza, A., Mimiaga, M., Saitz, R., & Bazzi, A. (2019). Strategies used by people who inject drugs to avoid stigma in healthcare settings. *Drug and Alcohol Dependence, 198*, 80–86. https://doi.org/10.1016/j.drugalcdep.2019.01.037

Breilh, J. (2010). Las tres 'S' de la determinación de la vida: 10 tesis hacia una visión crítica de la determinación social de la vida y la salud. In R. P. Nogueira (Ed.), *Determinação social da saúde e reforma sanitária* (pp. 87–125). Centro Brasileiro de Estudos de Saúde.

Brohan, E., Elgie, R., Sartorius, N., Thornicroft, G., & GAMIAN-Europe Study Group. (2010). Self-stigma, empowerment and perceived discrimination among people with schizophrenia in 14 European countries: The GAMIAN-Europe study. *Schizophrenia Research, 122*(1-3), 232–238. https://doi.org/10.1016/j.schres.2010.02.1065

Cañarte-Quimis, J. G., Villarreal-Calderón, L. A., & Villigua-Pincay, D. F. (2023). Prevención del consumo de estupefacientes y otras usos problematicos. *MQRInvestigar, 7*(4), 589–609. https://doi.org/10.56048/MQR20225.7.4.2023.589-609

Cazalis, A., Lambert, L., & Auriacombe, M. (2023). Stigmatization of people with addiction by health professionals: Current knowledge. A scoping review. *Drug and Alcohol Dependence Reports, 9*, 100196. https://doi.org/10.1016/j.dadr.2023.100196

Clinton, A., & Pollini, R. (2021). Using positive empathy interventions to reduce stigma toward people who inject drugs. *Frontiers in Psychology, 12*, 616729. https://doi.org/10.3389/fpsyg.2021.616729

Conrad, P. (1992). Medicalization and social control. *Annual Review of Sociology, 18*, 209–232.
Corrigan, P., Schomerus, G., Shuman, V., Kraus, D., Perlick, D., Harnish, A., Kulesza, M., Kane-Willis, K., Qin, S., & Smelson, D. (2017). Developing a research agenda for understanding the stigma of addictions Part I: Lessons from the mental health stigma literature. *The American Journal on Addictions, 26*(1), 59–66. https://doi.org/10.1111/ajad.12458
Corrigan, P. W. (2004). Target-specific stigma change: A strategy for impacting mental illness stigma. *Psychiatric Rehabilitation Journal, 28*(2), 113.
Cunningham, J. A., Sobell, L. C., & Chow, V. M. (1993). What's in a label? The effects of substance types and labels on treatment considerations and stigma. *Journal of Studies on Alcohol, 54*(6), 693–699. Recuperado en: http://nsuworks.nova.edu/cps_facarticles/798
Da Valle-Chervellera, C. A., Sundarrajan, M., & Gietzen, L. (2024). 3. Impact of provider obesity bias and stigma in Western medicine. *Pacific journal of health, 7*, 10. https://doi.org/10.56031/2576-215x.1036
El-Tantawy, A. M. A., Raya, Y. M., & Zaki, A. M. K. (2010). Depressive disorders among caregivers of schizophrenic patients in relation to burden of care and perceived stigma. *Current Psychiatry Reports, 17*(3), 15–25. https://encr.pw/iBume
Fernández, J. J. (2017). *Estigma en usuarios y usuarias de drogas. Estrategias para combatirlo.* Socidrogalcohol. Ponencia XIX Seminario RIOD.
Friedman, S. R., Williams, L. D., Guarino, H., Mateu-Gelabert, P., Krawczyk, N., Hamilton, L., Walters, S. M., Ezell, J. M., Khan, M., Di Iorio, J., Yang, L. H., & Earnshaw, V. A. (2021). 5. The stigma system: How sociopolitical domination, scapegoating, and stigma shape public health. *Journal of Community Psychology, 50*, 385. https://doi.org/10.1002/JCOP.22581
Gajardo, J., Espinosa, F., Goycolea, R., Oyarzún, M., Muñoz, I., Valdebenito, A., & Pezoa, C. (2022). Estigma hacia personas con enfermedad mental en estudiantes y profesores de terapia ocupacional. *Cadernos Brasileiros de Terapia Ocupacional, e30*, e3145. https://doi.org/10.1590/25268910.ctoAO24103145
Gajardo, J., Espinosa, F., Muñoz, I., Goycolea, R., Valdebenito, A., Oyarzún, M., & Pezoa, C. (2021). Traducción y análisis de validez de contenido del instrumento Opening Minds Scale for Healthcare Practitioners (OMS-HC) para la evaluación del estigma hacia la enfermedad mental en profesionales de la salud en Chile. *Revista Chilena de Neuro-Psiquiatría, 59*(2), 91–101. https://doi.org/10.4067/s0717-92272021000200091
Garpenhag, L., & Dahlman, D. (2021). Perceived healthcare stigma among patients in opioid substitution treatment: A qualitative study. *Substance Abuse Treatment, Prevention, and Policy, 16*(1), 81. https://doi.org/10.1186/s13011-021-00417-3
Goffman, E. (1963). *Stigma: Notes on the Management of Spoiled Identity*. Touchstone.
Guerrero, Z., Iruretagoyena, B., Parry, S., & Henderson, C. (2023). Anti-stigma advocacy for health professionals: A systematic review. *Journal of Mental Health, 33*, 394. https://doi.org/10.1080/09638237.2023.2182421
Hansen, G. (2019a). Estigma, consumo de drogas y usos problematicos: conceptos, implicaciones y recomendaciones. *Recuperado de:* https://riod.org/wp-content/uploads/2019/06/ESTIGMA-CONSUMO-DE-DROGAS-YUSOSPROBLEMATICOS.pdf
Hansen, G. (2019b). Estigma, consumo de drogas y adicciones. In *Conceptos, implicaciones y recomendaciones*. Consumo y Bienestar Social. RIOD.
Hatzenbuehler, M. L., & Link, B. G. (2014). Introduction to the special issue on structural stigma and health. *Social Science & Medicine, 103*, 1–6. https://doi.org/10.1016/j.socscimed.2013.12.017
Hatzenbuehler, M. L., Phelan, J. C., & Link, B. G. (2013). Stigma as a fundamental cause of population health inequalities. *American Journal of Public Health, 103*(5), 813–821.
Jones, E., Farina, A., Hastorf, A., Marcus, H., Miller, D., & Scott, R. (1984). *Social stigma: The psychology of marked relationships*. Freeman and Company.
Khazaee-Pool, M., Naghibi, S. A., Pashaei, T., & Ponnet, K. (2024). 2. Developing practical strategies to reduce addiction-related stigma and discrimination in public addiction treatment centers: A mixed-methods study protocol. *Addiction Science & ClinicalPractice, 19*, 40. https://doi.org/10.1186/s13722-024-00472-8

Kleinman, M. B., Anvari, M. S., Felton, J. W., Bradley, V. D., Belcher, A. M., Abidogun, T. M., Hines, A. C., Dean, D., Greenblatt, A. D., Wagner, M., Earnshaw, V. A., & Magidson, J. F. (2024). Reduction in substance use stigma following a peer-recovery specialist behavioral activation intervention. *International Journal of Drug Policy, 130*, 104511. https://doi.org/10.1016/j.drugpo.2024.104511

Knaak, S., Mantler, E., & Szeto, A. (2017). Mental illness-related stigma in healthcare: Barriers to access and care and evidence-based solutions. *Healthcare Management Forum, 30*, 111–116. https://doi.org/10.1177/0840470416679413

Link, B., & Phelan, J. (2001). Conceptualizing stigma. *Annual Review of Sociology, 27*, 363–385.

Link, B. G., Yang, L., Phelan, J. C., & Collins, P. (2004). Measuring mental illness stigma. *Schizophrenia Bulletin, 30*(3), 511–541.

Link, B. G., Struening, E. L., Rahav, M., Phelan, J. C., & Nuttbrock, L. (1997). On stigma and its consequences: Evidence from a longitudinal study of men with dual diagnoses of mental illness and substance abuse. *Journal of Health and Social Behavior*, 177–190.

Link, B. G., & Phelan, J. C. (2006). Stigma and its public health implications. *The Lancet, 367*(9509), 528–529.

Livingston, J. D., Milne, T., Fang, M. L., & Amari, E. (2012). The effectiveness of interventions for reducing stigma related to substance use disorders: A systematic review. *Addiction, 107*(1), 39–50. https://doi.org/10.1111/j.1360-0443.2011.03601.x

Lucas-Choez, M. M., Quijije-Segovia, S. K., Quiroz-Figueroa, M. S., & Lino-Conforme, Y. G. (2021). Actitudes del personal de salud ante la atención al paciente drogadicto. *Polo del Conocimiento: Revista Científico - Profesional, 6*(9), 1193–1213. https://doi.org/10.23857/pc.v6i9.3104

Madden, E., Prevedel, S., Light, T., & Sulzer, S. (2021). Intervention stigma toward medications for opioid use disorder: A systematic review. *Substance Use & Misuse, 56*, 2181–2201. https://doi.org/10.1080/10826084.2021.1975749

Magnan, E., Weyrich, M., Miller, M., Melnikow, J., Moulin, A., Servis, M., Chadha, P., Spivack, S., & Henry, S. G. (2023). Stigma against patients with substance use disorders among health care professionals and trainees and stigma-reducing interventions: A systematic review. *Academic Medicine, 99*(2), 221–231. https://doi.org/10.1097/acm.0000000000005467

McNeely, H. L., Nelson-Brantley, H., Teel, C., & Peterson, M. (2023). Role of stigma for health care professionals with nonmedical substance use. *Western Journal of Nursing Research, 45*, 833. https://doi.org/10.1177/01939459231187983

Michaels, P., López, M., Rüsch, N., & Corrigan, P. (2012). Constructs and concepts comprising the stigma of mental illness. *Psychology, Society, and Education, 4*, 183–194.

Mojtabai, R., Olfson, M., Sampson, N. A., Jin, R., Druss, B., Wang, P. S., Wells, K. B., Pincus, H. A., & Kessler, R. C. (2011). Barriers to mental health treatment: Results from the national comorbidity survey replication (NCS-R). *Psychological Medicine, 41*(8), 1751–1761. https://doi.org/10.1017/S0033291710002291

Moore, K. E., Johnson, J. E., Luoma, J. B., Taxman, F., Pack, R., & Corrigan, P. (2023). 3. A multi-level intervention to reduce the stigma of substance use and criminal involvement: A pilot feasibility trial protocol. *Health & Justice, 11*, 24. https://doi.org/10.1186/s40352-023-00224-x

Mora-Ríos, J., & Bautista, N. (2014). Estigma estructural, género e interseccionalidad. Implicaciones en la atención a la salud mental. *Salud mental, 37*(4), 303–312. https://www.medigraphic.com/pdfs/salmen/sam-2014/sam144d.pdf

Mota, T., Noto, R., & Santos, P. (2014). *Reduzindo o estigma entre usuários de Drogas: guia para profissionais e gestores*. Editora UFJF.

Muñoz, M., Pérez-Santos, E., Crespo, M. y Guillén, A. (2009). Estigma y enfermedad mental: análisis del rechazo social que sufren las personas con enfermedad mental.. Editorial Complutense SA.

Pedersen, D. (2005). Estigma y exclusión social en la enfermedad mental: Apunte para el análisis e investigación. *Revista de psiquiatria y salud mental Herminio Valdizan, 7*(1), 3–14.

Prado, F. C., Valenzuela, S., & Vidal Garcia, G. I. (2015). Usos problematicos juveniles ¿Delincuencia o enfermedad? Una mirada sociológica sobre la problemática. *RevIISE: Revista de Ciencias Sociales y Humanas, 7*(7), 23–32. https://ojs.unsj.edu.ar/index.php/reviise/article/view/68

Ronzani, T. M., Higgins-Biddle, J., & Furtado, E. F. (2009). Stigmatization of alcohol and other drug users by primary care providers in Southeast Brazil. *Social Science & Medicine, 69*(7), 1080–1084.

Rusch, N., Angermeyer, M. C., & Corrigan, P. W. (2005). Mental illness stigma: Concepts, consequences, and initiatives to reduce stigma. *European Psychiatry, 20*(8), 529–539.

Saunders-Adams, S., Hechmer, C., Peck, A., & Murray, M. M. (2020). Integrated care: Identifying and intervening with substance misuse in primary healthcare. In *The Routledge handbook of social work and addictive Behaviors* (pp. 436–452). Routledge.

Sibley, A. L., Colston, D. C., & Go, V. F. (2024). Interventions to reduce self-stigma in people who use drugs: A systematic review. *Journal of Substance Use and Addiction Treatment, 159*, 209284. https://doi.org/10.1016/j.josat.2023.209284

Valencia Arredondo, M. (2011). Aportes de los nuevos enfoques para la conformación de la salud pública alternativa. *Revista Facultad Nacional de Salud Pública, 29*, 85–93.

Van Boekel, L., Brouwers, E., Van Weeghel, J., & Garretsen, H. (2013). Stigma among health professionals towards patients with substance use disorders and its consequences for healthcare delivery: Systematic review. *Drug and Alcohol Dependence, 131*, 23–35.

Van Boekel, L. C., Brouwers, E. P., van Weeghel, J., & Garretsen, H. F. (2015). Stigmatisering van patiënten met een verslaving en de gevolgen voor de hulpverlening: een systematisch literatuuronderzoek [Stigma among health professionals towards patients with substance use disorders and its consequences for healthcare delivery: Systematic review]. *Tijdschrift voor Psychiatrie, 57*(7), 489–497. https://www.tijdschriftvoorpsychiatrie.nl/media/5/57-2015-7-artikel-vanboekel.pdf

Vázquez, A., & Stolkiner, A. (2009). Procesos de estigma y exclusión en salud: Articulaciones entre estigmatización, derechos ciudadanos, uso de drogas y drogadependencia. *Anuario de investigaciones, 16*, 295–303.

Vicario Cañas, A., & De la Villa Moral Jiménez, M. (2016). Actitudes hacia los trastornos mentales y su asociación percibida con delito: Estigma social. *Salud & Sociedad, 7*(3), 254–269. https://www.redalyc.org/pdf/4397/439749582002.pdf

Wakeman, S. E., Pham-Kanter, G., & Donelan, K. (2016). Attitudes, practices, and preparedness to care for patients with substance use disorder: Results from a survey of general internists. *Substance Abuse, 37*(4), 635–641. https://doi.org/10.1080/08897077.2016.1187240

Walters, S. M., Kerr, J., Cano, M., Earnshaw, V., & Link, B. (2023). Intersectional stigma as a fundamental cause of health disparities: A case study of how drug use stigma intersecting with racism and xenophobia creates health inequities for Black and Hispanic persons who use drugs over time. *Stigma and Health, 8*, 325. https://doi.org/10.1037/sah0000426

World Health Organization [WHO] (2005). Stigmatization and Access to Health Care in Latin America: Threats and Prospects.

Chapter 2
Stigma, Morality, and Intersectionality in Drug Use

Andrés Felipe Tirado-Otálvaro, Sandra Milena Velásquez-Vergara, and Edgar Orlando Arroyave-Álvarez

2.1 Introduction

Stigma was first conceptualized by Goffman (1986) as a devaluing attribute that discredits and generates contempt, and after this, Link and Phelan (2006) proposed that public stigma comes as a process that involves labeling, the construction of social stereotypes, the separation between labeled and unlabeled, and discrimination originated by an unequal power situation. However, research in the last two decades has deepened the conceptualization of stigma (Pescosolido & Martin, 2015), and some Latin American authors (Cassiani-Miranda et al., 2023) have proposed the concept of Stigma Discrimination Complex (SDC), which refers to stigma, not as a linear and hierarchical phenomenon, but as a network of dependent and determinant relationships in which aspects of the individual, social, and structural order are intimately linked, generating situations of exclusion.

Due to the social construction that opposes drug use with everything that is appreciated as good (Porter, 2020), it is common in almost all cultures that People who Use Drugs (PUD), especially those with Substance Use Disorder (SUD), are victims of public stigma (Corrigan et al., 2009), and individuals with this condition tend to be considered weak in character, incapable of making decisions, immoral,

A. F. Tirado-Otálvaro (✉)
Faculty of Nursing, Universidad Pontificia Bolivariana, Medellín, Colombia
e-mail: felipe.tirado@upb.edu.co

S. M. Velásquez-Vergara
Faculty of Nursing, Universidad de Antioquia, Medellín, Colombia
e-mail: sandra.velasquez3@udea.edu.co

E. O. Arroyave-Álvarez
Faculty of Social and Human Sciences, Universidad de Antioquia, Medellín, Colombia
e-mail: edgar.arroyave@udea.edu.co

T. Mota Ronzani (ed.), *Social Stigma and Drug Use*,
https://doi.org/10.1007/978-3-031-94813-8_2

and even dangerous (Can & Tanrıverdi, 2015; Yang et al., 2017), a situation that can have a direct and potentially harmful effect on their health (von Hippel et al., 2018).

On the other hand, intersectionality is a concept and a critical approach useful in the analysis of racial inequalities that have been expanded to other areas, allowing us to understand issues related to stigma and health, as it draws attention to power, privileges, and inequalities inherent to multiple interconnected social categories such as gender, race-ethnicity, the exercise of sexuality, social class, and gender dissidences, among others. In this sense, stigma and intersectionality essentially involve the power conferred by the social context (Else-Quest et al., 2023) and how these situations increase stigma and generate barriers to accessing healthcare services (Jackson-Best & Edwards, 2018).

Although values and emotions have been discussed in the sociological and political literature, the role of values and moral emotions in political decision-making has been poorly understood (Zampini, 2018). Therefore, this chapter addresses the stigma toward PUD from an intersectional perspective, framed in an analysis about how the moralistic view of the use of these substances generates multiple repercussions, linking different stigmatized conditions such as drug use and street dwelling (Tamayo et al., 2024; Vargas et al., 2021), living with HIV (Davila et al., 2018), being a woman and/or having a sexual orientation different from the binary (Vázquez & Panadero, 2020) or being a racialized person (Holland et al., 2024), among others, usually has implications in terms of access to health care, as in political-moral terms, decision-makers design laws that do not contradict the social imaginary constructed about drug use to not assume the risks that not doing so would bring for their careers, which translates into moralistic and exclusionary public policies (Tirado-Otálvaro et al., 2022).

2.2 Development of the Topic

2.2.1 Morality and Drug Use as a Political Issue

Human beings are conditioned by their beliefs, emotions, values, and moral principles (Lerkkanen & Storbjörk, 2023; Zampini, 2018). These social and cultural imprints are fundamental to understanding the surrounding reality and guiding both our behavior and the way we interpret the world that shapes our daily experiences. It is not only traces that influence our experiences, but they also generate a sensitivity or emotionality that guides our actions (Bargh, 2018). In this sense, society shapes our moral or ethical sensitivity and conditions our perception of the world.

The study of morality, understood as the set of principles that guide our behavior toward what is considered good or bad (Mosca et al., 2023), is especially relevant in the context of drugs, as the consumption of these substances is often seen as a moral failure (Holland et al., 2024), and has been widely questioned by organizations influenced by political, religious, clinical, military, or economic interests (Gargiulo,

2022) through prohibitionist policies that are usually aimed at controlling socially marginalized groups (Rybka et al., 2018).

Morality is constructed in interactions with others based on values, experiences, beliefs, emotions, and deliberations, which is why, in political debates, it is often confused with moralism (Zampini, 2018) to create moral codes that later become norms aimed at controlling socially prohibited behaviors (Guise et al., 2018). In this sense, Lerkkanen and Storbjörk (2023) argue that drug policy becomes a moral issue to legislate the issues that political actors consider to have implications for what they consider right or wrong based on their scale of values.

Models, norms, beliefs, and moral values shape our sensitivity, understood as the sensory reactions that generate a specific perception toward an object or human group, which can range from approach to rejection, indifference, or disapproval (Flaßpöhler, 2023). Therefore, behaviors considered morally questionable often provoke moral indignation (Stoljar, 2020). In this context, situations such as drug use, which can be perceived as a threat to social values and interests (Shiner & Winstock, 2015), activate emotional responses such as attraction or rejection that are difficult to modify. This occurs due to cognitive, emotional, moral, or political biases, which often prevail over scientific evidence (Zampini, 2018) and reflect the imprints of the learning acquired in our close affective environments during the process of socialization.

Recognition of close ties is usually based on empathetic sensitivity. When certain groups are perceived at a social level as morally different, opposed to our values, or even as a threat to our lifestyle, this empathetic sensitivity is withdrawn, generating a negative sensitivity. This is expressed through emotions of rejection, antipathy, dislike, hostility, disgust, or contempt, which can be reinforced or intensified by political, religious, or moral ideologies (Flaßpöhler, 2023).

Decision-makers selectively use scientific evidence to argue their moral positions (Zampini, 2018), this makes achieving changes in drug policies much more complex and favors the use of a prohibitionist and abstentionist discourse as a strategy of control and moral deterrence (Collins et al., 2012), supported by the arguments of medical and legal disciplines based on the dualism about good and evil, right and wrong (Liblik et al., 2024).

Despite this, public health decision-makers experience discomfort when talking about issues related to justice and power (Pauly et al., 2021), and when it comes to discussing issues like drug use, they prefer to handle a prohibitionist discourse that is better accepted by society to avoid being stigmatized as promoters of consumption, thus ensuring their stay in power, because in moral terms, it is fair that people obtain happiness and well-being if their actions are virtuous, or punishment and unhappiness if their actions are vicious (Tirado-Otálvaro et al., 2022).

To generate moral panics, politicians rely on the media because of their ability to mobilize emotions through a supposed crisis around drug use, the magnification of collective concerns, and the use of scapegoats through anecdotal sources without empirical evidence to redirect public sentiment toward normative and prohibitionist political responses, which not only produces serious difficulties for access to health services by PUDs but also turns decision-makers into moral entrepreneurs (Michaud et al., 2024), who through hygienist and paternalistic discourses that disregard individual freedoms and autonomy sustain punitive policies centered on the utopia of abstentionism to control the so-called social vices (Gargiulo, 2022).

2.2.2 *Intersectionality*

The stigma toward people who use drugs is connected with other forms of discrimination, such as racism, classism, and those linked with gender dissidences (Pauly et al., 2021), that are reflected in structural relations of capitalist domination and exploitation guided by the states for the control and exclusion of people who do not conform to hegemonic values, which are legitimized with segregating policies that criminalize difference (Livingston, 2013; Ronzani, 2018; Scambler, 2018; Shildrick, 2018).

In this sense, the theory of intersectionality allows approaching stigma from a macrostructural perspective that argues how the unequal distribution of wealth and power, being interconnected with conceptual categories such as gender, ethnicity, and social class, among others (Else-Quest et al., 2023), can increase stigma and generate barriers to access healthcare services (Jackson-Best & Edwards, 2018).

Next, we describe how the intersectionality between drug use, social class, racial-ethnic group, female gender, and gender dissidences increases stigma toward PUDs.

Drug Use and Social Class

There is no individual outside of the social; human beings are evolutionarily social, as Wilson (2012) affirms, tribal by nature. This means that individual and collective psychological processes are intimately connected by cultural traditions and social circumstances (Shiner & Winstock, 2015) in such a way that personal and social identity mutually adapt to create social categories to which individuals may or may not belong, according to socially accepted norms (Sibley et al., 2023).

Categorization is a cognitive process inherent to human beings, in which individuals recognize social attributes to place themselves in those with which they feel a greater affinity according to their own attitudes and those that others perceive from these groups. This is why it is a process with implications for personal identity, social identity, and group dynamics, as it involves social comparison, depersonalization, intra- and intergroup conflict, and collective behavior (Sibley et al., 2023). In addition to a moral hierarchical category, a social value (positive or negative) is an emotional expression of adherence or rejection of social groups by a society that establishes normative and regulatory criteria for what is perceived as good or bad. In summary, how we behave is mainly an action for others to validate these social values (Cohen, 2017).

Social categories are based on perceptions that allow the individual to distinguish "positive" (belonging) or "negative" (rejection) groups, which are differentiated according to the imprints acquired in a society, to orient themselves in the lifestyles that are considered more valuable or "more true" (Scandroglio et al., 2008). In this sense, attitudes toward drug use are mediated by structural factors, such as ethnicity or social class, which influence the behavior of individuals in the face of this phenomenon (Razaghi et al., 2023), including moralistic policies that reproduce and maintain the stigma toward PUD (Corrigan et al., 2017).

The war on drugs is actually a war on the poor (Cornelio & Lasco, 2020), as poverty ceases to be a matter of not having money to become a moral defect of the PUD, a situation that fits perfectly with a line of moral and prohibitionist political thought (Zampini, 2018).

Crack is a drug predominantly consumed by people with low economic income and mostly Black, which allowed it to be criminalized and classified as an addiction and a moral failure. However, opioid addiction in white people, with a high economic level, political influence, higher social status, and medical insurance, made it necessary to reconfigure the concept of addiction and be replaced by "opioid use disorder" so that the Center for Disease Control and Prevention (CDC) could understand it as a "treatable chronic disease" which can affect anyone, regardless of their ethnic group, age, gender, income level, religion, or social status (Pergolizzi & LeQuang, 2023). In other words, if opioid addiction had stayed in the world of street heroin and fentanyl and if those who consumed synthetic derivatives of opioids had been Black, poor, and without political power, possibly the consumption of these substances would continue to be treated as a crime or as a moral failure and not as it is currently defined, as a disease (Sibley et al., 2023).

Some exclusion practices increase based on social conditions and drug use, as occurs among street dwellers (Tamayo et al., 2024), and consumption is often associated with dirt, begging, and street life (Sibley et al., 2023). Considering the above, it is possible to argue that exclusion practices are based on traits qualified as negative by a society or by certain particular groups, against other groups or individuals who are not part of the values erected as unique or at least of greater ethical, moral, social, or cultural forces (Castro, 2006; Pineda, 2018).

Drug Use and Ethnic-Racial Group

Since the beginning of anti-drug policies in the twentieth century, racism has been present in the formulation and application of these regulations. Campaigns such as those implemented in Vancouver in 1920 against opium and those promulgated in the 60 s and 70 s resorted to racial stereotypes to instill fear in society, linking drug use with specific ethnic communities such as the Chinese in the case of opium and Blacks in the case of cocaine and marijuana (Michaud et al., 2024).

The criminalization of drug use and possession has been disproportionately directed toward racialized communities, especially Black, Indigenous people, and those living in poverty (Holland et al., 2024), through policies that increased the stigma, surveillance, and exclusion of these groups (Michaud et al., 2024), despite the fact that consumption figures do not show significant differences compared to those of white people (Holland et al., 2024).

Moralistic policies and institutionalized racism combine to disproportionately stigmatize and penalize Black people and other racialized communities, bringing serious implications to judicial terms and access to health services (Pergolizzi & LeQuang, 2023). For example, in Canada, there is an intergenerational marginalization of indigenous people who use drugs, as evidenced by the increase in arrests of this population (Leger et al., 2021). Similarly, Black women are disproportionately arrested compared with white women (Thomas et al., 2019). In fact, in the United States over the last 40 years, the number of incarcerated women exceeded that of men, and by 2018, Black women were twice as many as white women in prison (Sufrin & Knittel, 2021).

Racial discrimination increases the stigma associated with drug use (Pauly et al., 2021), and if being a woman, being pregnant, and being incarcerated are added to the above, it is even worse. Pregnant Black women are more likely to be tested for illicit substance use, even without their consent, during prenatal check-ups (Perritt, 2020). In the United States, 60% of Black women in prison have a diagnosis of substance use disorder, 70% have some mental health problem, and 82% have been victims of physical or sexual abuse (Sufrin & Knittel, 2021), situations that, added to being pregnant, increase the risk of losing custody of their children (Bleasdale et al., 2022), with the aggravating factor that once their children arrive at foster homes, being Black and children of imprisoned women, they stay longer in these places and receive lower quality services (Perritt, 2020).

Drug Use and Female Gender

Gender is a social construct that differentiates men from women in a patriarchal and heteronormative model, which also includes PUD (Gargiulo, 2022), and is used to identify social power relations between the sexes based on biological representations, especially in reference to procreation, reproduction, and division of labor (Lamas, 2022a). It has become a political tool used to encapsulate various collective fears, such as economic precariousness, access to health, and police violence, which are channeled to generate panic in the population, causing hatred to be directed towards the most vulnerable and disadvantaged communities (Butler, 2024).

The war on drugs, such as macrostructural issues such as racism, social class, feminism, and sexual orientation, has been attacked from moralistic positions that oppose rights over individual freedoms (Liblik et al., 2024), a situation in which the phenomenon under study has had a more severe impact on women. Since the 1980s, women have been more likely than men to be arrested for possession of small amounts of drugs; figures represent an increase in arrests for women of 200% in contrast to 40% for men (Sufrin & Knittel, 2021).

On the other hand, sexuality as a political issue organized in unequal power systems that reward or blame individuals depending on their condition, has been more drastic in questioning and condemning women about experimentation with psychoactive substances, the regulation of their sexual behaviors, and the medicalization of "social vices" and "perverse pleasures" (Gargiulo, 2022), in this sense women who use drugs are seen as bad women or as "the embodiment of contaminated bodies" (Ettorre, 2017) because culturally the woman's environment should be the home and they are expected to be good mothers, wives, or daughters (Tamayo et al., 2024), which means having "correct" or "respectable" behaviors, since they are in charge of taking care of the children and the home (Harris et al., 2022), a situation that is reflected in the loss of family and social support, with consequences such as an increase in the number of relapses, imprisonment, mental illnesses, and the uprooting of motherhood (Bleasdale et al., 2022), which contributes to women hiding their consumption, delaying the request for therapeutic help, which generally hinders timely access to treatment and support, generating greater consequences at a personal, family, work, and social level (Harris et al., 2022).

Gender continues to be understood as a representation of sexual differences, which define what is considered characteristic of men and women. The masculinization of men's bodies and the feminization of women's bodies imply the construction of pre-established discourses about the roles of men and women, as well as the internalization of unfair cultural constructions, which are installed in the collective unconscious, where women generally occupy social positions inferior to those of men (Lamas, 2022a).

There were also differences in the reasons for consumption regarding gender roles and social pressures. Men, due to the mandates and expectations of hegemonic masculinity, may feel greater social pressure to demonstrate strength or resistance through drug use, while in women, consumption makes their morality questioned and they are labeled as "shameless" (Sibley et al., 2023), despite the fact that their consumption may be a way of escaping stress, violence, or discrimination related to their gender, derived from the multiple roles they must carry out: caregiver, employee, student, economic provider of the home, among others (Litherland et al., 2022).

Violence against women represents an unequal exercise of power in asymmetric social contexts in which gender inequity is present (Ferrer-Pérez & Bosch-Fiol, 2019; Restrepo et al., 2021). Women who use drugs are more stigmatized than men, and if factors such as street habitation are added, discrimination increases (Tamayo et al., 2024), as some of them must resort to sex work to get money for consumption (Holland et al., 2024) which makes them more vulnerable to being victims of sexual violence (Souza et al., 2016).

Drug use increases the risk of gender-based violence against women by 1.95 times (Rivera-Rivera et al., 2021), either because in these scenarios men seek to drug women to take advantage of their condition of vulnerability and defenselessness when under the effects of these substances (Sibley et al., 2023) or because patriarchal justice protects male aggressors and blames women for this situation (Gargiulo, 2022).

Obstetric violence is another form of violence against women using drugs. Pregnant women who use drugs, even before their children are born, are discriminated against and labeled as bad mothers, have difficulty accessing prenatal care, and when they do, are often persuaded by health professionals to abort (Golichenko et al., 2024). The impact of gender in the war on drugs is evident not only with the number of women in prison, which in the case of Russia amounts to 70% (Margo, 2020), but also with other forms of criminalization of reproduction, pregnancy, and parenting because these women are considered unfit for the roles they are socially expected to assume (Sufrin & Knittel, 2021).

The intersectionality between drug use, being a woman, being pregnant, and being in prison involves the convergence of multiple historical, racialized, and gender issues that generate multiple consequences for them and their families (Sufrin & Knittel, 2021) such as higher rates of interpersonal violence, physical and/or sexual abuse, mental health problems, loss of custody of children (Bleasdale et al., 2022), multiple obstacles to accessing health services, including access to treatment for their drug dependence (Knittel et al., 2020), shackling during childbirth (Sufrin & Knittel, 2021), the prohibition of the father or another family member being present during birth (Goshin et al., 2020; Vedam et al., 2019) and barriers to breastfeeding (Sufrin & Knittel, 2021), in addition to difficulties in accessing employment, housing, and education services for those who have already served their sentences (Bleasdale et al., 2022) and mistreatment by justice system employees for those who reenter the prison system (Thomas et al., 2019).

Drug Use, Gender Dissidence, and Social Class

The hegemonic clinical-biologist discourse has addressed sexuality with a stigmatizing and moralistic view toward people with dissident sexual practices, labeling them as "deviant" or "inappropriate" or classifying them as "dysfunctions" or "disorders" (Gargiulo, 2022), and given that the process of stigma construction also involves power relations, people who use drugs and who are also gender dissidents receive greater discrimination (Tamayo et al., 2024).

The LGBTIQ+ population, especially trans people who use drugs and live on the streets, are more vulnerable to mistreatment and discrimination based on their sexual and/or gender identity (Ecker et al., 2020), which increases the risk of mental disorders, such as anxiety and depression (LoSchiavo et al., 2020), and hinders their access to health services (Fraser et al., 2019).

Social and political inequalities in the sex/gender system, according to Lamas (2022b), have to do with the beliefs that guide human behavior and materialize in inequalities in access to education, the labor market, and political participation. This could be explained by systemic racism that, through various forms of violence, such as the promotion of collective fear toward political debate on gender issues and anything that challenges binarism and the patriarchal order, makes non-binary and trans people, particularly those of Black race and who use drugs, much more vulnerable to being victims of different types of violence and even murder (Butler, 2024).

2.3 Final Considerations

This chapter discusses how stigma toward people who use drugs is configured in a complex network of dependent and determinant relationships in which individual, social, and structural issues intervene and link with each other, generating situations of exclusion.

Analyzing the issue from an intersectional perspective that involves multiple stigmatizations, derived from the union of different depreciated characteristics or conditions, added to the design and application of moralistic, prohibitionist, and non-inclusive policies, results in the execution of discrimination and exclusion actions against people who do not conform to the hegemonic values of this society.

The text highlights how structural inequalities, crossed by issues of gender, ethnicity, and social condition, are linked with the Stigma Discrimination Complex (CED), increasing the vulnerability of people who use drugs and limiting the guarantee of their fundamental rights, including the right to health. These realities demand a reevaluation of current drug policies and a shift toward approaches that, not only from a discursive point of view but also from the executive, are based on human rights, social justice, and respect for difference.

The war on drugs failed (Leger et al., 2021), and this forced us not only to develop better methodological tools to analyze the role of morality in decision-making (Guise et al., 2018; Tirado-Otálvaro et al., 2022), as well as evidence-based strategies aimed at reducing stigma toward PUD, but also to design and implement real policies that intervene in macrostructural factors such as access to decent housing, education, health, employment, recreation and sports, improvement of living conditions, equitable distribution of resources, solidarity, and ethics (Pauly et al., 2021), with a differential gender approach that recognizes PUD as subjects of rights (Gargiulo, 2022).

References

Bargh, J. (2018). *¿Por qué hacemos lo que hacemos?* Ediciones B.

Bleasdale, J., Morse, D. S., Cerulli, C., Hordes, M., Wilson, K., Gabriel, S. J., & Przybyla, S. M. (2022). Women's motivators to engage in opioid use disorder treatment while enrolled in an opioid intervention court. *Substance Use & Misuse, 57*(7), 1035–1042. https://doi.org/10.1080/10826084.2022.2058704

Butler, J. (2024). Ideología de género y miedo a la destrucción. In J. Butler (Ed.), *¿Quién teme al género?* (pp. 11–51).

Can, G., & Tanrıverdi, D. (2015). Social functioning and internalized stigma in individuals diagnosed with substance use disorder. *Archives of Psychiatric Nursing, 29*(6), 441–446. https://doi.org/10.1016/j.apnu.2015.07.008

Cassiani-Miranda, C. A., Ronzani, T. M., & Tirado-Otálvaro, A. F. (2023). Stigmatization in people who use drugs: Causes, consequences, and intervention. In O. Scoppetta et al. (Eds.), *Mental health & addiction: An integrated care in Latin America* (pp. 57–88). CDS Press. Humber College Institute of Technology and Advanced Learning.

Castro, V. S. (2006). La psicología social de las relaciones intergrupales: Modelos e hipótesis. *Actualidades en psicología, 20*(107), 45–71.

Cohen, S. (2017). *Demonios populares y pánicos morales*. Gedisa.

Collins, S. E., Clifasefi, S. L., Logan, D. E., Samples, L. S., Somers, J. M., & Marlatt, G. A. (2012). Current status, historical highlights and basic principles of harm reduction. In G. A. Marlatt, M. E. Larimer, & K. Witkiewitz (Eds.), *Harm reduction: Pragmatic strategies for managing high risk behaviors* (2nd ed., pp. 3–35). The Guilford Press.

Cornelio, J., & Lasco, G. (2020). Morality politics: Drug use and the Catholic Church in The Philippines. *Open Theology, 6*(1), 327–341. https://doi.org/10.1515/opth-2020-0112

Corrigan, P. W., Kuwabara, S. A., & O'Shaughnessy, J. (2009). The public stigma of mental illness and drug addiction: Findings from a stratified random sample. *Journal of Social Work, 9*(2), 139–147. https://doi.org/10.1177/1468017308101818

Corrigan, P. W., Schomerus, G., Shuman, V., Kraus, D., Perlick, D., Harnish, A., Kulesza, M., Kane-Willis, K., Qin, S., & Smelson, D. (2017). Developing a research agenda for reducing the stigma of addictions, part II: Lessons from the mental health stigma literature. *The American Journal on Addictions, 26*(1), 67–74. https://doi.org/10.1111/ajad.12436

Davila, J. A., Cabral, H. J., Maskay, M. H., Marcus, R., Yuan, Y., Chisolm, N., Belton, P., McKeithan, L., & Rajabuin, S. (2018). Risk factors associated with multi-dimensional stigma among people living with HIV/AIDS who are homeless/unstably housed. *AIDS Care, 30*(10), 1335–1340. https://doi.org/10.1080/09540121.2018.1484069

Ecker, J., Aubry, T., & Sylvestre, J. (2020). Pathways into homelessness among LGBTQ2S adults. *Journal of Homosexuality, 67*(11), 1625–1643. https://doi.org/10.1080/00918369.2019.1600902

Else-Quest, N. M., French, A. M., & Telfer, N. A. (2023). The intersectionality imperative: Calling in stigma and health research. *Stigma and Health, 8*(3), 269–278. https://doi.org/10.1037/sah0000397

Ettorre, E. (2017). Feminist autoethnography, gender, and drug use: "Feeling about" empathy while "storying the I". *Contemporary Drug Problems, 44*(4), 356–374. https://doi.org/10.1177/0091450917736160

Ferrer-Pérez, V. A., & Bosch-Fiol, E. (2019). El Género en el Análisis de la Violencia contra las Mujeres en la Pareja: De la "Ceguera" de Género a la Investigación Específica del Mismo. *Anuario de Psicologia Juridica, 29*(1), 69–76. https://doi.org/10.5093/apj2019a3

Flaßpöhler, S. (2023). *Sensible. Sobre la sensibilidad moderna y los límites de lo tolerable*. Herder.

Fraser, B., Pierse, N., Chisholm, E., & Cook, H. (2019). LGBTIQ+ homelessness: A review of the literature. *International Journal of Environmental Research and Public Health, 16*(15), 2677. https://doi.org/10.3390/ijerph16152677

Gargiulo, R. d. P. D. (2022). Usos de drogas, biocodificación del género, y sexualidades disidentes-minoritarias. Entre el pánico moral y la narcotización de la sexualidad. *Cultura y Droga, 27*(33), 33. https://doi.org/10.17151/culdr.2022.27.33.6

Goffman, E. (1986). *Stigma: Notes on the management of spoiled identity* (2nd ed.).

Golichenko, M., Chu, S. K. H., & Lehman, R. (2024). Maternal health and human rights impacts of Russian drug policy. *International Journal of Gynaecology and Obstetrics: The Official Organ of the International Federation of Gynaecology and Obstetrics, 164*(1), 358–363. https://doi.org/10.1002/ijgo.15214

Goshin, L. S., Sissoko, D. R. G., Stringer, K. L., Sufrin, C., & Byrnes, L. (2020). Stigma and US nurses' intentions to provide the standard of maternal care to incarcerated women, 2017. *American Journal of Public Health, 110*(S1), S93–S99. https://doi.org/10.2105/AJPH.2019.305408

Guise, A., Melo, J., Mittal, M. L., Rafful, C., Cuevas-Mota, J., Davidson, P., Garfein, R. S., & Werb, D. (2018). A fragmented code: The moral and structural context for providing assistance with injection drug use initiation in San Diego, USA. *The International Journal on Drug Policy, 55*, 51–60. https://doi.org/10.1016/j.drugpo.2018.02.009

Harris, M. T. H., Laks, J., Stahl, N., Bagley, S. M., Saia, K., & Wechsberg, W. M. (2022). Gender dynamics in substance use and treatment: A women's focused approach. *The Medical Clinics of North America, 106*(1), 219–234. https://doi.org/10.1016/j.mcna.2021.08.007

Holland, A., Etches, S., & Gander, S. (2024). Drug decriminalization: The importance of policy change for the health and wellbeing of children and youth in Canada. *Paediatrics & Child Health, 29*(2), 87–89. https://doi.org/10.1093/pch/pxad006

Jackson-Best, F., & Edwards, N. (2018). Stigma and intersectionality: A systematic review of systematic reviews across HIV/AIDS, mental illness, and physical disability. *BMC Public Health, 18*, 1–19. https://doi.org/10.1186/s12889-018-5861-3

Knittel, A. K., Zarnick, S., Thorp, J. M., Amos, E., & Jones, H. E. (2020). Medications for opioid use disorder in pregnancy in a state women's prison facility. *Drug and Alcohol Dependence, 214*, 108159. https://doi.org/10.1016/j.drugalcdep.2020.108159

Lamas, M. (2022a). Complejidad y claridad en torno al concepto "género". In M. Lamas (Ed.), *Imensiones de la Diferencia. Género y Política* (Vol. 1, pp. 137–165). CLACSO.

Lamas, M. (2022b). Uso, dificultades y posibilidades de la categoría género. In M. Lamas (Ed.), *Dimensiones de la Diferencia. Género y Política* (Vol. 1, pp. 75–110). CLACSO.

Leger, P., Hamilton, A., Bahji, A., & Martell, D. (2021). Policy brief: CSAM in support of the decriminalization of drug use and possession for personal use. *Canadian Journal of Addiction, 12*(1), 13–15. https://doi.org/10.1097/CXA.0000000000000101

Lerkkanen, T., & Storbjörk, J. (2023). Debating the drug policy in Sweden: Stakeholders' moral justifications in media 2015–2021. *Contemporary Drug Problems, 50*(2), 269–293. https://doi.org/10.1177/00914509231159394

Liblik, S. A., Cunha, T. R. d., Liblik, C. S. d. F. K., Biscioni, D. N., & Girardi, D. R. (2024). Ética en el uso de psicodélicos: La definición de las drogas ilícitas bajo la óptica de la bioética crítica. *Salud Colectiva, 20*, e4630. https://doi.org/10.18294/sc.2024.4630

Link, B. G., & Phelan, J. C. (2006). Stigma and its public health implications. *The Lancet, 367*(9509), 528–529.

Litherland, S., Miller, P. G., & Hyder, S. (2022). Illicit drug use and male barroom aggression among members of the Australian construction industry: Associations with personality and masculinity factors. *Drug and Alcohol Review, 41*(6), 1463–1474. https://doi.org/10.1111/dar.13498

Livingston, J. D. (2013). *Mental illness-related structural stigma: The downward spiral of systemic exclusion final report*. Mental Health Commission of Canada.

LoSchiavo, C., Krause, K. D., Singer, S. N., & Halkitis, P. N. (2020). The confluence of housing instability and psychosocial, mental, and physical health in sexual minority young adults: The P18 cohort study. *Journal of Health Care for the Poor and Underserved, 31*(4), 1693–1711. https://doi.org/10.1353/hpu.2020.0127

Margo, G. (2020). Policing and sentencing practices in Russia and their impacts on women who use drugs. In J. Buxton, G. Margo, & L. Burger (Eds.), *The impact of global drug policy on women: Shifting the needle* (pp. 113–121). Emerald Publishing Limited. https://doi.org/10.1108/978-1-83982-882-920200017

Michaud, L., Kolla, G., Rudzinski, K., & Guta, A. (2024). Mapping a moral panic: News media narratives and medical expertise in public debates on safer supply, diversion, and youth drug use in Canada. *The International Journal on Drug Policy, 127*, 104423. https://doi.org/10.1016/j.drugpo.2024.104423

Mosca, A., Miuli, A., Mancusi, G., Chiappini, S., Stigliano, G., De Pasquale, A., Di Petta, G., Bubbico, G., Pasino, A., Pettorruso, M., & Martinotti, G. (2023). To bridge or not to bridge: Moral Judgement in cocaine use disorders, a case-control study on human morality. *Social Neuroscience, 18*(5), 271. https://doi.org/10.1080/17470919.2023.2242096

Pauly, B., Revai, T., Marcellus, L., Martin, W., Easton, K., & MacDonald, M. (2021). «The health equity curse»: Ethical tensions in promoting health equity. *BMC Public Health, 21*(1), 1567. https://doi.org/10.1186/s12889-021-11594-y

Pergolizzi, J., & LeQuang, J. A. K. (2023). How opioids changed what we thought about addiction and the implications for public health: An editorial. *Cureus, 15*(6), e40181. https://doi.org/10.7759/cureus.40181

Perritt, J. (2020). #WhiteCoatsForBlackLives—Addressing physicians' complicity in criminalizing communities. *The New England Journal of Medicine, 383*(19), 1804–1806. https://doi.org/10.1056/NEJMp2023305

Pescosolido, B. A., & Martin, J. K. (2015). The stigma complex. *Annual Review of Sociology, 41*, 87–116. https://doi.org/10.1146/annurev-soc-071312-145702

Pineda, E. (2018). Las heridas del racismo: Efectos psicosociales de la discriminación racial en las personas afrodescendientes en américa latina. *Iberoamérica Social: Revista-red de estudios sociales, 6*(11), 46–64.

Porter, L. B. (2020). Harm reduction and moral desert in the context of drug policy. *Health Care Analysis: HCA: Journal of Health Philosophy and Policy, 28*(4), 362–371. https://doi.org/10.1007/s10728-020-00411-z

Razaghi, E., Farhoudian, A., Pilevari, A., Noroozi, A., Hooshyari, Z., Radfar, R., & Malekinejad, M. (2023). Identification of the socio-cultural barriers of drug addiction treatment in Iran. *Heliyon, 9*(5), e15566. https://doi.org/10.1016/j.heliyon.2023.e15566

Restrepo, E. G., Cardona, D., & Otálvaro, A. F. T. (2021). La violencia contra las mujeres en Colombia, un desafío para la salud pública en cuanto a su prevención, atención y eliminación. *CES Derecho, 12*(1), 1. https://doi.org/10.21615/cesder.12.1.9

Rivera-Rivera, L., Natera-Rey, G., Séris-Martínez, M., Leyva-López, A., Zavala-Arciniega, L., Ortega-Ceballos, P. A., Reynales-Shigematsu, L. M., Rivera-Rivera, L., Natera-Rey, G., Séris-Martínez, M., Leyva-López, A., Zavala-Arciniega, L., Ortega-Ceballos, P. A., & Reynales-Shigematsu, L. M. (2021). Encodat 2016: Violencia de pareja y uso de tabaco, alcohol y drogas. Nuevos retos para la salud mental. *Salud Pública de México, 63*(5), 630–640. https://doi.org/10.21149/12288

Ronzani, T. M. (2018). *Drugs and social context: Social perspectives on the use of alcohol and other drugs*. Springer.

Rybka, L. N., Nascimento, J. L. d., & Guzzo, R. S. L. (2018). Os mortos e feridos na "guerra às drogas": Uma crítica ao paradigma proibicionista. *Estudos de Psicologia (Campinas), 35*, 99–109. https://doi.org/10.1590/1982-02752018000100010

Scambler, G. (2018). Heaping blame on shame: 'Weaponising stigma' for neoliberal times. *The Sociological Review, 66*(4), 766–782. https://doi.org/10.1177/0038026118778177

Scandroglio, B., Martínez, J. S. L., & Sebastián, C. S. J. (2008). La Teoría de la Identidad Social: Una síntesis crítica de sus fundamentos, evidencias y controversias [Social identity theory: A critical synthesis of its bases, evidence and controversies.]. *Psicothema, 20*(1), 80–89.

Shildrick, T. (2018). Lessons from Grenfell: Poverty propaganda, stigma and class power. *The Sociological Review, 66*(4), 783–798. https://doi.org/10.1177/0038026118777424

Shiner, M., & Winstock, A. (2015). Drug use and social control: The negotiation of moral ambivalence. *Social Science & Medicine, 1982*(138), 248–256. https://doi.org/10.1016/j.socscimed.2015.06.017

Sibley, A. L., Baker, R., Levander, X. A., Rains, A., Walters, S. M., Nolte, K., Colston, D. C., Piscalko, H. M., Schalkoff, C. A., Bianchet, E., Chen, S., Dowd, P., Jaeb, M., Friedmann, P. D., Fredericksen, R. J., Seal, D. W., & Go, V. F. (2023). «I am not a junkie»: Social categorization and differentiation among people who use drugs. *The International Journal on Drug Policy, 114*, 103999. https://doi.org/10.1016/j.drugpo.2023.103999

Souza, M. R. R. d., Oliveira, J. F. d., Chagas, M. C. G., & Carvalho, E. S. d. S. (2016). Género, violencia y la vida em la calle: Experiencias de mujeres que tienen problemas de drogadicción. *Revista Gaúcha de Enfermagem, 37*, e59876.

Stoljar, N. (2020). Disgust or dignity? The moral basis of harm reduction. *Health Care Analysis: HCA: Journal of Health Philosophy and Policy, 28*(4), 343–351. https://doi.org/10.1007/s10728-020-00412-y

Sufrin, C. B., & Knittel, A. (2021). Health care and social justice implications of incarceration for pregnant people who use drugs. *International Review of Psychiatry (Abingdon, England), 33*(6), 557–571. https://doi.org/10.1080/09540261.2021.1887097

Tamayo, S., Hernández, E. M., & Tirado-Otálvaro, A. F. (2024). Estigma hacia habitantes de calle, consumo de drogas y género. Consecuencias en derechos humanos y salud pública. *Diversitas, 20*(1), Art. 1. https://doi.org/10.15332/22563067.10229

Thomas, K., Wilson, J. L., Bedell, P., & Morse, D. S. (2019). «They didn't give up on me»: A women's transitions clinic from the perspective of re-entering women. *Addiction Science & Clinical Practice, 14*(1), 12. https://doi.org/10.1186/s13722-019-0142-8

Tirado-Otálvaro, A. F., Castaño-Perez, G. A., & Yepes-Delgado, C. E. (2022). The meaning of stigma about illegal drug use and its contribution to public policymaking in Colombia. *International Journal of Mental Health and Addiction, 22*, 1797. https://doi.org/10.1007/s11469-022-00959-y

Vargas, M. G., Ramírez, E. M. H., Salazar, M. J. O., Otálvaro, A. F. T., Bedoya, J. S. E., Morales, D. R. Z., Cañas, L. D., & Agudelo, L. M. S. (2021). Emociones, creencias y actitudes de personal asistencial hacia habitantes de calle que usan drogas. *Revista Facultad Nacional de Salud Pública, 39*(3), e344658–e344658. https://doi.org/10.17533/udea.rfnsp.e344658

Vázquez, J. J., & Panadero, S. (2020). Meta-stereotypes among women living homeless: Content, uniformity, and differences based on gender in Madrid, Spain. *Journal of Community Psychology, 48*(5), 1316–1326. https://doi.org/10.1002/jcop.22327

Vedam, S., Stoll, K., Taiwo, T. K., Rubashkin, N., Cheyney, M., Strauss, N., McLemore, M., Cadena, M., Nethery, E., Rushton, E., Schummers, L., Declercq, E., & GVtM-US Steering Council. (2019). The giving voice to mothers study: Inequity and mistreatment during pregnancy and childbirth in the United States. *Reproductive Health, 16*(1), 77. https://doi.org/10.1186/s12978-019-0729-2

von Hippel, C., Brener, L., & Horwitz, R. (2018). Implicit and explicit internalized stigma: Relationship with risky behaviors, psychosocial functioning and healthcare access among people who inject drugs. *Addictive Behaviors, 76*, 305–311. https://doi.org/10.1016/j.addbeh.2017.08.036

Wilson, E. (2012). *La conquista social de la tierra*. Debate.

Yang, L., Wong, L. Y., Grivel, M. M., & Hasin, D. S. (2017). Stigma and substance use disorders: An international phenomenon. *Current Opinion in Psychiatry, 30*(5), 378–388. https://doi.org/10.1097/YCO.0000000000000351

Zampini, G. F. (2018). Evidence and morality in harm-reduction debates: Can we use value-neutral arguments to achieve value-driven goals? *Palgrave Communications, 4*(1), 62. https://doi.org/10.1057/s41599-018-0119-3

Chapter 3
Poverty, Gender, Drug Use, and Stigma: An Intersectional Discussion from the Perspective of Homeless Women

Weverton Corrêa Netto, Gabriel Martins Silva, Aldo Tomassini, Alexandre Aranha Arbia, Marina Fernandes Toledo Lourenço, Viviane Souza Pereira, and Telmo Mota Ronzani

3.1 Introduction

Stigma was initially defined by Goffman (1980) as a deeply depreciative attribute that leads to the devaluation of the social identity of its bearers, leading to a loss of social status for stigmatized individuals. Understanding that "what is needed, in reality, is a language of relations and not of attributes" (Goffman, 1980, p. 13), the author already highlighted that the problem of stigma is not in the mark and the individual who possesses it, but in the processes and social relations through which certain marginalized groups are stigmatized due to their categorization.

Link and Phelan (2001) proposed a definition of stigma as the convergence of the components of *labeling*, its connection with a *negative stereotype*, the *separation* of the stigmatized group by the stereotype, and the consequent *loss of social status* and *discrimination* of the same in a situation of *power* that would allow the occurrence

W. C. Netto
Postgraduate Program in Collective Health, Universidade Federal de Juiz de Fora, Juiz de Fora, Brazil
e-mail: weverton.correa@estudante.ufjf.br

G. M. Silva · T. M. Ronzani (✉)
Department of Psychology, Universidade Federal de Juiz de Fora, Juiz de Fora, Brazil
e-mail: telmo.ronzani@ufjf.br

A. Tomassini
Faculty of Psychology, Universidad de la República, Montevideo, Uruguay
e-mail: Aldo.Tomassini@imm.gub.uy

A. A. Arbia · V. S. Pereira
School of Social Work, Universidade Federal de Juiz de Fora, Juiz de Fora, Brazil
e-mail: alexandre.arbia@ufjf.br; vivianesouza.pereira@ufjf.br

M. F. T. Lourenço
Postgraduate Program of Social Psychology, Universidade de São Paulo, Sao Paulo, Brazil

T. Mota Ronzani (ed.), *Social Stigma and Drug Use*,
https://doi.org/10.1007/978-3-031-94813-8_3

of stigma. Central to this definition is the dependence of stigma on political, economic, and social power inequality between groups, responsible for the impact of stigma in relation to disadvantages in various aspects of the life of the stigmatized group. In a similar line of discussion, Parker (2013) emphasizes the need to rethink stigma as a social process directly linked to power and domination, that is, as a phenomenon that plays a fundamental role in the production and reproduction of social inequalities that impact the health of certain groups. As a *fundamental cause of health inequities* (Link et al., 2018), understanding stigma requires reference to the totality of social relations in a given space and historical moment, reflecting on how some groups are in a position of disadvantage, exploitation, and oppression.

The understanding of stigma and its functionality proposed by these authors allows tracing its connections with the broader structures responsible for determining social inequalities, allowing the analysis of the influence of these on the stigmatization of certain groups based on categories such as race, gender, class, and drug use, as well as the effects that simultaneous belonging to multiple structurally marginalized groups can have on the phenomenon of stigma. However, most studies on stigma focus on the consequences associated with only one form of stigma in isolation, with only recent recognition of the need to consider the consequences of possessing multiple stigmatized identities on stigma outcomes in various domains of life (Williams & Fredrick, 2015). For this, the adoption of an intersectional look presents great contributions.

Intrinsically linked to the thought of Black feminism, *intersectionality* seeks to understand the interconnection of different systems of oppression and how their intertwining determines disadvantages or privileges for people whose identity is characterized by the intersection of multiple social categories, with the ultimate goal of promoting social justice (Else-Quest et al., 2023). It refers to the critical idea that socially constructed categories, such as, for example, race, gender, and class do not operate as unitary and mutually exclusive entities but as reciprocally constructed phenomena that shape individual experience and social inequalities among groups through the complex combination of structures of oppression (Collins, 2015). Therefore, in dealing with how power and inequity are related to the social categories that construct identity and to the social structures that produce inequalities based on the devaluation of certain identities, intersectionality constitutes an "imperative" for the study of stigma (Else-Quest et al., 2023).

The concept of *intersectional stigma* has been recently used in the literature to characterize the convergence of multiple stigmatized identities in a person or group and the way in which the intersection between different forms of stigma impacts vulnerable groups (Turan et al., 2019). The justification for the use of the concept is that current stigma models do not consider that identities do not occur in isolation, but that individuals have simultaneously multiple identities that, when taken in relation to existing power structures, influence the phenomenon of stigma due to the possibility of intersection of more than one socially devalued category. Thus, for groups with multiple stigmatized identities, the experience of stigma related to one aspect of their identity would be linked to the experience of other stigmas, whose combined negative effects can be either additive or result from more complex interactions (Turan et al., 2019).

Women living on the streets, the focus of the chapter, constitute a group that evidences the intersection of stigmas and oppressions (Thomas & Menih, 2022). Like men living on the streets, they face the impacts of poverty stigma, racism, and drug use stigma. However, intersecting these stigmas, women living on the streets also suffer the effects of unequal gender relations in society. Gender-based oppression is visible through violence present in their life trajectories as a common causal factor for living on the streets among women, and reproduced daily on the streets, where being a woman increases the chances of victimization. They also have worse physical and mental illness compared to men living on the street, deal with difficulties and prejudices for the exercise of motherhood on the streets, face with the lack of infrastructure for menstrual health care, are more stigmatized for drug use, and are made invisible in policies for the homeless (Coldibelli et al., 2022; Phipps et al., 2019; Thomas & Menih, 2022).

3.2 Poverty, Drugs, and Racism: The Stigmatization of the Homeless Population

The homeless population is one of the most widely stigmatized groups in society, with stigma being one of the main social determinants of their health (Canham et al., 2024). Among the negative outcomes associated with stigma for the homeless, examples include dehumanization and inferior treatment; the barriers faced in accessing housing and health services; violence and systematic discrimination by the general population, by professionals, and by institutions, which generate social isolation and the withdrawal from seeking care; the internalization of stigma and feelings of humiliation, shame, and self-blame; psychological suffering and mental health problems; among others (Canham et al., 2024). The stigma of the homeless is the result of the conjunction of multiple socially stigmatized characteristics present in this group, such as poverty and substance use, as well as the potential simultaneous membership in other marginalized groups, such as ethnic-racial minorities and women.

The stigmatization of poverty is a historical phenomenon that, in the context of capitalism, is linked to constructions of the social identity of poor people based on notions of value and personal merit (Pauly, 2014). This is evident in the generic representations of these individuals as "vagabonds," "lazy," "sick," and "dangerous" (Moura Jr. & Ximenes, 2016). The understanding of stigma as a fundamental cause of social inequities (Link et al., 2018), with socioeconomic inequality as one of its most harmful expressions, highlights the role of poverty stigma in perpetuating domination and oppression. When recognized through a stigmatized social identity, poor people are seen as the cause of social problems and as guilty of their own situation, in an ideological inversion responsible for masking the real causes of the production and reproduction of poverty in society, found in capitalism and in the unequal concentration of wealth intrinsic to its development (Moura Jr. & Ximenes, 2016).

In Latin America and the Caribbean, despite a decline in extreme poverty rates, economic disparities and income concentration continue to rise (Economic Commission for Latin America and the Caribbean [CEPAL], 2023). While the wealthiest 10% concentrate a significant portion of income, the poorest live in extreme deprivation, with hunger and food insecurity reaching alarming levels (United Nations Organization for Food and Agriculture [FAO], 2023). In countries of the Organization for Economic Cooperation and Development (OECD), the increase in housing prices, especially in metropolitan regions, aggravates the situation, with the cost of living rising and wages remaining stagnant, contributing to the impoverishment of the population (OECD, n.d.). This scenario reflects a historical process that, in many cases, associates economic liberalism with the emergence of extremist ideologies. The deterioration of living conditions generates discontent, leading individuals to formulate simplistic explanations that blame certain vulnerable groups for economic and social crises, fueling stigma. In this context of deepening social inequalities, there has been a recent increase in the homeless population in Latin American countries, such as Uruguay (Ministry of Social Development [MIDES], 2023) and Brazil (Brazil, 2023).

Despite the variation of definitions and ways of measuring homelessness among different countries and regions, the situation of extreme poverty is a structuring aspect of the definitions. The homeless are the "poorest among the poor," enduring the effects of precarious living conditions on the streets and stigma more pervasively than other impoverished groups, either by the greater visibility they have living on the streets, by the association of their bodies with dirt, given the difficulty of access to personal hygiene in this context, by the belief reinforced by the media that these people display disruptive behaviors or by their association with other stigmatized conditions (Phelan et al., 1997). Frequently, homeless people are subject to stigmatizing discourses that reinforce negative stereotypes about who they are and why they are in this situation (Canham et al., 2024).

One of the ways in which the stigma of poverty can manifest itself is through blaming the homeless for the situation they live in. Although accumulated evidence shows that homelessness is predominantly caused by structural factors of capitalism, such as poverty, unemployment, the absence of affordable housing and effective social security systems, shared explanations of the phenomenon based on individual characteristics and behaviors of the homeless persist in society (Bramley & Fitzpatrick, 2017; Vázquez et al., 2018). Attributing responsibility to individuals due to stigma fosters discriminatory attitudes toward homeless people by groups with greater economic power through the opposition of "us" (productive and deserving) against "them" (unproductive, undeserving, and dangerous), as well as the society's disengagement with the problem by not seeing it as a failure of the current economic model but as individual failure (Belcher & Deforge, 2012). Thus, stigma shapes the formulation of political responses and limits social change (Belcher & Deforge, 2012).

However, the stigmatization of the homeless is not a unique function of poverty. It results from the intersection of multiple stigmas that contribute to the oppression of the homeless and the perpetuation of inequities through the interplay of these stigmas at different levels and through various mechanisms (Pauly, 2014). The homeless are also stigmatized due to substance use and face discrimination based on race, gender, and the intersection of other systems of oppression (Canham et al., 2024). Thus, for homeless individuals with multiple devalued social identities, such as Black homeless women who use drugs, the impact of stigma results from the accumulation and intersection of different stigmas, often exacerbating their vulnerability beyond the sum of each individual stigma's effects.

Drug use is another significant source of stigma for the homeless. Although drug use is highly prevalent among the homeless, including in the form of substance use disorders (SUD), not all homeless individuals use drugs. Furthermore, study designs typically overestimate the prevalence of SUD among the homeless (Mayock & O'Shaughnessy, 2023). Often, drug use among the homeless is a response to traumatic experiences in their life histories and to the harsh living conditions on the streets, including hunger, cold, sleep deprivation, constant vigilance, and chronic stress (Moreira et al., 2024). In this context, drugs serve as a potential coping strategy for total vulnerability and the suffering of street life. Even when use is prior to becoming homeless, the experience in this environment can influence the establishment of more harmful consumption patterns and expose individuals to greater risks. However, due to stigma, substance use is seen as the reason for these people being homeless and as an individual problem, again blaming the homeless and disregarding the weight of the contextual factors involved both in the determination of homelessness and drug use and dependence (Mayock & O'Shaughnessy, 2023).

Using the concept of intersectional stigma, we can analyze how the intersection of poverty and drug use stigma influences state responses to homeless drug users. According to Ximenes et al. (2018), repressive policies encompassed by the ideology of the "War on Drugs" are not truly directed at substances but at representatives of the most vulnerable and subaltern classes—namely, poor and non-white individuals. By simultaneously carrying the social identities of being poor and drug users, the homeless are historically perceived through the stereotype of a dangerous class and criminalized for their situation. Through the intersection of these stigmas, various hygienist and extremely violent interventions against the homeless are legitimized with the aim of "cleaning" urban space and in the name of supposed public safety (Ximenes et al., 2018). Such actions end up perpetuating the stigma and vulnerability of the homeless.

Directly aligned with this discussion is the issue of the ethnic-racial profile of the homeless and its relations with stigma. In Brazil, as seen in other countries with regard to the overrepresentation of Black people and ethnic-racial minorities among the homeless, administrative records show that Black individuals make up 68% of the homeless population (more than double the proportion of white individuals), despite representing 55.5% of the total population (Brazil, 2023). Although the use of official data may underestimate the number of Black people among the homeless, considering that, due to intersectional stigma, they may face even greater barriers to accessing services, these statistics make visible how stigma and structural racism affect the unequal distribution of risks for homelessness among different ethnic-racial groups (Fowle, 2022). Explanations for the greater vulnerability of Black people to homelessness due to stigma and structural racism can be found, for example, in the historical economic and social inequities between white and Black people, housing segregation, restricted access to adequate housing, the criminalization and mass incarceration of Black populations under the "War on Drugs" and in the focus of homelessness policies on immediate individual causes rather than structural causes (Fowle, 2022; Verissimo et al., 2021).

In addition to the increased risk for homelessness, racism reinforces the intersectional stigma faced by homeless people. Studies such as those by Markowitz and Syverson (2019) and Verissimo et al. (2021) show that the experience of stigma and discrimination differs for Black people living on the streets. They are perceived as more dangerous by others and face greater discrimination than other subgroups of the homeless due to the overlap of multiple stigmatized identities. Oliveira et al. (2023) highlight the heightened vulnerability of Black people and women living on the streets to violence, emphasizing the potential role of intersectional stigma in legitimizing violence and perpetuating inequities and oppressive processes. In this sense, the next section focuses on the particular impact of gender in the intersectional stigma faced by women living on the streets.

3.3 Gender on the Streets: The Stigma of Homeless Women

The daily life and forms of stigma that affect women living on the streets must be understood from the historical-social construction of this population. In the context of deepening and consolidation of the capitalist mode of production, it stands out, particularly, the way in which gender roles were shaped to serve as supports to the sphere of reproduction of the emerging order. In general, the capitalist mode of production, by imposing a sexual division of labor and establishing gender roles, places a division of work tasks outside the home (Federeci, 2017). This structure creates a strong power relationship that is often intersected by violence and various forms of abuse and exploitation. Women, in addition to the formal workday, are responsible for the care of the home, children, elderly or sick family members, and other tasks. And, as reproducers of human labor, they also assume the function of guaranteeing the conditions for the realization of production itself. The home and life need to be in order so that men can carry out their external work with tranquility, and this has been traditionally seen as a female responsibility (Davis, 2013).

Although oppression against women is not original to capitalism, its dynamics structurally require *machismo* and patriarchy as sustaining forces. In 2018, the Brazilian Institute of Geography and Statistics (IBGE) found that 30.4% of homicides against women occurred within their own homes, while the rate among men was 11.2% (IBGE, 2018). Data from the International Labor Organization (ILO) (2024) indicate that for 75% of men in the labor market, women make up 48.5%.

Meanwhile, housework occupies 21.3 h per week for women and 11.7 h for men. Women's wages are 20.7% lower, and the unemployment rate is 50% higher. The data frame represents to some extent the living conditions of women and the multiple exploitations present in their lives, frequent motivators for women, in their search for survival, to end up on the streets.

Despite historically being a minority in homelessness statistics, the increase in the number of women living on the streets has been observed worldwide (Phipps et al., 2019), accompanying the increase in the number of the homeless in general. The "feminization" of the homelessness and the consequent greater visibility of women in this context in recent years reflect the effect of the intersection of systems of oppression—not reduced only to gender—in the configuration of inequities and systematic disadvantages for women, as observed in the consistent associations between domestic violence, childhood abuse, economic dependence and exploitation, and homelessness among women (Bretherton, 2023). Trauma, abusive relationships, exploitation, broken bonds, and drug use are common factors that motivate the move to the streets among women. Also contributing to this situation are extreme socioeconomic conditions, which leave poor women with no option but to live on the street to ensure their survival. It is noteworthy that this process does not necessarily occur abruptly. Most of the time, it occurs gradually after the rupture with family and work institutions and the exhaustion of available resources. This is a process that is even more intensified for Black women, who, due to structural racism, have a greater vulnerability to end up on the streets due to domestic violence, higher probability of living in conditions of poverty and in communities with high rates of violence, in addition to having less access to resources to deal with crises (Bullock et al., 2020).

Despite the greater visibility gained by women living on the streets in recent years, according to Löfstrand and Quilgars (2016), the generalized stereotypes about the homeless as a predominantly male population and widely visible in public spaces were responsible for masking and minimizing the presence of women on the streets for a long time. Influenced by intersectional stigma, the invisibility of women living on the streets is also linked to the perception of deviation from gender roles and cultural norms about being a woman founded on patriarchy. This perspective is consistent with the *intersectional invisibility hypothesis* (Purdie-Vaughns & Eibach, 2008), which proposes that people belonging to multiple marginalized groups are socially made invisible because they are not "prototypes" of any particular social category. Women living on the streets deviate from both the hegemonic representations of women, linked to the domestic environment, and the homeless, associated with the male sex and visible presence on the streets, having their experiences silenced within these two groups. In addition, intersectional stigma and attempts to manage it lead women to experience more "hidden" forms of homelessness, as they seek precarious living arrangements with families and friends, remove their presence from public view on the streets, and avoid male-dominated services (Löfstrand & Quilgars, 2016).

Life on the streets puts women in a situation of great fragility and exposure in all areas. Women face the countless difficulties that exist for all homeless people, however, when experiencing the streets as women, gender is a component that complicates and amplifies the inherent risks of this space and reinforces their stigmatization (Esmeraldo & Ximenes, 2022). Women living on the streets suffer not only the same material and social deprivations as men but also experience specific forms of violence related to their gender. The streets are predominantly a male space, which generates dynamics of subordination and violence against women. Often, these women depend on affective or sexual relationships to obtain basic resources or ensure their protection, which perpetuates unequal power relations. The patriarchal dynamics experienced in the domestic environment are updated in the gender inequalities present on the streets, adding layers to the processes of domination and oppression of women living on the streets and influencing how they are represented.

It is a consensus in the literature that violence constitutes a structuring element of the lives of women living on the streets, both before and after they end up on the streets. Living on the streets is already considered a traumatic experience in itself and involves great exposure to violence. However, the intersection of being a woman and being on the streets makes these women even more vulnerable to all types of violence, whether physical, sexual, or symbolic, perpetrated by other men living on the streets, by state agents, or by service professionals (Silva et al., 2022). For example, in the study by Oliveira et al. (2023), the chance of women living on the streets suffering some type of violence was 42 times greater than that of men. As a result of disproportionate victimization and the traumas suffered, women living on the streets suffer more in terms of their mental health than men in the same situation, such as from anxiety, depression, and post-traumatic stress (Phipps et al., 2019). Usually, substance use appears as a strategy to cope with psychological suffering and as a form of protection against the risk of being violated by allowing them to stay alert and vigilant, constituting a means of adapting to reality and an alternative to dealing with dangers (Moreira et al., 2024).

But if, on one hand, drug use serves as a defense and escape from the harmful circumstances in which these women are inserted, on the other hand, it makes them more susceptible to sexually transmitted diseases, unwanted pregnancy, and to suffer abuses and violence on the streets (Coldibelli et al., 2022). Added to this, drug use reinforces the intersectional stigma of women living on the streets (Thomas & Menih, 2022). Being a behavior linked to the male universe, the use of drugs by women living on the streets violates normative and socially constructed standards about femininity, which confine women to the domestic sphere and the maternal role. By breaking with these representations, women living on the streets who use drugs are even more stigmatized for their use than men, being seen as promiscuous, irresponsible, criminal, morally condemnable, and guilty for their situation (Medeiros et al., 2017). In this sense, they suffer from a "triple" stigmatization: for transgressing the social role of women, for using drugs, and for living on the streets (a "fourth" dimension of racial stigma can also be added).

The overlap of multiple stigmas and vulnerabilities in the daily lives of women living on the streets legitimizes prejudiced attitudes and punitive institutional interventions, especially in pregnancy and motherhood (Santos et al., 2024). Women living on the streets are immediately labeled as "bad mothers" and incapable of exercising motherhood or even criminalized and blamed for the use of substances during pregnancy, without the slightest consideration of the context of extreme social vulnerability in which these women, mostly Black and extremely poor, live. There are common reports of interventions implemented by the State that violate the reproductive rights of women living on the streets, such as the compulsory separation of mothers and babies already in maternity, even when the mother expresses the desire for the child and the search for alternatives to ensure their care (Santos et al., 2024). Also, women living on the streets with children are the object of control and surveillance by professionals, suffering stigmatization and discrimination for not conforming to the dominant notions of a "good mother." State interventions, instead of empowering them, usually reinforce control dynamics that perpetuate cycles of marginalization and vulnerability.

As another implication of intersectional stigma and the invisibility of women living on the streets, there is also the non-existence of public policies specifically directed at women in this situation and their particularities, except when related to pregnancy (Esmeraldo & Ximenes, 2022). In this case, it is the presence of one or more children that is the main determinant of service provision, and not the needs of the women. The existing services for the homeless are marked by access barriers for women living on the streets, by the absence of a gender focus and attention to victims of violence, and by the institutional violence perpetrated by professionals who stigmatize and neglect their needs, seeing women living on the streets as dependent and vulnerable (Löfstrand & Quilgars, 2016). The stigmatization by professionals distances women from the services and points to the need for care in the way women living on the streets are made visible. Barriers in access to treatment for problems related to the use of alcohol and other drugs and TUS, due to previous experiences of discrimination based on the intersection of stigmas, the underlying misogyny in these environments, the majority presence of men in these spaces, the fear of having their children taken away, as well as the lack of coordination of services, also hinder the meeting of the needs of this group and perpetuate their cycle of oppression (Thomas & Menih, 2022). To illustrate the impacts of intersectional stigma, some data about the reality of women living on the streets in Uruguay and Brazil are presented below.

3.4 Women Living on the Streets in Uruguay and in Brazil

In recent years, the issue of homelessness in Uruguay has gained increasing visibility, particularly in urban areas such as Montevideo. According to recent data from MIDES (2023), 2756 people were recorded in this condition in Montevideo, with 1375 living outdoors and 1381 in night shelters or contingency shelters. This increase represents a 24% growth compared to 2021, with a particularly alarming 49.5% rise among those sleeping outdoors, compared to a 6.6% increase in night shelters. Although the homeless population is predominantly composed of young and adult men, the proportion of women has increased, reaching 8.7% among those sleeping outdoors in 2023. These data indicate a change in the profile of people affected by this issue.

Furthermore, it is worth noting that, within this population, certain groups are overrepresented, such as Afro-descendants, indigenous people, and transgender individuals. Transgender individuals, in particular, represent only 0.03% of the total population but constitute 0.8% of those who sleep outdoors and 1.6% of those who are in night shelters. These data highlight the existence of structural patterns of discrimination that disproportionately affect these populations. In the case of women, the increase in their participation in the homeless population highlights their greater vulnerability, as they face not only the precariousness of living on the street but also multiple forms of gender violence and social stigmatization. However, the report does not provide additional details on gender-related issues.

Additionally, it is important to consider the dynamics of aggression experienced by people living on the streets. According to available data, the main aggressors of those who sleep outdoors are other people in the same situation (31.9%), followed by the police (30%) and by neighbors or passers-by who are not homeless (17.9%). Also, substance use is an important element in this reality. Since 2020, base paste has become the most consumed substance among this population, reported by 77% of respondents in 2023, surpassing alcohol (53.3%) and marijuana (47.5%). The use of cocaine, although less frequent, also experienced a notable increase of almost 10 percentage points between 2020 and 2023, being consumed by a quarter of the homeless population (MIDES, 2023).

Although the MIDES Program for Attention to People in Homeless Situations has played a role in providing night shelters, its limitations are evident, especially when it comes to serving women who use substances. The current shelters do not contemplate the particular needs of these women, who often show reluctance to access these spaces for fear of being separated from their children or suffering violence and abuse in them. Thus, Uruguay has implemented specific programs aimed at women in homeless situations, particularly those with children. In this sense, there is a program that has 15 shelters intended for single-parent families led by women. This differentiated approach aims to address the specific needs of women in homeless situations, who face both social exclusion and the responsibility of caring for minors (Evans Penela, 2020). However, despite the existence of these measures, it is evident that challenges persist. In addition, there are also civil society initiatives that try to offer alternatives to this vulnerable population. One example is the collective Not Everything Is Lost (NITEP), which emerged in 2018 with the aim of combating prejudice against people experiencing homelessness. NITEP fights for the dignity of these people and seeks to empower them through active participation in assemblies and cooperative projects (Guevara & González, 2022). Although their resources are limited, these initiatives have managed to generate support spaces and community networks for women seeking to escape precariousness and violence. The COVID-19 pandemic has further exacerbated this reality, increasing the violence and social exclusion that these women face.

In Uruguay, women experiencing homelessness face vulnerabilities common to this population in other countries, including a life history marked by abuse, problematic substance use, gendered experiences on the streets, and greater barriers to accessing social assistance and healthcare services. Analogous to this reality, Brazil presents a hostile environment for women experiencing homelessness, particularly regarding the forms of violence encountered in this context. According to the Ministry of Human Rights and Citizenship (MDHC), in a report built from the Federal Government's data systems, women represent only 13% of the total number of people living on the streets but account for 40% of the reported cases of violence (Brazil, 2023). Transgender women represent the most frequent gender identity among the victims who had this field filled out. The most reported forms of violence were physical (88%) and psychological (14%), with the probable perpetrators of the violence being unknown to the victims (39%).

In order to illustrate this reality, a cut was made from the *Census and Diagnosis of the Homeless Population of Juiz de Fora* (Pereira et al., 2023), carried out in November 2022. The Census data indicates that 147 women are homeless, accounting for approximately 18.3% of the city's homeless population. Of these, 26 women responded to the diagnostic questionnaire. The average age of the respondents was 44.11 years (SD = 15.22). The majority were Black women (69.3%), heterosexual (76.9%), literate (88.5%), and had education up to the elementary school level (57.7%). Most respondents reported having been on the streets for more than 5 years (38.5%), followed by 1–2 years (26.9%). When asked about the frequency of sleeping on the streets in the last month, many stated they had slept on the streets every day during this period (79.2%). The primary reason reported for sleeping on the streets was conflict or the breakdown of family ties (53.84%). Other common reasons included: release from the prison system (34.6%), substance use (34.6%), dismissal/unemployment (19.2%), and threats/violence (19.2%). The interviewees also reported having slept in private homes before becoming homeless (73.1%). Most have used or are currently using government shelters (92%). Among the women who had worked before becoming homeless (65.38%), informal employment was the most common (58.8%).

Regarding health issues, two women reported being pregnant (9.5%) and are both receiving prenatal care through the Unified Health System (SUS). The most reported health conditions were substance use (57.7%), physical injuries (50%), lung diseases (30.8%), oral diseases (30.8%), hypertension (19.2%), and HIV (19.2%). However, few women reported having access to treatment for these conditions: substance use (0%), physical injuries (7.7%), lung diseases (11.5%), oral diseases (15.4%), with the exception of treatment for hypertension (15.4%) and HIV (19.2%). Regarding the consumption of substances in the context of the streets, 83.3% of the interviewees reported using some substance. Among them, the most consumed substances in the month prior to the interview were: tobacco (95%), alcohol (60%), crack cocaine (35%), and marijuana/hashish (30%). The trend of consumption of these substances followed the frequency of use in the week prior to the interview: daily consumption of tobacco (70%), daily consumption of alcohol (25%), daily consumption of crack cocaine (15%), and daily consumption of marijuana/hashish (5%). The primary reasons reported for substance use were seeking relief from the suffering caused by life on the streets (20%) and curiosity/desire (20%).

Most of the interviewees stated they had suffered some type of violence on the streets (80.8%). The most commonly reported types of violence included verbal abuse, humiliation, and discrimination (81%), physical assault (61.9%), robbery/theft (61.9%), having belongings discarded (57.1%), shooting/stabbing (23.8%), being forcibly removed from the streets (14.3%), and sexual abuse (9.5%). Other people living on the streets were the authors of the most frequent violence in the reports (75%), followed by people passing by the streets (52.6%), police (36.8%), residents of the surrounding area (31.6%), drug dealers (26.3%), merchants (21.1%), private security (21.1%), and municipal guards (10.5%).

The data highlight the intersectional stigma faced by women experiencing homelessness in Juiz de Fora. Coldibelli et al. (2022) emphasize that in the reality of women living on the streets, violence, extreme poverty, drug use, and health conditions are intertwined in a dynamic of living on the streets, where each of these elements influences the other, with violence being the central axis of this dynamic. The health conditions of these women highlight the barriers to accessing healthcare services, as evidenced by the untreated conditions presented. Generally, these barriers stem from the way women experiencing homelessness are treated by healthcare providers: their concerns and health needs are often neglected, and they do not receive care that is suitable for their circumstances (Souza et al., 2016). The high levels of substance use foster discussions about its role in the daily lives of these women. However, the impact of the illicit status of certain drugs and the stigma associated with their use are often more harmful than the substances themselves (Souza et al., 2016), as they can legitimize violence against this population.

The violent daily life experienced by women living on the streets is also demonstrated in the exposed data. The life story of these women is commonly crossed by violence, whether it is violence suffered or exposed to in childhood or violence exercised by intimate partners and family members in adulthood. In both cases, the main perpetrator of violence is the male figure present in the context. Also, the search for protection against violence often constitutes the reason why women are forced to leave their homes and go to the streets (Silva et al., 2022; Souza et al., 2016). However, despite this escape, the streets also present themselves as a dangerous space, where there is violence associated with stigma, which dehumanizes the victim. The data reflect this reality when they indicate that most of the interviewed women stated they had suffered some form of discrimination and physical aggression on the streets. The fact that other people living on the streets and people passing by the streets were the main perpetrators of violence shows that the constant violation continues on the streets. It is important to note that the legitimacy of violence, as well as other forms of violation reported, is justified by intersectional stigma. The stigmas associated with race, women drug users, and the situation of living on the streets compose this scenario.

3.5 Final Considerations

This chapter sought to briefly discuss how intersectional stigma affects women living on the streets and deepens their vulnerability due to the overlap of oppressions based on gender, poverty, race, and drug use. The intersection of these stigmas not only renders the existence of homeless women invisible but also legitimizes various forms of violence against their bodies, perpetuated by the general population, professionals, and the State. This creates barriers that hinder their access to essential services. The effects of stigma on their health and in the direction of State interventions point to the urgent need for the development of policies that, acknowledging the harmful impacts of intersectional stigma, are more equitable and attentive to the particularities of the needs of these women. In this regard, there is a critical need for increased investment in programs that provide access to healthcare, harm reduction, and social assistance. Additionally, public policies should adopt an intersectional approach that addresses the specific needs of these women, ensuring their access to housing, protection from violence, and trauma-informed care. Finally, the establishment of safe spaces for homeless women and their children should be prioritized in public policy, with a focus on defending the rights of women experiencing homelessness.

References

Belcher, J. R., & DeForge, B. R. (2012). Social stigma and homelessness: The limits of social change. *Journal of Human Behavior in the Social Environment, 22*(8), 929–946.

Bramley, G., & Fitzpatrick, S. (2017). Homelessness in the UK: Who is most at risk? *Housing Studies, 33*(1), 96–116.

Brasil (2023). População em Situação de Rua: Diagnóstico com base nos dados e informações disponíveis em registros administrativos e sistemas do Governo Federal.. Ministério dos Direitos Humanos e Cidadania.

Bretherton, J. (2023). Gender. In J. Bretherton & N. Pleace (Eds.), *The Routledge handbook of homelessness* (pp. 147–157). Routledge.

Bullock, H. E., Reppond, H. A., Truong, S. V., & Singh, M. R. (2020). An intersectional analysis of the feminization of homelessness and mothers' housing precarity. *Journal of Social Issues, 76*(4), 835–858.

Canham, S. L., Weldrick, R., Erisman, M., McNamara, A., Rosa, J. N., Siantz, E., Casucci, T., & McFarland, M. M. (2024). A scoping review of the experiences and outcomes of stigma and discrimination towards persons experiencing homelessness. *Health & Social Care in the Community, 2024*, 2060619.

Coldibelli, L. P., Paiva, F. S., & Batista, C. R. (2022). Gênero, pobreza e políticas públicas nas trajetórias de mulheres em situação de rua. In I. V. Ximenes, A. F. L. Esmeraldo, & C. E. E. Filho (Eds.), *Viver nas Ruas: Trajetórias, Desafios e Resistências* (pp. 285–308). Expressão Gráfica e Editora.

Collins, P. H. (2015). Intersectionality's definitional dilemmas. *Annual Review of Sociology, 41*, 1–20.

Comissão Econômica para a América Latina e Caribe. (2023). *Panorama Social da América Latina e Caribe 2023: Resumo Executivo*. CEPAL.

Davis, A. (2013). *Mulheres, Raça e Classe*. Plataforma Gueto.
Else-Quest, N. M., French, A. M., & Telfer, N. A. (2023). The intersectionality imperative: Calling in stigma and health research. *Stigma and Health, 8*(3), 269–278.
Esmeraldo, A. F. L., & Ximenes, V. M. (2022). Mulheres em Situação de Rua: Implicações Psicossociais de Estigmas e Preconceitos. *Psicologia: Ciência e Profissão, 42*, 1–15.
Evans Penela, T. (2020). La relevancia de la temporalidad en los estudios y políticas sobre situación de calle: Un análisis de secuencias de asistencias a refugios para personas sin hogar en Uruguay. *Revista de Ciencias Sociales, 29*(45), 135–164.
Federeci, S. (2017). *Calibã e a Bruxa*. Editora Elefante.
Fowle, M. Z. (2022). Racialized homelessness: A review of historical and contemporary causes of racial disparities in homelessness. *Housing Policy Debate, 32*(6), 940–967.
Goffman, E. (1980). *Estigma: Notas sobre a Manipulação da Identidade Deteriorada* (3rd ed.). Zahar Editores. (Trabalho original publicado em 1963).
Guevara, A., & González, T. (2022). «Trinchera de cuidados» Formas de vivir, convivir y cuidar en colectivo en situación de calle. *Encuentros Latinoamericanos (segunda época), 6*(1), 57–72.
Instituto Brasileiro de Geografia e Estatística. (2018). Estatísticas de gênero: indicadores sociais das mulheres no Brasil.. IBGE.
Link, B. G., & Phelan, J. C. (2001). Conceptualizing stigma. *Annual Review of Sociology, 27*(1), 363–385.
Link, B. G., Phelan, J. C., & Hatzenbuehler, M. L. (2018). Stigma as a fundamental cause of health inequality. In B. Major, J. F. Dovidio, & B. G. Link (Eds.), *The Oxford handbook of stigma, discrimination and health* (pp. 56–67). Oxford University Press.
Löfstrand, C. H., & Quilgars, D. (2016). Cultural images and definitions of homeless women: Implications for policy and practice at the European level. In P. Mayock & J. Bretherton (Eds.), *Women's homelessness in Europe* (pp. 41–73). Palgrave Macmillan.
Markowitz, F. E., & Syverson, J. (2019). Race, gender, and homelessness stigma: Effects of perceived blameworthiness and dangerousness. *Deviant Behavior, 42*(7), 919–931.
Mayock, P., & O'Shaughnessy, B. (2023). Homelessness and substance use. In J. Bretherton & N. Pleace (Eds.), *The Routledge handbook of homelessness* (pp. 35–47). Routledge.
Medeiros, K. T., Maciel, S. C., & Sousa, P. F. (2017). A Mulher no Contexto das Drogas: Representações Sociais de Usuárias em Tratamento. *Paidéia (Ribeirão Preto), 27*, 439–447.
Ministerio de Desarrollo Social. (2023). *Relevamiento de personas en situación de calle en Montevideo: Informe 2023*. Dirección Nacional de Transferencias y Análisis de Datos (DINTAD) & Dirección Nacional de Protección Social (DNPS).
Moreira, A. L. C., Alves, N. S. S., Macêdo, M. L., Reis, A. E. S. F., Holanda, N. V., & Conceição, M. I. G. (2024). The hidden face of the moon: Unveiling the minutiae of a Black Woman's experience on the streets. *Trends in Psychology, 32*, 505–524.
Moura, J. F., Jr., & Ximenes, V. M. (2016). A identidade social estigmatizada de pobre: uma constituição opressora. *Fractal: Revista De Psicologia, 28*(1), 76–83.
Oliveira, G. C. M., Martins, A. C., Pazini, D. S., Paula, E. E. P., Nunes, L. C., & Freitas, E. D. (2023). Tipificação e fatores associados à ocorrência de violência em pessoas em situação de rua em um município de Minas Gerais, Brasil. *Ciência & Saúde Coletiva, 28*(6), 1607–1617.
Organização das Nações Unidas para Alimentação e Agricultura. (2023). *World food and agriculture—Statistical yearbook 2023*. FAO.
Organização Internacional do Trabalho. (2024, 8 de Março). *A longa e sinuosa estrada rumo à igualdade de gênero*. https://www.ilo.org/pt-pt/resource/news/artigo-de-opiniao-longa-e-sinuosa-estrada-rumo-igualdade-de-genero
Organização para a Cooperação e Desenvolvimento Econômico. (n.d.). *Housing*. https://www.oecd.org/en/topics/housing.html
Parker, R. (2013). Interseções entre Estigma, Preconceito e Discriminação na Saúde Pública Mundial. In S. Monteiro & W. Villella (Eds.), *Estigma e saúde* (pp. 25–46). Editora FIOCRUZ.

Pauly, B. (2014). Homelessness, stigma, and health. In W. C. Cockerham, R. Dingwall, & S. R. Quah (Eds.), *The Wiley Blackwell encyclopedia of health, illness, behavior, and society*. John Wiley & Sons.

Pereira, V. S., Arbia, A. A., Ferreira, A. M., Ribeiro, L. C., Castro, M. M. C., & Ronzani, T. M. (2023). *Censo e Diagnóstico da População Adulta de Juiz de Fora (MG): Relatório Final*. UFJF.

Phelan, J., Link, B. G., Moore, R. E., & Stueve, A. (1997). The stigma of homelessness: The impact of the label "homeless" on attitudes toward poor persons. *Social Psychology Quarterly, 60*(4), 323–337.

Phipps, M., Dalton, L., Maxwell, H., & Cleary, M. (2019). Women and homelessness, a complex multidimensional issue: Findings from a scoping review. *Journal of Social Distress and the Homeless, 28*(1), 1–13.

Purdie-Vaughns, V., & Eibach, R. P. (2008). Intersectional invisibility: The distinctive advantages and disadvantages of multiple subordinate-group identities. *Sex Roles, 59*(5–6), 377–391.

Santos, K. C. C. D., Marques, L. S. S., Gonçalves, M. T., Soledade, M. M. S., Santos, J. G. S., & Oliveira, J. F. (2024). Maternidade e maternagem em situação de rua: revisão integrativa. *Ciência & Saúde Coletiva, 29*, e010982023.

Silva, M. L., Bousfield, A. B. S., Silva, A. B., Giacomozzi, A. I., Leandro, M., & Cavaler, C. M. (2022). Violence for women experiencing homelessness. *PSICO, 53*(1).

Souza, M. R. R., Oliveira, J. F., Chagas, M. C. G., & Carvalho, E. S. S. (2016). Gênero, violência e viver na rua: vivências de mulheres que fazem uso problemático de drogas. *Revista Gaúcha de Enfermagem, 37*(3), e59876.

Thomas, N., & Menih, H. (2022). Negotiating multiple stigmas: Substance use in the lives of women experiencing homelessness. *International Journal of Mental Health and Addiction, 20*, 2973–2992.

Turan, J. M., Elafros, M. A., Logie, C. H., Banik, S., Turan, B., Crockett, K. B., Pescosolido, B., & Murray, S. M. (2019). Challenges and opportunities in examining and addressing intersectional stigma and health. *BMC Medicine, 17*, 7.

Vázquez, J. J., Panadero, S., & Zúñiga, C. (2018). Attributions about homelessness in homeless and domiciled people in Madrid, Spain: "Why are they homeless people?". *The American Journal of Orthopsychiatry, 88*(2), 236–247.

Verissimo, A. D. O., Henley, N., Gee, G. C., Davis, C., & Grella, C. (2021). Homelessness and discrimination among US adults: The role of intersectionality. *Journal of Social Distress and Homelessness, 32*(1), 1–15.

Williams, S. L., & Fredrick, E. G. (2015). One size may not fit all: The need for a more inclusive and intersectional psychological science on stigma. *Sex Roles, 73*, 384–390.

Ximenes, V., Paiva, F. S., Moura, J. F., Jr., & Costa, P. H. A. (2018). Drugs and poverty: Interfaces of oppression in the capitalist world. In T. M. Ronzani (Ed.), *Drugs and social contexts: Social perspectives on the use of alcohol and other drugs* (pp. 49–61). Springer.

Chapter 4
Stigma in Vulnerable Drug-Using Populations: Migrants, Incarcerated Individuals, and Women

Bárbara González Amado, Carolina Gorlero, Raquel Gallego, and Víctor José Villanueva-Blasco

4.1 Introduction

The term "stigma," understood as a complex process by which people or groups are seen as different, less desirable, or intelligent, or dangerous (Goffman, 1963), has traditionally accompanied drug users, especially when they carry the label of a vulnerable population, such as migrants or incarcerated individuals. This double categorization carries a double stigma (Fountain, 2009), which can negatively affect their social integration and their interpersonal relationships (Livingston et al., 2012), increase discrimination (Douglass et al., 2023) and their mental health problems (Garcini et al., 2016; Kartal & Kiropoulos, 2016), and lead to a poor overall quality of life. From a gender perspective, the predominant emphasis on substance use by men has focused on care designed for this population, thus neglecting the need for

B. G. Amado
Valencian International University, Valencia, Spain
e-mail: barbara.gonzaleza@professor.universidadviu.com

C. Gorlero
International Society of Substance Use Professionals (ISSUP) – Argentina, Buenos Aires, Argentina

R. Gallego
Women's Information Center, Vigo, Spain

V. J. Villanueva-Blasco (✉)
Valencian International University, Valencia, Spain

Research Network in Primary Care of Addictions (RIAPAd), Madrid, Spain

International Society of Substance Use Professionals (ISSUP), Madrid, Spain

International Center for Technology Transfer in Addictions (ITTC), Valencia, Spain
e-mail: vjvillanueva@universidadviu.com

T. Mota Ronzani (ed.), *Social Stigma and Drug Use*,
https://doi.org/10.1007/978-3-031-94813-8_4

attention toward women and their particular circumstances. This disparity has contributed to the invisibility of the problems that women face in relation to drug use.

4.2 Stigma in Migrant Drug-Using Population

The stigma toward the migrant drug-using population is a complex phenomenon. Migrants, generally defined as those who reside outside their country of origin for more than 12 months (United Nations DESA, 1998), often face multiple forms of discrimination, increasing their vulnerability if they are also drug users. These are populations often subjected to situations of xenophobia and discrimination, often characterized by lack of employment and a home, which can lead to isolation and lack of access to services that provide support for their mental and physical health (WHO, 2023).

When we talk about migrants in vulnerable situations, we refer to those people who cannot effectively exercise their human rights and are at greater risk of violations and abuses (UN IOM, 2019). This can occur, especially, in situations of forced migration; that is, when there is a migratory movement that, although its triggering factors can be diverse, involves force, compulsion, or coercion (UN IOM, 2019).

Some situations of forced migration often lead to seeking asylum in host countries. When applying for asylum, refugees seek protection in other countries due to conflicts and persecutions in their place of origin, which makes returning dangerous for their life or freedom. The term "refugee" is a legal concept that provides certain safeguards to those who qualify under this condition (UNHCR, 2011). According to the Convention on the Status of Refugees (1951), a refugee is a person who, fearing persecution for reasons such as race, religion, nationality, membership of a social group, or political opinions, cannot or does not wish to return to their country (Convention on the Status of Refugees, [UN], 1951).

These clarifications are important when considering the situation of vulnerable migrants and distinguishing what happens with asylum seekers or refugees. Migrating is a human right (Universal Declaration of Human Rights, art. 13), and international organizations emphasize the importance of avoiding oversimplified assumptions that every migrant is in a vulnerable situation (Mosler Vidal & Laczko, 2022). There are migratory journeys that improve the quality of life of people, increase their contact networks, and favor access to a better job or education, among other issues. However, in many countries, negative social representations associated with migrants function as major barriers when accessing fundamental human rights, and the stigma that falls on them can generate psychological distress and obstruct the processes of integration in the host communities (Gorlero et al., 2021).

This situation is even more complex for those who, in addition to being migrants, are drug users. Drug use, along with the condition of being a migrant and other stigmatized identities such as gender, race, or ethnicity, amplifies the negative impact on mental health and social relationships of those who possess multiple stigmatized identities (Douglass et al., 2023; Saleh et al., 2023). In addition, migrants who use drugs are often categorized as deviant individuals, with an inferior status, are seen as weak and guilty of the situation in which they find themselves, which exacerbates their marginalization (Douglass et al., 2023).

This vulnerability is aggravated in many cases, especially when migrants face socioeconomic barriers, isolation, and lack of employment, factors that worsen both their physical and mental health (WHO, 2023). In fact, access to a job and favorable working conditions facilitate the inclusion of migrants, which reduces situations of discrimination and social stigmatization (Li et al., 2014) and promotes an improvement in mental health (Porter & Haslam, 2005).

Likewise, migratory processes are often modulated by variables of various kinds that can pose a risk factor for addiction (Aleer et al., 2023). Migratory stress and trauma are determining factors in the onset and perpetuation of substance use (Kronick et al., 2023). This is particularly so in the case of forced migrations, asylum seekers, and refugees. Studies like that of Horyniak et al. (2016) highlight that post-traumatic stress disorder (PTSD) is more prevalent among refugees than in the local population. This stress is intensified by the long stay in refugee camps, exposure to risky situations during the journey, such as arrests or kidnappings, and continuous exposure to trauma (Porter & Haslam, 2005). Likewise, many of the forced migrants have been direct or indirect victims of potentially traumatic or stressful situations, such as deprivation, violence in its different forms, tortures, deaths, family separations, and loss of friendships (Horyniak et al., 2016), among other things. All of this usually predisposes these populations to the development of mental disorders. Also, the comorbidity between mental disorders and substance use is common, especially when substance use is employed as a coping strategy in response to trauma, socio-structural barriers, and the process of forced migration (Saleh et al., 2023).

To this are added the challenges of acculturation or apprehension to the new culture of the destination country and marginalization, which generates greater risks of mental health problems such as depression, anxiety, and increased substance use as a coping mechanism (Garcini et al., 2016; Saleh et al., 2023). The worst consequences in mental health (greater anxious and depressive symptomatology) are those that are related to the processes of marginalization, that is, when the possibility of maintaining the culture of origin and participating in the host country is small. This translates into situations of community isolation, invisibility, loss of rights, and separation from family and friends (Garcini et al., 2016). In general, acculturation stress has been identified as a risk factor in the development of mental health problems, such as emotional distress or anguish (Garcini et al., 2016), post-traumatic stress (Kartal & Kiropoulos, 2016), and alcohol and other drug use.

Stigma also acts as a significant barrier to the access of migrant and refugee people to health and social support services (Horyniak et al., 2016), as well as to mental health and addiction treatment, often for fear of rejection or deportation (EUDA, 2023). Those migrants who use illegal drugs face a greater stigma, affecting the quality of the health services they receive and increasing the dropout rates from treatment (Douglass et al., 2023). Likewise, treatment programs are often not culturally adapted to meet their needs, which increases the dropout rate from these (Fountain, 2009).

In fact, stigma is one of the barriers that weighs most in the explanation of access to treatment for SUD in migrants, both men (Lindert et al., 2021) and women, along with shame (Douglass et al., 2023). Other factors that reduce access to health benefits may be related to barriers such as language or, even, being in an irregular situation, with the fear of deportation, not being able to hold residence rights in the destination country, or losing custody of their children, among other issues (EUDA, 2023).

To reduce stigma toward drug-using migrants, strategies such as educational and awareness programs have been implemented, proving to be effective in reducing prejudices (Horyniak et al., 2016). From a preventive point of view, early identification of risk factors and the provision of appropriate support through health services are fundamental to preventing substance abuse in the migrant population. An individualized approach to each particular case allows designing a response adjusted to the needs of each person, thus increasing the probability of effectiveness (Alegría et al., 2017).

On the other hand, interventions with migrant population that can improve the treatment of substance use and, therefore, reduce the stigma associated with their condition as consumers must be culturally sensitive and adapted to minority racial or ethnic groups (Banks et al., 2023; WHO, 2023), thus recognizing the right to health of refugee and migrant populations. Culturally adapting an intervention implies understanding individual and community experiences, as well as cultural and migratory backgrounds of the target population, to capture their worldview and values (Bernal et al., 2009; Jarvis & Kirmayer, 2023). Evidence has shown that this type of intervention makes treatments more accessible and better adjusted, increasing participation rates (Pinedo et al., 2018) and their effectiveness(Lauricella et al., 2016). In addition, culturally sensitive treatment programs, which address both migration-related traumas and substance use, are fundamental to improving retention rates in treatments and facilitating rehabilitation (Fountain, 2009).

In light of the above, it is essential that institutions promote equitable access to health services for the migrant population who use drugs, considering both the problems derived from the migratory process and the effects of stigma. Culturally sensitive interventions, which address the role of stigma as a key barrier to access to treatment, along with public health policies based on equity and justice, can facilitate reintegration and improve the quality of life of these vulnerable populations (Banks et al., 2023; WHO, 2023).

4.3 Stigma in People Deprived of Liberty Who Use Drugs

The intersectionality of multiple stigmatized identities that often accompanies this population, such as inmates and drug users, negatively affects their mental health (Novo et al., 2017), their self-esteem (Ahern et al., 2007), and adherence to treatments, as well as promotes the internalization of socially ingrained stereotypes about criminality (Newman & Crowell, 2021). Additionally, stigma can hinder access to medical care and rehabilitation programs within prisons, which increases the chances of relapse after release (Binswanger et al., 2011). In fact, in prison contexts, stigma can manifest as discriminatory treatment by prison staff or other inmates. This can include restricted access to rehabilitation programs and social segregation within the prison (Binswanger et al., 2012).

The comorbidity between substance use and mental disorders in prisons is quite common. Around 50% of the prison population has some SUD comorbid with other mental disorders (Bukten et al., 2024; EMCDDA, 2015). The dual condition of inmates who also have one or more mental disorders increases their social stigmatization compared to those individuals deprived of freedom who do not have any type of mental disorder, which again, can lead to worse recovery rates, worse treatment outcomes, and loss of job opportunities (Tremlin & Beazley, 2024).

Among the consequences of deprivation of liberty is the difficulty for these individuals to integrate socially, reducing their participation in society, making it difficult to obtain employment, causing family uprooting, and increasing the likelihood of recidivism (Tomaz et al., 2023). Likewise, outside of prison, the stigma persists, affecting access to employment, housing, and health services, perpetuating a cycle of social exclusion that increases the risk of criminal recidivism and relapse into drug use (Fazel et al., 2017).

On the other hand, the lack of adequate treatment for drug addiction during imprisonment increases the chances of criminal recidivism and relapses (Fazel et al., 2017). In fact, the implementation of evidence-based treatment programs within prisons has proven to be effective in reducing stigma. Pharmacological strategies, such as opioid maintenance treatment and harm reduction, have shown positive results in reducing drug use, increasing the chances of attending treatment and staying in it after prison, and improving opportunities for social reintegration (Hedrich et al., 2012). These programs help to reconfigure the perception of drug use, treating it as just another health problem, which contributes to the reduction of stigma. On the other hand, therapeutic communities are one of the most effective interventions with inmates to reduce recidivism and prevent relapses (Aslan, 2018; De Andrade et al., 2018), and cognitive-behavioral therapy is the most effective in reducing alcohol and other substance use (Doyle et al., 2019). For their part, interventions based on acceptance and commitment therapies manage to reduce self-stigma, while motivational interviewing and the life experiences of other individuals with SUDs are effective in reducing social stigma and stereotypes of the general population (Livingston et al., 2012).

In the field of public policy, some countries have adopted restorative justice approaches that focus on rehabilitation rather than punishment. These approaches have been effective in mitigating stigma and offer ex-offenders an opportunity to reintegrate into society constructively (Bazemore & Stinchcomb, 2004). In short, effective interventions in prison and healthcare assistance once they are free facilitate the social integration of ex-offenders with substance addiction and reduce the chances of recidivism. This is why political and institutional efforts should be primarily directed at facilitating access for these populations to health services, and the establishment of adherence to specific multi-level treatments (combining pharmacological treatment with psychosocial and follow-up outside of prison), with the aim of minimizing future risks and improving the quality of life of these people once in the community. Likewise, given the high comorbidity between mental disorders and substance use, interventions must be robust and flexible, addressing the different dual pathologies frequently present in this population.

4.4 Stigma in Women Who Use Drugs

Historically, drug use has been seen as a topic mainly associated with men, but epidemiological trends show that, in some countries, women are using certain drugs at the same level or in greater proportion than men. The non-medical use of controlled prescription drugs, synthetic drugs, and opioids demonstrates how drug use patterns are changing. The prevalence of tranquilizer use is higher among women than among men in almost all countries where data is available. And this pattern is valid not only in the general population but also among high school and university students (i.e., OAS-CICAD, 2019; OEDA, 2023).

Even so, drug use in women remains largely invisible, and the offer of specific treatments for them continues to be very limited, largely due to the strongly established social stigma in relation to women with a drug use problem (Fonseca et al., 2021).

The stigma toward women who use drugs is a complex phenomenon that operates, at least, on two interrelated levels: on the one hand, gender stigma, and on the other, the stigma associated with substance use. This intersection favors the prevalence of social environments of discrimination and exclusion that not only affect the social and family life of women but also have direct implications on their access to health services and treatment and in the perpetuation of the violation of their rights (UNODC, 2016).

4.4.1 Gender Stigma and Drug Use Stigma

Gender stigma is deeply rooted in social expectations that define the traditional roles assigned to women. Socially, they are expected to assume the role of caregivers and to be responsible for maintaining family cohesion (Ng & Indran, 2021). When a woman does not meet these expectations, as is the case with drug use, social judgment is considerably more severe than toward men who display the same behavior.

Vázquez and Stolkiner (2009), in their reading of Goffman (2006), reflect that one of the main effects of stigmatization is its ability to produce specific groups of citizens who see their rights fulfillment limited, such as the right to health care. In this sense, various research has pointed out that women face more barriers than men to start treatment. Motyka et al. (2022) agree in identifying several of these barriers, which can be summarized as: (a) a higher degree of disapproval and rejection from the environment, which translates into less social and/or family support; (b) greater family pressure not to start or quickly end treatment, since the traditional caregiver role takes precedence over her recovery, prioritizing the care of children or household chores; (c) the fear that, by making their consumption explicit, they could lose the custody of their children or other relatives in their care; and, (d) the lack of adaptation of treatment services to their particular needs, such as the lack of adequate resources for child care and the scarce social support.

These studies highlight how the stigma associated with substance use and traditional gender roles generates additional obstacles for women, who face a more intense emotional and social burden, making their access to treatment services more difficult in an equitable and sustained manner. Apsley et al. (2022) identified that social and logistical stigma is a predominant factor that prevents women from seeking treatment. This includes concerns about how participation in treatment programs could negatively affect their jobs or generate unfavorable social judgments in their communities. But, in addition, as Ortiz and Silva (2005) and Chacón (2017) mention, health workers are not free from stigmatizing people with drug use in general and women in particular. The stigma is reproduced in different health and social services. These stigmas, although not necessarily made explicit in direct care, are present in health contexts and generate negative effects on the possibility of establishing trust bonds (Acuña & Bolis, 2005; RIOD, 2019).

The United Nations Office on Drugs and Crime (UNODC, 2016) highlights that women who use drugs are seen as moral transgressors, which intensifies their stigmatization. Unlike men, women are expected to maintain a standard of moral behavior and care that, when broken, generates greater rejection, both socially and within the family. The stigmatization associated with feelings of shame and guilt due to the transgression of the gender role is greater in women who use drugs. Therefore, when considering their care, it is necessary to take into account fundamental axes, such as concern for treatment confidentiality, exposure to traumas such as violence and abuse, the scarce social network and the phenomenon of invisible consumption relegated to the domestic sphere, greater social deterioration (telescoping), low support from family and friends, and less economic independence on many occasions (Greenfield et al., 2010; IMUS, 2001; Rawat et al., 2021; RIOD, 2019; SAMHSA, 2011).

On the other hand, as Mota et al. (2014) express, self-stigma is the experience of alienation that substance users suffer when internalizing certain negative stereotypes that are related to substance use. Ariel et al. (2016) found that self-stigma is a common problem in substance users, which is explained by the attribution of the responsibility of addiction to the substance user themselves. Recent studies have documented the impact of self-stigma on women with drug use. This internalization of social prejudices reduces self-esteem and generates strong social isolation. According to Motyka et al. (2022), self-stigma is related to lower rates of treatment seeking, as women fear being judged or discriminated against by health professionals and their communities. This cycle of isolation and self-stigma perpetuates substance use and decreases the chances of recovery.

4.4.2 Impact on Access to Treatment

Stigma and self-stigma have a direct impact on women‘s access to treatment services. According to the UNODC (2016), women who use drugs find a much more limited treatment offer, and it is poorly adapted to their specific needs. This marginalization has serious consequences, as when women manage to ask for help, they usually arrive at more severe stages of substance use and with fewer possibilities of engaging in treatment and achieving a recovery. In addition, women face additional barriers, such as the lack of specialized services that integrate and address factors like gender violence, child care, and complex family dynamics (Fonseca et al., 2021; Pujal et al., 2020). These obstacles not only reduce their access to treatment but also perpetuate social exclusion and vulnerability. IMUS (2001) and SAMHSA (2011) argue that it is essential to adapt treatment services to address the particular needs of women, offering comprehensive support that contemplates both their physical and emotional health.

The lack of a gender approach in treatment perpetuates the exclusion of women from the health system (UNODC, 2004). In this sense, a review by Public Health Ontario (2024) concluded that participation in support groups can help reduce self-stigma and increase women‘s willingness to seek treatment. Women who attend these groups tend to experience lower levels of self-stigma, which improves their access to health services, promotes social integration, and improves treatment adherence rates.

4.4.3 Perpetuation of Rights Violations

The stigma and criminalization of women who use drugs not only affects their health but also perpetuates the violation of their rights. The Inter-American Commission for Drug Abuse Control (CICAD, 2019) points out that punitive policies toward drug use tend to criminalize these women, exposing them to social exclusion and institutional abuse. Stigmatization and criminalization reinforce a cycle of marginalization that is difficult to break.

4.4.4 Violence and Mental Health

Gender violence, combined with the stigma associated with drug use, has a devastating impact on women's mental health. According to various studies, women who face stigmatization and violence are more likely to use drugs as a coping strategy in the face of adversity, which perpetuates the cycle of consumption and stigmatization (Livingston et al., 2012). Also, stigma not only manifests itself in social discrimination but also, as mentioned, in self-stigma, contributing to the emergence of mental health disorders such as depression, anxiety, and PTSD. Self-stigma generates additional barriers to treatment access. Motyka et al. (2022) point out that women with high levels of self-stigma are less likely to disclose their drug use, which limits their ability to access appropriate treatment services.

4.5 Destigmatization of Women with Substance Use Disorder in Latin America. An OAS-CICAD Initiative

As described, research and clinical experience have shown that women respond better to treatments centered on their needs. In fact, women show better clinical outcomes when they undergo their treatment in centers that have programs exclusively for them than when they do so in mixed programs (UNODC, 2016). It is important that women-centered treatments include programs that address trauma and incorporate specific components for them and their families, such as nurseries, prenatal care, and workshops that include female health topics, among others. From this perspective, OAS-CICAD has been implementing, since 2023, initiatives that seek to support the destigmatization of women with SUD in the Americas.

On the one hand, exchanges with the national anti-drug commissioners and the agencies responsible for drug policies in several countries in the region show a clear shortage of treatment centers with programs specifically designed for women. This lack of specialized services also extends to care for adolescents, and particularly female adolescents, which is particularly worrying, given that young people continue to be the most vulnerable group to drug use worldwide (UNODC, 2023). Finally, there is a lack of information about the availability of services for children in treatment centers, which significantly limits the ability of women who are mothers or caregivers to access and maintain their treatment. The absence or lack of awareness of these services can act as a significant structural barrier in their recovery process and reinforce stigma.

In line with these challenges, OAS-CICAD has implemented an initiative aimed at the destigmatization of women with SUD that focused on the development of two documents that emerged from collaborative work with representatives from various countries during the subregional workshops on "Women, drugs and stigma." These workshops identified key recommendations to reduce stigma and improve access to treatment for women with SUD. Both documents underline that stigma continues to be one of the main barriers that hinder women's access to adequate health and treatment services, largely due to the social gender expectations placed on them.

Among the main initiatives proposed in these documents, the importance of training health professionals, media, educators, and the community in general on the use of non-stigmatizing language stands out. This includes making visible and eliminating practices that perpetuate stigma and hinder women's access to necessary services. Awareness strategies are also recommended that promote a broader understanding of the rights and needs of women with SUD. Measures to improve the infrastructure of care services are also highlighted, including spaces that allow for child care and comprehensive support for women.

Finally, the recommendations propose the creation of intersectoral alliances and the promotion of public policies that ensure the sustainability of these initiatives in the long term, with the aim of facilitating the recovery and social integration of women affected by substance use.

4.6 Final Considerations

Migrants, refugees, and people deprived of their liberty face multiple stigmatized identities, which affect their psychological well-being and quality of life. Contextual and personal barriers limit their access to substance abuse treatments and health services. The intersection between drug use, the condition of being a migrant or prisoner, and other stigmatized identities increases their vulnerability and stigma, making it essential that institutions guarantee their rights, especially equal access to health. Interventions must be culturally sensitive and address not only drug use but also factors such as employment, housing, social support, and personal relationships. In addition, early detection of dual pathologies allows for comprehensive and effective treatments.

Women who use drugs face an additional gender stigma, which limits their access to health, increases violence, and reinforces exclusion. Highlighting their specific needs and designing interventions with a gender focus is crucial for improving adherence to treatment and the effectiveness of interventions.

In conclusion, public health policies should adopt a gender approach, reduce self-stigma, and eliminate structural barriers, facilitating access to adapted treatments that improve the well-being and social reintegration of these vulnerable populations.

References

Acuña, C., & Bolis, M. (2005). La estigmatización y el acceso a la atención de salud en América Latina: Amenazas y perspectivas. In 29° *Congreso de la Academia Internacional de Derecho y Salud Mental*. París, Francia.

Ahern, J., Stuber, J., & Galea, S. (2007). Stigma, discrimination and the health of illicit drug users. *Drug and Alcohol Dependence, 88*(2–3), 188–196. https://doi.org/10.1016/j.drugalcdep.2006.10.014

Aleer, E., Alam, K., Rashid, A., Mohsin, M., & Eacersall, D. (2023). Substance abuse amongst refugee youth: A scoping review. *Current Addiction Reports, 10*, 594–609. https://doi.org/10.1007/s40429-023-00502-6

Alegría, M., Álvarez, K., & DiMarzio, K. (2017). Immigration and mental health. *Current Epidemiology Reports, 4*, 145–155. https://doi.org/10.1007/s40471-017-0111-2

Apsley, H. B., Vest, N., Knapp, K. S., Santos-Lozada, A., Gray, J., Hard, G., & Jones, A. A. (2022). Non-engagement in substance use treatment among women with an unmet need for treatment: A latent class analysis on multidimensional barriers. *Drug and Alcohol Dependence, 242*, 109715. https://doi.org/10.1016/j.drugalcdep.2022.109715

Ariel, R., Gallo, V., Soledad, M., & Ruth, A. (2016). Estigma internalizado en consumidores de drogas en Córdoba, Argentina. *Acta de Investigación Psicológica, 6*(2), 2404–2411. https://doi.org/10.1016/j.aipprr.2016.06.003

Asamblea General de las Naciones Unidas. (1951). *Convención sobre el estatuto de los refugiados*. https://www.acnur.org/sites/default/files/2023-05/Convencion_1951.pdf

Aslan, L. (2018). Doing time on a TC: How effective are drug-free therapeutic communities in prison? A review of the literature. *Therapeutic Communities: The International Journal of Therapeutic Communities, 39*(1), 26–34. https://doi.org/10.1108/TC-10-2017-0028

Banks, D. E., Brown, K., & Saraiya, T. C. (2023). "Culturally responsive" substance use treatment: Contemporary definitions and approaches for minoritized racial/ethnic groups. *Current Addiction Reports, 10*, 422–431. https://doi.org/10.1007/s40429-023-00489-0

Bazemore, G., & Stinchcomb, J. B. (2004). A civic engagement model of reentry: Involving community through service and restorative justice. *Federal Probation, 68*(2), 14.

Bernal, G., Jiménez-Chafey, M. I., & Domenech-Rodríguez, M. M. (2009). Cultural adaptation of treatments: A resource for considering culture in evidence-based practice. *Professional Psychology: Research and Practice, 40*(4), 361–368. https://doi.org/10.1037/a0016401

Binswanger, I. A., Nowels, C., Corsi, K. F., Glanz, J., Long, J., Booth, R. E., & Steiner, J. F. (2012). Return to drug use and overdose after release from prison: A qualitative study of risk and protective factors. *Addiction Science & Clinical Practice, 7*(1), 3. https://doi.org/10.1186/1940-0640-7-3

Binswanger, I. A., Redmond, N., Steiner, J. F., & Hicks, L. S. (2011). Health disparities and the criminal justice system: An agenda for further research and action. *Journal of Urban Health, 89*(1), 98–107. https://doi.org/10.1007/s11524-011-9614-1

Bukten, A., Virtanen, S., Hesse, M., Chang, Z., Kvamme, T. L., Thylstrup, B., Tverborgvik, T., Skjaervo, I., & Stavseth, M. R. (2024). The prevalence and comorbidity of mental health and substance use disorders in Scandinavian prisons 2010-2019: A multi-nacional register study. *BMC Psychiatry, 24*(1), 95. https://doi.org/10.1186/s12888-024-05540-6

Chacón, S. (2017). *Estigma hacia personas con consumo problemático de drogas en equipos de tratamiento en Santiago de Chile*. Pontificia Universidad Católica de Chile. https://sergiochacon.cl/wp-content/uploads/2019/09/TESIS-SERGIO-CHACON_ESTIGMA-Y-DROGAS_versi%C3%B3n-empaste-corregida.pdf

Comisión Interamericana para el Control del Abuso de Drogas (OEA-CICAD). (2019). *Informe sobre el consumo de drogas en las Américas*. https://www.gub.uy/junta-nacional-drogas/sites/junta-nacional-drogas/files/documentos/noticias/Informe%20sobre%20el%20consumo%20de%20drogas%20en%20las%20Am%C3%A9ricas%202019.pdf

De Andrade, D., Ritchie, J., Rowlands, M., Mann, E., & Hides, L. (2018). Substance use and recidivism outcomes for prison-based drug and alcohol interventions. *Epidemiologic Reviews, 40*(1), 121–133. https://doi.org/10.1108/TC-10-2017-0028

Douglass, C. H., Win, T. M., Goutzamanis, S., Lim, M. S. C., Block, K., Onsando, G., Hellard, M., Higgs, P., Livingstone, C., & Horyniak, D. (2023). Stigma associated with alcohol and other drug use among people from migrant and ethnic minority groups: Results from a systematic

review of qualitative studies. *Journal of Immigrant and Minority Health, 25*(6), 1402–1425. https://doi.org/10.1007/s10903-023-01468-3
Doyle, M. F., Shakeshaft, A., Guthrie, J., Snijder, M., & Butler, T. (2019). A systematic review of evaluations of prison-based alcohol and other drug use behavioural treatment for men. *Australian and New Zealand Journal of Public Health, 43*(2), 120–130. https://doi.org/10.1111/1753-6405.12884
European Monitoring Center for Drug and Drug Addiction [EMCDDA]. (2015, May 31). *Perspectives on drugs. Comorbidity of substance use and mental disorders in Europe.* https://www.euda.europa.eu/publications/pods/comorbidity-substance-use-mental-health_en
European Union Drugs Agency [EUDA]. (2023). *Las personas migrantes y las drogas: respuestas sanitarias y sociales.* https://www.euda.europa.eu/publications/mini-guides/migrants-and-drugs-health-and-social-responses_es
Fazel, S., Yoon, I. A., & Hayes, A. J. (2017). Substance use disorders in prisoners: An updated systematic review and meta-regression analysis in recently incarcerated men and women. *Addiction, 112*(10), 1725–1739. https://doi.org/10.1111/add.13877
Fonseca, F., Robles-Martínez, M., Tirado-Muñoz, J., Alías-Ferri, M., Mestre-Pintó, J. I., Coratu, A. M., & Torrens, M. (2021). A gender perspective of addictive disorders. *Current Addiction Reports, 8*, 89–99. https://doi.org/10.1007/s40429-021-00357-9/
Fountain, J. (2009). *Issues surrounding drug use and drug services among the Black Caribbean communities in England.* National Treatment Agency. https://citeseerx.ist.psu.edu/document?repid=rep1&type=pdf&doi=c1ebd36c58491b807eda366676fde573f3fdc4f2
Garcini, L. M., Murray, K. E., Zhou, A., Klonoff, E. A., Myers, M. G., & Elder, J. P. (2016). Mental health of undocumented immigrant adults in the United States: A systematic review of methodology and findings. *Journal of Immigrant & Refugee Studies, 14*(1), 1–25. https://doi.org/10.1080/15562948.2014.998849
Goffman, E. (1963). *Stigma notes on the management of spoiled identity.* Prentice Hall.
Goffman, E. (2006). *Estigma. La identidad deteriorada* (1st ed.). Amorrortu.
Gorlero, C., Finkelstein, L., Pérez Caraballo, G., Durruty, L., & Serafini, L. (2021). *Manual de Salud Mental y Apoyo Psicosocial para la Atención de la Población Migrante y Refugiada en la República Argentina.* Organización Internacional para las Migraciones (OIM), Ciudad Autónoma de Buenos Aires. https://argentina.iom.int/sites/g/files/tmzbdl901/files/documents/Manual-de-Salud-Mental-y-Apoyo-Psicosocial.pdf
Greenfield, S. F., Back, S. E., Lawson, K., & Brady, K. T. (2010). Substance abuse in women. *Psychiatric Clinics of North America, 33*(2), 339–355. https://doi.org/10.1016/j.psc.2010.01.004
Hedrich, D., Alves, P., Farrell, M., Stöver, H., Møller, L., & Mayet, S. (2012). The effectiveness of opioid maintenance treatment in prison settings: A systematic review. *Addiction, 107*(3), 501–517. https://doi.org/10.1111/j.1360-0443.2011.03676.x
Horyniak, D., Melo, J. S., Farrell, R. M., Ojeda, V. D., & Strathdee, S. A. (2016). Epidemiology of substance use among forced migrants: A global systematic review. *PLoS One, 11*(7), e0159134. https://doi.org/10.1371/journal.pone.0159134
Instituto de Medicina (IMUS) Committee on Understanding the Biology of Sex and Gender Differences. (2001). *Exploring the biological contributions to human health: Does sex matter?* National Academies Press. https://www.ncbi.nlm.nih.gov/books/NBK222288/
International Organization for Migration. (2019). *International migration law: Glossary on migration.* https://publications.iom.int/system/files/pdf/iml_34_glossary.pdf
Jarvis, G. E., & Kirmayer, L. J. (2023). Global migration: Moral, political and mental health challenges. *Transcultural Psychiatry, 60*(1), 5–12. https://doi.org/10.1177/13634615231162282
Kartal, D., & Kiropoulos, L. (2016). Effects of acculturative stress on PTSD, depressive and anxiety symptoms among refugees resettled in Australia and Austria. *European Journal of Psychotraumatology, 7*(S1), 28711. https://doi.org/10.3402/ejpt.v7.28711

Kronick, R., Jarvis, G. E., & Kirmayer, L. J. (2023). Migrant mental health: Immigrants, refugees and displaced persons. In A. Tasman, M. B. Riba, T. Schutze, C. H. Ng, C. A. Alfonso, D. Lecic-Tosevski, S. Kanba, R. D. Alarcón, & D. Ndetei (Eds.), *Psychiatry* (5th ed.). Springer.

Lauricella, M., Valdez, J. K., Okamoto, S. K., Helm, S., & Zaremba, C. (2016). Culturally grounded prevention for minority youth populations: A systematic review of the literature. *Journal of Primary Prevention, 37*, 11–32. https://doi.org/10.1007/s10935-015-0414-3

Li, J., Chang, S. S., Yip, P. S., Li, J., Jordan, L. P., Tang, Y., Hao, Y., Huang, X., Yang, N., Chen, C., et al. (2014). Mental wellbeing amongst younger and older migrant workers in comparison to their urban counterparts in Guangzhou city, China: A cross-sectional study. *BMC Public Health, 14*, 1280.

Lindert, J., Neuendorf, U., Nata, M., & Schäfer, I. (2021). Escaping the past and living in the present: A qualitative exploration of substance use among Syrian male refugees in Germany. *Conflict and Health, 15*(26), 1–11. https://doi.org/10.1186/s13031-021-00352-x

Livingston, J. D., Milne, T., Fang, M. L., & Amari, E. (2012). The effectiveness of interventions for reducing stigma related to substance use disorders: A systematic review. *Addiction, 107*(1), 39–50. https://doi.org/10.1111/j.1360-0443.2011.03601.x

Mosler Vidal, E., & Laczko, F. (2022). *Migration and the SDGs: Measuring progress—An edited volume*. Organización Internacional para las Migraciones. https://publications.iom.int/books/migration-and-sdgs-measuring-progress-edited-volume

Mota, T., Noto, R., & Santos, P. (2014). *Reduzindo o estigma entre usuários de drogas: Guia para profissionais e gestores*. Editora UFJF.

Motyka, M. A., Al-Imam, A., Haligowska, A., & Michalak, M. (2022). Helping women suffering from drug addiction: Needs, barriers, and challenges. *International Journal of Environmental Research and Public Health, 19*(21), 14039.

Newman, B. N., & Crowell, K. A. (2021). The intersectionality of criminality and substance use self-stigmas. *American Psychological Association, 8*(2), 212–222. https://doi.org/10.1037/sah0000293

Ng, R., & Indran, N. (2021). Societal perceptions of caregivers linked to culture across 20 countries: Evidence from a 10-billion-word database. *PLoS One, 16*(7), e0251161. https://doi.org/10.1371/journal.pone.0251161

Novo, M., Pereira, A., Vázquez, M. J., & Amado, B. G. (2017). Adaptación a la prisión y ajuste psicológico en una muestra de internos en centros penitenciarios. *Acción Psicológica, 14*(2), 113–128. https://doi.org/10.5944/ap.14.2.20784

Observatorio Español sobre Drogas [OEDA]. (2023). *Encuesta sobre alcohol y drogas en España 1995–2022 [EDADES]*. Observatorio Español sobre Drogas. Delegación del Gobierno para el Plan Nacional sobre Drogas. https://pnsd.sanidad.gob.es/profesionales/sistemasInformacion/sistemaInformacion/encuestas_EDADES.htm

Ortiz, N., & Silva, M. (2005). Significados y contradicciones del fenómeno de las drogas: drogas lícitas e ilícitas en Chile. *Revista Latino-Americana de Enfermagem, 13*, 903–911. https://www.scielo.br/j/rlae/a/KvnZQSdF6Kz3BNbnDfbyDcB/

Pinedo, M., Zemore, S., & Rogers, S. (2018). Understanding barriers to specialty substance abuse treatment among Latinos. *Journal of Substance Abuse Treatment, 94*, 1–8. https://doi.org/10.1016/j.jsat.2018.08.004

Porter, M., & Haslam, N. (2005). Predisplacement and postdisplacement factors associated with mental health of refugees and internally displaced persons. A meta-analysis. *JAMA, 294*(5), 602–612. https://doi.org/10.1001/jama.294.5.602

Public Health Ontario. (2024). *Evidence for strategies that address substance-use related stigma*. Public Health Ontario. https://www.publichealthontario.ca/-/media/Documents/E/2024/evidence-strategies-substance-use-related-stigma.pdf

Pujal, M., Calatayud, M., & Amigot, P. (2020). Subjetividad, desigualdad social y malestares de género: una relectura del DSM-V. *Revista Internacional de Sociología, 78*(2), 155–170. https://doi.org/10.3989/ris.2020.78.2.18.113

Rawat, H., Petzer, S. L., & Gurayah, T. (2021). Effects of substance use disorder on women's roles and occupational participation. *South African Journal of Occupational Therapy, 51*(1), 54–62. https://doi.org/10.17159/2310-3833/2021/vol51n1a8

Red Iberoamericana de Organizaciones No Gubernamentales que trabajan en Drogas y adicciones (RIOD). (2019). *Estigma, consumo de drogas y adicciones*. https://riod.org/wp-content/uploads/2019/06/ESTIGMA-CONSUMO-DE-DROGAS-Y-ADICCIONES.pdf

Saleh, E. A., Lazaridou, F. B., Klapprott, F., Wazaify, M., Heinz, A., & Kluge, U. (2023). A systematic review of qualitative research on substance use among refugees. *Addiction, 118*, 218–253. https://doi.org/10.1111/add.16021

Substance Abuse and Mental Health Services Administration (SAMHSA). (2011). *Addressing the needs of women and girls: Core competencies for mental health and substance abuse service professionals*. U.S. Department of Health and Human Services. https://www.samhsa.gov

Tomaz, V., Moreira, D., & Cruz, O. S. (2023). Criminal reactions to drug-using offenders: A systematic review of the effect of treatment and/or punishment on reduction of drug use and/or criminal recidivism. *Frontiers in Psychiatry, 14*, 935755. https://doi.org/10.3389/fpsyt.2023.935755

Tremlin, R. C., & Beazley, P. (2024). A systematic review of offender mental health stigma: Commonality, psychometric measures and differential diagnosis. *Psychology, Crime and Law, 30*(2), 125–149. https://doi.org/10.1080/1068316X.2022.2072842

United Nations Department of Economic and Social Affairs [UN DESA]. (1998). *Recommendations on statistics of international migration. Revision 1*. United Nations. https://unstats.un.org/unsd/publication/SeriesM/SeriesM_58rev1E.pdf

United Nations High Commissioner for Refugees. (2011). *Handbook and guidelines on procedures and criteria for determining refugee status* (HCR/1P/4/enG/Rev. 3). https://www.acnur.org/sites/default/files/2023-05/Convencion_1951.pdf

United Nations Office on Drugs and Crime (UNODC). (2004). *Substance abuse treatment and care for women: Case studies and lessons learned*. https://www.unodc.org/docs/treatment/Toolkits/Women_Treatment_Case_Studies_E.pdf

United Nations Office on Drugs and Crime. (2016). *Outcome document of the 2016 United Nations General Assembly Special Session on the World Drug Problem*. https://www.unodc.org/documents/postungass2016/outcome/V1603301-E.pdf

United Nations Office on Drugs and Crime (UNODC). (2016). *Guidelines on drug prevention and treatment for girls and women*. UNODC. https://www.unodc.org/documents/drug-prevention-and-treatment/unodc_2016_drug_prevention_and_treatment_for_girls_and_women_E.pdf

United Nations Office on Drugs and Crime (UNODC). (2023). *World drug report*. UNODC. https://www.unodc.org/unodc/en/data-and-analysis/world-drug-report-2023.html

Vázquez, A., & Stolkiner, A. (2009). Procesos de estigma y exclusión en salud. Articulaciones entre estigmatización, derechos ciudadanos, uso de drogas y drogadependencia. *Anuario de Investigaciones, vol. XVI*, Facultad de Psicología, Universidad de Buenos Aires. Disponible en el Repositorio Digital Institucional de la Universidad de Buenos Aires.

World Health Organization. [WHO]. (2023). *Mental Health of refugees and migrants risk and protective factors and access to care*. World Health Organization. https://www.who.int/publications/i/item/9789240081840.

Chapter 5
Stigma and Diagnostic Overshadowing in People with Mental Disorder and Substance Addiction

Concepción Martínez-Martínez, Leticia Olave, Vicente Gea-Caballero, and Víctor José Villanueva-Blasco

5.1 Introduction

The civil rights movement in the United States during the 1950s and 1960s spurred the fight against racial discrimination toward the African American population and promoted equality in political and socio-health fields. In this context, Congress passed the Community Mental Health Act of 1963 (CMHA, Public Law 88–164), which marked the beginning of the deinstitutionalization of people with mental disorders and intellectual disabilities through the closure of chronic psychiatric hospitals and their replacement with community centers. Simultaneously, social psychology began to investigate cognitive biases that influenced healthcare. Routh and King (1972) identified that social class biased judgment about the need for psychological help, while Yamamoto et al. (1967) observed that therapists'

C. Martínez-Martínez
Universitat de València, València, Spain
e-mail: concepcion.martinez-martinez@uv.es

L. Olave
Complutense University of Madrid, Madrid, Spain
e-mail: leticiaolave@ucm.es

V. Gea-Caballero
Valencian International University, Valencia, Spain
e-mail: vagea@universidadviu.com

V. J. Villanueva-Blasco (✉)
Valencian International University, Valencia, Spain

Research Network in Primary Care of Addictions (RIAPAd), Madrid, Spain

International Society of Substance Use Professionals (ISSUP), Madrid, Spain

International Center for Technology Transfer in Addictions (ITTC), Valencia, Spain
e-mail: vjvillanueva@universidadviu.com

T. Mota Ronzani (ed.), *Social Stigma and Drug Use*,
https://doi.org/10.1007/978-3-031-94813-8_5

ethnocentrism reduced the sessions offered to minority patients. Additionally, studies like those of Philips (1967) and Kanne (2013) highlighted that symptoms like hyperactivity or anxiety were erroneously attributed to intellectual disability, ignoring their origin in underlying mental health problems.

5.2 Stigma and Mental Health

Cognitive biases are inherent to the individual. Making a value judgment about the personal and structural characteristics of an individual or group allows us to make quick decisions about whether or not to interact. However, sometimes these patterns of interpreting reality can lead us to erroneous conclusions and make incorrect judgments that determine the development of stigma. Stigma refers to a mark or attribute that contributes to the bearer being recognized, singled out, and socially ostracized (Goffman, 1963). It is a social construct that is forged from interpersonal relationships and is characterized by its dynamism, as it fluctuates according to the culture, education, and morality of each society at a given historical moment (Pedersen, 2005).

The conceptual model of attribution processes and danger assessment applied to the stigma of mental illness examines the relationships that occur between causal attributions of control, personal responsibility, familiarity, and dangerousness, and the likelihood of different emotional responses, both discriminatory and helpful, toward people with mental disorders (Fig. 5.1).

Familiarity with mental disorders positively impacts emotional responses. Individuals with previous contact with people with mental disorders are more likely to offer their help. In relation to the attribution of control, people tend to avoid helping those with mental disorders when they perceive that the cause of the disorder is under their control, i.e., they attribute responsibility for what happens to them (e.g., their situation is derived from having consumed toxic substances). In these cases, if the person is considered dangerous and unpredictable, fear and even anger responses will appear, generating avoidance and segregation reactions. On the other hand, if

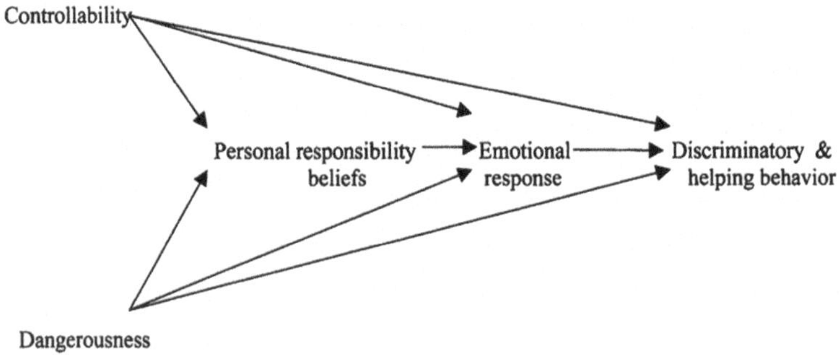

Fig. 5.1 Attribution processes and danger assessment in stigma and discrimination in mental disorder. Source: Own elaboration based on Corrigan et al. (2003)

the person is not considered responsible for what happens to them, the emotion that will arise is pity, and the desire to help will increase (Corrigan et al., 2003).

In the case of people with mental disorders, the most common stereotypes and prejudices associated with belonging to this group are dangerousness, unpredictability, and the existence of conflictual backgrounds. To the common stereotypes and prejudices observed in relation to mental disorders in general, specific stereotypes are added for SUD. Individuals who consume toxic substances are considered more dangerous and unpredictable than people with other mental disorders such as depression; and people who consume cocaine are considered less capable of making decisions than people with schizophrenia, depression, or dependence on alcohol; holding them more responsible for the condition they suffer from (Yang et al., 2017). This is partly due to the association of drug use with criminality (Warburton et al., 2005) and the simplistic identification that using drugs is equivalent to using heroin or crack, or the equivalent to "junkie" as a pejorative term, and the idea that these cause a lot of harm to society (Radcliffe & Stevens, 2008).

5.3 Stigma in the Healthcare Context

Discrimination and social distance are manifested in barriers to access to healthcare (Corrigan et al., 2017). In addition, when patients perceive certain attitudinal barriers from healthcare professionals, they tend to seek treatment less (Disability Rights Commission, 2006; Mojtabai et al., 2011). The study conducted by Wakeman et al. (2016) found that the majority of specialized care health professionals (97%) and primary care professionals (95%) considered that patients with SUD were more difficult to attend to than the average patient. Among the findings, Wakeman et al. (2016) highlight that 12% of specialized care professionals believe that someone who uses drugs is committing a crime and deserves to be punished. Despite the fact that it has been observed that having more favorable attitudes toward patients with SUD is associated with a higher probability of performing clinical practice. However, people with SUD continue to endure stigma when accessing the health system (Cazalis et al., 2023). Many avoid the use of resources for addiction treatment due to the belief that these units are for "junkies." They do not want to be seen by acquaintances or to be associated with labels that discredit them in society and to themselves; as they internalize these stereotypes, their self-image is damaged to the point of defining themselves as "social trash," "source of contamination," and "a danger to other members of society" (Radcliffe & Stevens, 2008).

This may be one of the reasons why, despite having effective treatments for addictions, only 7.1% of people with SUD or AUD participating in a study conducted in 26 countries had received treatment during the last year (Degenhardt et al., 2010). The study conducted by Clement et al. (2015) revealed that only 25% of people with alcohol use disorders participated in detoxification programs. In addition, people who perceived greater stigma toward their peers with alcohol use disorders were less likely to use alcoholism treatment programs and to participate in sterile syringe programs.

Considering how stereotypes, discrimination, and social distance in the healthcare context affect behavior, there are several types of stigma that can occur in the care of people with mental illness or addictions: social or public stigma, structural/institutional stigma, provider stigma, vicarious stigma, and courtesy stigma.

5.4 Stigma and Diagnostic Masking in Mental Disorders and SUD

When the stigmatizing attitudes of the healthcare professional toward a particular group interfere in the clinical process, we can talk about diagnostic masking (Shefer et al., 2014). Diagnostic masking refers to the negative bias that influences the clinician and makes it difficult for him to contemplate the possibility of the existence of other concurrent disorders (Kanne, 2013). This can occur when the main diagnosis has a great presence, as is the case with mental disorders, and masks other possible secondary diagnoses, attributing symptoms and signs to the disorder previously diagnosed (Jones et al., 2008). Kanne (2013) also points out that it is common for symptoms and behaviors that may be due to another mental problem to be attributed to the already established mental disorder without considering that several diagnoses can occur simultaneously.

In this regard, the multimorbidity of mental disorder and SUD with physical diseases is very common. The study conducted by Wu et al. (2018), in which 211,880 patients participated, confirmed not only that people with SUD were more likely than the general population to suffer from chronic diseases in a comorbid way, but also, the prevalence of SUD increased as the number of medical conditions increased (1 diagnosis 14.3%, 2–3 diagnoses 21.2%, and 4–9 diagnoses 32.5%). They also found that the main associated physical diseases were hypertension, arthritis, type 1 or 2 diabetes, chronic kidney disease, asthma, chronic obstructive pulmonary disease, ischemic heart disease, cancer, and viral hepatitis B or C.

People with mental disorder have a life expectancy 10–20 years lower than that of the general population. This difference is mostly due to mortality caused by preventable physical diseases (Nordentoft et al., 2013; World Health Organization [WHO], 2022). When analyzing why these differences in morbidity and mortality several causes are found. First, socioeconomic conditions. We cannot forget that people with mental disorder and SUD have higher rates of unemployment, poverty, low literacy, etc., which makes it difficult to lead a healthy lifestyle (Kirkbride et al., 2024). Second, there is structural stigma, which hinders access to healthcare (Corrigan, 2000). Third, there are health problems derived from the metabolic alterations produced by psychiatric medication (Fiorillo & Sartorius, 2021). And finally, another important factor especially concerning healthcare professionals is diagnostic masking (Thornicroft et al., 2007). Patients report not being believed when they go to healthcare service professionals seeking help. The diagnosis is present as a barrier in communication, and sometimes it is not considered that there may be truth in their complaints, or these are attributed to "their problems" of mental health. Even when they present physical symptoms, it is considered that they are faking, exaggerating, or that their symptoms have a psychosomatic origin (Cunningham, Imlach, Haitana, et al., 2023; Raven, 2017; Shefer et al., 2014).

Diagnostic masking leads to a series of injustices in healthcare with significant consequences for individuals. In 2022, the Joint Commission issued a sentinel alert to warn about the importance of diagnostic masking in health disparities. Not surprisingly, different authors agree that, during the interaction of health professionals with people with physical, intellectual disabilities, history of substance abuse, mental disorders, etc., a diagnostic masking can occur that results in a diagnostic error and, as a consequence, a delay in the start of treatment, with the repercussions for health that this may cause (Cunningham, Imlach, Lockett, et al., 2023; Schuller et al., 2023; The Joint Commission, 2022).

Diagnostic masking also affects trust. If during the consultation healthcare professionals do not speak directly with the patient, do not try to use alternative forms of communication when it is difficult, or do not check if the understanding of the information has been correct, patients may perceive a lack of interest or fear in the professional, so they choose not to tell their problems, they may even choose not to seek healthcare when they need it (Disability Rights Commission, 2006). In the study conducted by Mojtabai et al. (2011), 97.4% of respondents reported that they did not seek treatment for mental health due to attitudinal or evaluative barriers on the part of the professionals who attend to them.

Although sometimes it is not easy to establish appropriate communication due to the presence of psychiatric symptoms, the labels that often accompany them, "dangerous" and "unpredictable" (Corrigan et al., 2017), increase the possibility of not dedicating the necessary time to perform the physical examination and anamnesis exhaustively. This leads to important information being overlooked with the risk of masking concomitant problems (Skeie, 2024).

Another reason for diagnostic masking among health professionals is the belief that there is a "drug-seeking behavior" on the part of the patient. When a patient with a previous history of substance use goes to the emergency services seeking help for inability to control pain, the likelihood of being misdiagnosed is very high (Bean et al., 2022; Cunningham, Imlach, Haitana, et al., 2023). This mistrust is greater for people with SUD or at risk of it, but it also extends to people with other mental disorders (Cunningham, Imlach, Lockett, et al., 2023).

5.5 Dual Pathology, Stigma, and Diagnostic Masking

Dual diagnosis, or pathology, is spoken of when there is comorbidity of a psychiatric diagnosis along with a SUD. Various studies show a high comorbidity with schizophrenia (Westermeyer, 2006), anxiety and depression disorders (Compton et al., 2007), bipolar disorder (Hunt et al., 2016; Léda-Rêgo et al., 2023; Preuss et al., 2021), severe personality disorders (Verheul, 2001), and with Attention Deficit Hyperactivity Disorder (ADHD) (Groenman et al., 2017; Özgen et al., 2021).

Dual patients present greater difficulties in their detection, diagnosis, and treatment, greater psychopathological and psychosocial severity, a lower functional capacity, a greater use of health and social resources, and worse adherence to treatments (Farren et al., 2012; González-Pinto et al., 2006, 2010; Grau-López et al., 2014; Lagerberg et al., 2010; Torrens et al., 2012). Therefore, if studies like that of Wakeman et al. (2016) with healthcare professionals show that they considered patients with SUD to be more difficult to attend to than the average patient, patients with dual pathology still pose a greater challenge. This can lead to processes of structural stigma or provider stigma toward dual patients. In such a way that exposure to stigma, discrimination, and social distance can be even greater than in patients with only mental disorder or only SUD. Likewise, they can be configured as barriers in the access and maintenance in the health network of a population that, due to its dual diagnosis and all the implications derived from it, shows greater vulnerability.

On the other hand, in people with dual pathology, it is common for one pathology to mask the other. It is often difficult to distinguish the coincident symptoms of addictive disorders and various mental disorders, which makes diagnosis difficult. This often happens with bipolar disorder, attention deficit/hyperactivity disorder (ADHD), and substance use (Albanese et al., 2006; Goldberg et al., 2008; Muhammad et al., 2023). Likewise, personality disorders have a high comorbidity in patients with bipolar disorder and SUD, which further complicates the differential diagnosis between the traits of a personality disorder, manifestations of a SUD, and bipolar disorder (Arias et al., 2017; Levin & Hennessy, 2004; Stewart & El-Mallakh, 2007). These considerations can make it difficult to detect substance use during an initial examination in the emergency department or after hospital admission. Having an appropriate diagnosis in relation to the use/abuse of toxic substances can change the patient's prognosis, so it is important to review the history and ask about previous symptoms so that important data is not overlooked (Albanese et al., 2006). For example, the study conducted by Stewart and El-Mallakh (2007) found that 67% of the sample had been misdiagnosed with a bipolar disorder when they actually met criteria for a Substance-Induced Mood Disorder.

The diagnosis of SUD and ADHD in the adult population is very complex since it requires a retrospective diagnosis, and there are no specific diagnostic criteria for adults in the DSM 5 (American Psychiatric Association, 2013). Added to this is that, generally, addiction specialists do not usually assess ADHD or do not pay enough attention to this disorder by prioritizing other psychiatric pathologies (Levin & Upadhyaya, 2007). Additionally, among the factors that can influence diagnostic masking in dual pathology between SUD and ADHD, Levin and Upadhyaya (2007) point out: (a) similar symptomatology in various psychiatric pathologies that are confused with ADHD; (b) symptomatology similar to that of ADHD in people with an intoxication or in withdrawal from a substance; (c) the use of screening instruments without concluding with a clinical diagnosis; and (d) the simulation of ADHD symptoms to obtain secondary gains, such as stimulant medication. In short, knowing the possible comorbidity between different mental disorders and substance use is crucial for diagnostic masking since the concurrence of alterations influences the clinical presentation of the disorder, its course, and the therapeutic approach (Arias et al., 2017).

5.6 Stigma and Diagnostic Masking in Adolescents with Dual Pathology

Epidemiological studies in the adolescent population that begin treatment for SUD reflect that between 60% and 88% of cases present dual pathology with another comorbid psychiatric diagnosis (Chan et al., 2008). From the inverse perspective, among the adolescents admitted to psychiatric units, the rate of SUD reaches 70% (Niethammer & Frank, 2007); while among those who are in outpatient follow-up for a psychiatric disorder, the rate of SUD is between 10% and 16%.

Psychiatric emergencies in young people who use substances have been increasing in recent years (Castillo Yzquierdo et al., 2023; Herbert et al., 2015; Mascaraque & Aduna, 2014). Despite this, there are few studies where dual pathology in adolescents is addressed. In the study by Matali et al. (2016), in which psychiatric emergencies of adolescents with dual pathology were analyzed, several differences were found in terms of medical attention and the clinical picture of these patients compared to young people with mental disorder without SUD. These authors found that the group of adolescents with dual pathology presented a higher comorbidity with conduct disorders and cannabis use, more social problems, a higher frequency of emergencies, a higher admission rate, and less connection to the care network. These differences imply the need to use a large number of resources to manage patients with dual diagnoses in healthcare services compared to other users. In addition, in some groups of adolescents, stigma can be increased by transgender and gender diversity issues (Mezzalira et al., 2022; White Hughto et al., 2015). So, just like it was proposed with adult dual patients, it can lead to processes of structural stigma or provider stigma toward these dual adolescents.

Mental disorders that show greater comorbidity with SUD in adolescents are disruptive behavior disorders (Chan et al., 2008), attention deficit hyperactivity disorder (ADHD) (Groenman et al., 2017; Özgen et al., 2021), and mood disorders (Chan et al., 2008). As in adults, the overlap of some symptoms of SUD with these mental disorders can generate diagnostic masking. For example, ADHD symptoms often go unnoticed in young people with SUD due to overlap, and vice versa, SUD is not detected among patients with ADHD (McAweeney et al., 2010). That is, these adolescents may find their diagnosis and adequate healthcare hindered as a result of diagnostic masking.

5.7 Final Considerations

The stigma surrounding mental disorders, substance use disorders (SUD), and, especially, dual pathology affects various social levels and requires a cross-cutting approach. From the health field, structural stigma and provider stigma are key factors in health inequities, as pointed out by the National Institute on Drug Abuse (NIDA). To combat it, the Mental Health Commission of Canada (MHCC, 2023) suggests strategies such as continuously training professionals, developing inclusive policies, involving people with lived experience in program design, and ensuring resources for patients and professionals. Additionally, initiatives like Open Minds Stigma and The Working Mind (Knaak et al., 2015; Ungar & Knaak, 2013) seek to reduce stigma in institutions. In clinical practice, the importance of language is highlighted, with resources like the Addictionary® to promote a stigma-free vocabulary, and the use of strategies such as active listening, shared decision-making, and the creation of respectful environments are essential to generate trust and avoid therapeutic pessimism. Likewise, the use of standardized interviews, diagnostic reviews, and alerts in complex cases can improve diagnostic accuracy and treatment. It is also questioned whether the separation of services for addictions and mental health contributes to diagnostic masking, underlining the need for adequate time and resources for a comprehensive assessment.

References

Albanese, M. J., Clodfelter, R. C. J., Pardo, T. B., & Ghaemi, S. N. (2006). Underdiagnosis of bipolar disorder in men with substance use disorder. *Journal of Psychiatric Practice, 12*(2), 124–127. https://doi.org/10.1097/00131746-200603000-00010

American Psychiatric Association. (2013). *Diagnostic and statistical manual of mental disorders* (5th ed.). American Psychiatric Publishing.

Arias, F., Szerman, N., Vega, P., Mesías, B., Basurte, I., & Rentero, D. (2017). Trastorno bipolar y trastorno por uso de sustancias. Estudio Madrid sobre prevalencia de patología dual. *Adicciones, 29*(3), 186–194. https://www.redalyc.org/pdf/2891/289151752006.pdf

Bean, D. J., Dryland, A., Rashid, U., & Tuck, N. L. (2022). The determinants and effects of chronic pain stigma: A mixed methods study and the development of a model. *The Journal of Pain, 23*(10), 1749–1764. https://doi.org/10.1016/j.jpain.2022.05.006

Castillo Yzquierdo, G. C., Rodríguez del Rosario, C. Z., & Leyva Castells, A. (2023). Urgencias psiquiátricas en niños y adolescentes. *Revista Cubana de Pediatría, 95*. http://scielo.sld.cu/scielo.php?pid=S0034753120230001000020&script=sci_arttext&tlng=pt

Cazalis, A., Lambert, L., & Auriacombe, M. (2023). Stigmatization of people with addiction by health professionals: Current knowledge. A scoping review. *Drug and Alcohol Dependence Reports, 9*, 100196. https://doi.org/10.1016/j.dadr.2023.100196

Chan, Y. F., Dennis, M. L., & Funk, R. R. (2008). Prevalence and comorbidity of major internalizing and externalizing problems among adolescents and adults presenting to substance abuse treatment. *Journal of Substance Abuse Treatment, 34*(1), 14–24. https://doi.org/10.1016/j.jsat.2006.12.031

Clement, S., Schauman, O., Graham, T., Maggioni, F., Evans-Lacko, S., Bezborodovs, N., Morgan, C., Rüsch, N., Brown, J. S., & Thornicroft, G. (2015). What is the impact of mental health-related stigma on help-seeking? A systematic review of quantitative and qualitative studies. *Psychological Medicine, 45*(1), 11–27. https://doi.org/10.1017/S0033291714000129

Compton, W. M., Thomas, Y. F., Stinson, F. S., & Grant, B. F. (2007). Prevalence, correlates, disability, and comorbidity of DSM-IV drug abuse and dependence in the United States. Results from the national epidemiologic survey on alcohol and related conditions. *Archives of General Psychiatry, 64*, 566–576. https://doi.org/10.1001/archpsyc.64.7.830

Corrigan, P. W. (2000). Mental health stigma as social attribution: Implications for research methods and attitude change. *Clinical Psychology: Science and Practice, 7*(1), 48–67. https://doi.org/10.1093/clipsy.7.1.48

Corrigan, P., Markowitz, F. E., Watson, A., Rowan, D., & Kubiak, M. A. (2003). An attribution model of public discrimination towards persons with mental illness. *Journal of Health and Social Behavior, 44*(2), 162–179. https://doi.org/10.2307/1519806

Corrigan, P., Schomerus, G., Shuman, V., Kraus, D., Perlick, D., Harnish, A., Kulesza, M., Kane-Willis, K., Qin, S., & Smelson, D. (2017). Developing a research agenda for understanding the stigma of addictions part I: Lessons from the mental health stigma literature. *The American Journal on Addictions, 26*(1), 59–66. https://doi.org/10.1111/ajad.12458

Cunningham, R., Imlach, F., Haitana, T., Every-Palmer, S., Lacey, C., Lockett, H., & Peterson, D. (2023). It's not in my head: A qualitative analysis of experiences of discrimination in people with mental health and substance use conditions seeking physical healthcare. *Frontiers in Psychiatry, 14*, 1285431. https://doi.org/10.3389/fpsyt.2023.1285431

Cunningham, R., Imlach, F., Lockett, H., Lacey, C., Haitana, T., Every-Palmer, S., Clark, M. T. R., & Peterson, D. (2023). Do patients with mental health and substance use conditions experience discrimination and diagnostic overshadowing in primary care in Aotearoa New Zealand? Results from a national online survey. *Journal of Primary Health Care, 15*(2), 112–121. https://doi.org/10.1071/HC23015

Degenhardt, L., Dierker, L., Chiu, W. T., Medina-Mora, M. E., Neumark, Y., Sampson, N., Alonso, J., Angermeyer, M., Anthony, J. C., Bruffaerts, R., de Girolamo, G., de Graaf, R., Gureje, O., Karam, A. N., Kostyuchenko, S., Lee, S., Lépine, J.-P., Levinson, D., Nakamura, Y., et al. (2010). Evaluating the drug use 'gateway' theory using cross-national data: Consistency and associations of the order of initiation of drug use among participants in the WHO World Mental Health Surveys. *Drug and Alcohol Dependence, 108*(1–2), 84–97. https://doi.org/10.1016/j.drugalcdep.2009.12.001

Disability Rights Commission. (2006). Equal treatment: Closing the gap: A formal investigation into physical health inequalities experienced by people with learning disabilities and/or mental health problems. https://disability-studies.leeds.ac.uk/wp-content/uploads/sites/40/library/DRC-Health-FI-main.pdf

Farren, C. K., Hill, K. P., & Weiss, R. D. (2012). Bipolar disorder and alcohol use disorder: A review. *Current Psychiatry Reports, 14*, 659–666. https://doi.org/10.1007/s11920-012-0320-9

Fiorillo, A., & Sartorius, N. (2021). Mortality gap and physical comorbidity of people with severe mental disorders: The public health scandal. *Annals of General Psychiatry, 20*, 52. https://doi.org/10.1186/s12991-021-00374-y

Goffman, E. (1963). *Stigma: Notes on the management of spoiled identity*. Touchstone.

Goldberg, J. F., Garno, J. L., Callahan, A. M., Kearns, D. L., Kerner, B., & Ackerman, S. H. (2008). Overdiagnosis of bipolar disorder among substance use disorder inpatients with mood instability. *The Journal of Clinical Psychiatry, 69*(11), 1751–1757. https://doi.org/10.4088/JCP.v69n1110

González-Pinto, A., Mosquera, F., Alonso, M., López, P., Ramírez, F., Vieta, E., & Baldessarini, R. J. (2006). Suicidal risk in bipolar I disorder patients and adherence to longterm lithium treatment. *Bipolar Disorders, 8*, 618–624. https://doi.org/10.1111/j.1399-5618.2006.00368.x

González-Pinto, A., Reed, C., Novick, D., Bertsch, J., & Haro, J. M. (2010). Assessment of medication adherence in a cohort of patients with bipolar disorder. *Pharmacopsychiatry, 43*, 263–270. https://doi.org/10.1055/s-0030-1263169

Grau-López, L., Roncero, C., Daigre, C., Miquel, L., Barral, C., Gonzalvo, B., Collazos, F., & Casas, M. (2014). Observational study on medications prescribed to dual-diagnosis outpatients. *Journal of Addiction Medicine, 8*(2), 84–89. https://doi.org/10.1097/ADM.0000000000000024

Groenman, A. P., Janssen, T. W. P., & Oosterlaan, J. (2017). Childhood psychiatric disorders as risk factor for subsequent substance abuse: A meta-analysis. *Journal of the American Academy of Child and Adolescent Psychiatry, 56*(7), 556–569. https://doi.org/10.1016/j.jaac.2017.05.004

Herbert, A., Gilbert, R., González-Izquierdo, A., & Li, L. (2015). Violence, self-harm and drug or alcohol misuse in adolescents admitted to hospitals in England for injury: A retrospective cohort study. *BMJ Open, 5*(2), e006079. https://doi.org/10.1136/bmjopen-2014-006079

Hunt, G. E., Malhi, G. S., Cleary, M., Lai, H. M. X., & Sitharthan, T. (2016). Comorbidity of bipolar and substance use disorders in national surveys of general populations, 1990–2015: Systematic review and meta-analysis. *Journal of Affective Disorders, 206*, 321–330. https://doi.org/10.1016/j.jad.2016.06.051

Jones, S., Howard, L., & Thornicroft, G. (2008). 'Diagnostic overshadowing': Worse physical health care for people with mental illness. *Acta Psychiatrica Scandinavica, 118*(3), 169–171. https://doi.org/10.1111/j.1600-0447.2008.01211.x

Kanne, S. (2013). Diagnostic overshadowing. In F. R. Volkmar (Ed.), *Encyclopedia of autism spectrum disorders* (pp. 938–940). Springer. https://doi.org/10.1007/978-1-4419-1698-3_398

Kirkbride, J. B., Anglin, D. M., Colman, I., Dykxhoorn, J., Jones, P. B., Patalay, P., Pitman, A., Soneson, E., Steare, T., Wright, T., & Griffiths, S. L. (2024). The social determinants of mental health and disorder: Evidence, prevention and recommendations. *World Psychiatry, 23*(1), 58–90. https://doi.org/10.1002/wps.21160

Knaak, S., Patten, S., & Ungar, T. (2015). Mental illness stigma as a quality-of-care problem. *The Lancet Psychiatry, 2*(10), 863–864. https://doi.org/10.1016/S2215-0366(15)00382-X

Lagerberg, T. V., Larsson, S., Sundet, K., Hansen, C. B., Hellvin, T., Andreassen, O. A., & Melle, I. (2010). Treatment delay and excessive substance use in bipolar disorder. *Journal of Nervous and Mental Disease, 198*, 628–633. https://doi.org/10.1097/NMD.0b013e3181ef3ef4

Léda-Rêgo, G., Studart-Bottó, P., Sarmento, S., Cerqueira-Silva, T., Bezerra-Filho, S., & Miranda-Scippa, Â. (2023). Psychiatric comorbidity in individuals with bipolar disorder: Relation with clinical outcomes and functioning. *European Archives of Psychiatry and Clinical Neuroscience, 273*(5), 1175–1181. https://doi.org/10.1007/s00406-023-01562-5

Levin, F. R., & Hennessy, G. (2004). Bipolar disorder and substance abuse. *Biological Psychiatry, 56*(10), 738–748. https://doi.org/10.1016/j.biopsych.2004.05.008

Levin, F. R., & Upadhyaya, H. P. (2007). Diagnosing ADHD in adults with substance use disorder: DSM-IV criteria and differential diagnosis. *The Journal of Clinical Psychiatry, 68*(7), e18. https://doi.org/10.4088/jcp.0707e18

Mascaraque, P. S., & Aduna, O. V. G. (2014). Urgencias en psiquiatría infantil. *Pediatria Integral, 18*(5), 312–319. https://www.pediatriaintegral.es/wp-content/uploads/2014/xviii05/04/312-319.pdf

Matali, J. L., Andión, O., Pardo, M., Iniesta, R., Serrano, E., & San, L. (2016). Adolescentes y diagnóstico dual en el servicio de urgencias psiquiátricas. *Adicciones, 28*(2), 71–79. https://doi.org/10.20882/adicciones.783

McAweeney, M., Rogers, N. L., Huddleston, C., Moore, D., & Gentile, J. P. (2010). Symptom prevalence of ADHD in a community residential substance abuse treatment program. *Journal of Attention Disorders, 13*(6), 601–608. https://doi.org/10.1177/1087054708329973

Mental Health Commission of Canada. (2023). *Dismantling structural stigma in health care. An implementation guide to making real change for and with people living with mental health problems or illnesses and/or substance use concerns.* Mental Health Commission of Canada. https://mentalhealthcommission.ca/structural-stigma/dismantling-structural-stigma-in-health-care-implementation-guide/

Mezzalira, S., Scandurra, C., Mezza, F., Miscioscia, M., Innamorati, M., & Bochicchio, V. (2022). Gender felt pressure, affective domains, and mental health outcomes among transgender and gender diverse (TGD) children and adolescents: A systematic review with developmental and clinical implications. *International Journal of Environmental Research and Public Health, 20*(1), 785. https://doi.org/10.3390/ijerph20010785

Mojtabai, R., Olfson, M., Sampson, N. A., Jin, R., Druss, B., Wang, P. S., Wells, K. B., Pincus, H. A., & Kessler, R. C. (2011). Barriers to mental health treatment: Results from the national comorbidity survey replication (NCS-R). *Psychological Medicine, 41*(8), 1751–1761. https://doi.org/10.1017/S0033291710002291

Muhammad, N., Murugesan, B., Singal, P., Antai, A., & Jain, L. (2023). Diagnostic dilemma of differentiating attention-deficit/hyperactivity disorder (ADHD) from mood disorders and other common psychiatric illnesses in substance use patient population. *Cureus Journal of Medical Science, 15*(4). https://doi.org/10.7759/cureus.37372

Niethammer, O., & Frank, R. (2007). Prevalence of use, abuse and dependence on legal and illegal psychotropic substances in an adolescent inpatient psychiatric population. *European Child & Adolescent Psychiatry, 16*(4), 254–259. https://doi.org/10.1007/s00787-006-0597-5

Nordentoft, M., Wahlbeck, K., Hällgren, J., Westman, J., Ösby, U., Alinaghizadeh, H., Gissler, M., & Laursen, T. M. (2013). Excess mortality, causes of death and life expectancy in 270,770 patients with recent onset of mental disorders in Denmark, Finland and Sweden. *PLoS One, 8*(1), e55176. https://doi.org/10.1371/journal.pone.0055176

Özgen, H., Spijkerman, R., Noack, M., Holtmann, M., Schellekens, A., Dalsgaard, S., van den Brink, W., & Hendriks, V. (2021). Treatment of adolescents with concurrent substance use disorder and attention-deficit/hyperactivity disorder: A systematic review. *Journal of Clinical Medicine, 10*(17), 3908. https://doi.org/10.3390/jcm10173908

Pedersen, D. (2005). Estigma y exclusión social en la enfermedad mental: Apunte para el análisis e investigación. *Revista de psiquiatria y salud mental Herminio Valdizan, 7*(1), 3–14.

Philips, I. (1967). Psychopathology and mental retardation. *American Journal of Psychiatry, 124*(1), 29–35. https://doi.org/10.1176/ajp.124.1.29

Preuss, U. W., Schaefer, M., Born, C., & Grunze, H. (2021). Bipolar disorder and comorbid use of illicit substances. *Medicina, 57*(11), 11. https://doi.org/10.3390/medicina57111256

Radcliffe, P., & Stevens, A. (2008). Are drug treatment services only for «thieving junkie scumbags»? Drug users and the management of stigmatised identities. *Social Science & Medicine, 67*(7), 1065–1073. https://doi.org/10.1016/j.socscimed.2008.06.004

Raven, M. C. (2017). *Diagnostic overshadowing dangers*. Patient Safety Network. https://psnet.ahrq.gov/web-mm/diagnostic-overshadowing-dangers

Routh, D. K., & King, K. M. (1972). Social class bias in clinical judgment. *Journal of Consulting and Clinical Psychology, 38*(2), 202–207. https://doi.org/10.1037/h0032620

Schuller, J., Cavenaile, J.-C., & Briganti, G. (2023). Somatic management of psychiatric patients in the emergency department. *Psychiatria Danubina, 35*(2), 341–346. https://europepmc.org/article/med/37800253

Shefer, G., Henderson, C., Howard, L. M., Murray, J., & Thornicroft, G. (2014). Diagnostic overshadowing and other challenges involved in the diagnostic process of patients with mental illness who present in emergency departments with physical symptoms—A qualitative study. *PLoS One, 9*(11), e111682. https://doi.org/10.1371/journal.pone.0111682

Skeie, I. (2024). Health improvements needed in persons with mental disorders and substance use disorders. Helsa til folk med psykiske lidelser og rusmiddellidelser må bedres. *Tidsskrift for den Norske laegeforening: tidsskrift for praktisk medicin, ny raekke, 144*(1), 0650. https://doi.org/10.4045/tidsskr.23.0650

Stewart, C., & El-Mallakh, R. (2007). Is bipolar disorder overdiagnosed among patients with substance abuse? *Bipolar Disorders, 9*(6), 646–648. https://doi.org/10.1111/j.1399-5618.2007.00465.x

The Joint Commission. (2022). Diagnostic overshadowing among groups experiencing health disparities. *Sentinel Event Alert, 65*. https://www.jointcommission.org/-/media/tjc/documents/

resources/patient-safety-topics/sentinel-event/sea-65-diagnostic-overshadowing-6-16-22-final.pdf. Accessed 8 June 2024.

Thornicroft, G., Rose, D., & Kassam, A. (2007). Discrimination in health care against people with mental illness. *International Review of Psychiatry (Abingdon, England), 19*(2), 113–122. https://doi.org/10.1080/09540260701278937

Torrens, M., Rossi, P. C., Martínez-Riera, R., Martínez-Sanvisens, D., & Bulbena, A. (2012). Psychiatric co-morbidity and substance use disorders: Treatment in parallel systems or in one integrated system? *Substance Use & Misuse, 47*, 1005–1014. https://doi.org/10.3109/10826084.2012.663296

Ungar, T., & Knaak, S. (2013). The hidden medical logic of mental health stigma. *Australian & New Zealand Journal of Psychiatry, 47*(7), 611–612. https://doi.org/10.1177/0004867413476758

Verheul, R. (2001). Co-morbidity of personality disorders in individuals with substance use disorders. *European Psychiatry, 16*(5), 274–282. https://doi.org/10.1016/S0924-9338(01)00578-8

Wakeman, S. E., Pham-Kanter, G., & Donelan, K. (2016). Attitudes, practices, and preparedness to care for patients with substance use disorder: Results from a survey of general internists. *Substance Abuse, 37*(4), 635–641. https://doi.org/10.1080/08897077.2016.1187240

Warburton, H., Turnbull, P. J., & Hough, M. (2005). *Occasional and controlled heroin use*. Joseph Rowntree Foundation.

Westermeyer, J. (2006). Comorbid schizophrenia and substance abuse: A review of epidemiology and course. *The American Journal on Addictions, 15*, 345–355. https://doi.org/10.1080/10550490600860114

White Hughto, J. M., Reisner, S. L., & Pachankis, J. E. (2015). Transgender stigma and health: A critical review of stigma determinants, mechanisms, and interventions. *Social Science & Medicine, 1982*(147), 222–231. https://doi.org/10.1016/j.socscimed.2015.11.010

Wu, L. T., Zhu, H., & Ghitza, U. E. (2018). Multicomorbidity of chronic diseases and substance use disorders and their association with hospitalization: Results from electronic health records data. *Drug and Alcohol Dependence, 192*, 316–323. https://doi.org/10.1016/j.drugalcdep.2018.08.013

World Health Organization. (2022). *World mental health report: Transforming mental health for all*. World Health Organization. https://iris.who.int/bitstream/handle/10665/356119/9789240049338-eng.pdf?sequence=1

Yamamoto, J., James, Q. C., Bloombaum, M., & Hattem, J. (1967). Racial factors in patient selection. *American Journal of Psychiatry, 124*(5), 630–636. https://doi.org/10.1176/ajp.124.5.630

Yang, L. H., Wong, L. Y., Grivel, M. M., & Hasin, D. S. (2017). Stigma and substance use disorders: An international phenomenon. *Current Opinion in Psychiatry, 30*(5), 378–388. https://doi.org/10.1097/YCO.0000000000000351

Chapter 6
Stigma and Behavioral Addictions: Problematic Gambling and Video Game Addiction

Víctor José Villanueva-Blasco, Dalila Eslava Pérez, and Antonio Rial-Boubeta

6.1 Introduction

Gambling Disorder (American Psychological Association [APA], 2013; World Health Organization [WHO], 1992) and, more recently, Gaming Disorder (video game addiction) (WHO, 2022) have been recognized by the scientific community as behavioral addictions. Both issues are topics of increasing scientific and social interest for two decades, and their relevance from a public health perspective is observed both at the epidemiological level and in their specific consideration in the design of public policies.

However, these behavioral addictions have not received the same attention as substance addictions in relation to stigma. And yet, they are not exempt from this phenomenon, although with some particularities that distinguish it from the stigma associated with substance addictions. In fact, substance addictions generate more stigma than other physical or mental conditions (Kilian et al., 2021), so it is worth asking to what extent this is extrapolated to behavioral addictions. There is no

V. J. Villanueva-Blasco (✉)
Valencian International University, Valencia, Spain

Research Network in Primary Care of Addictions (RIAPAd), Madrid, Spain

International Society of Substance Use Professionals (ISSUP), Madrid, Spain

International Center for Technology Transfer in Addictions (ITTC), Valencia, Spain
e-mail: vjvillanueva@universidadviu.com

D. E. Pérez
Valencian International University, Valencia, Spain
e-mail: dalila.eslava@universidadviu.com

A. Rial-Boubeta
University of Santiago de Compostela, Santiago de Compostela, Spain
e-mail: antonio.rial.boubeta@usc.es

T. Mota Ronzani (ed.), *Social Stigma and Drug Use*,
https://doi.org/10.1007/978-3-031-94813-8_6

specific theory that explains why non-substance addictions are associated with the phenomenon of stigma. However, some authors have turned to theories commonly used to understand stigma in diseases (Casale et al., 2023; Hing et al., 2015; Peter et al., 2018) to offer a conceptual approach. These are the attribution theory (Weiner, 1986; Weiner et al., 1988) and the danger appraisal hypothesis (Corrigan et al., 2003).

6.1.1 Attribution Theory

The attribution theory (Weiner, 1995) holds that, depending on whom or what the cause and control of a disease are attributed to, the person's responsibility in their condition is judged. If it is considered that the person is the one who has control, they are perceived as responsible; on the other hand, if it is attributed to genetic or contextual factors, responsibility decreases. When it is considered that someone is responsible for their disease, it can generate anger and the desire for punishment, manifesting in stigmatizing behaviors.

In the case of non-substance addictions, they are perceived as more controllable than physical diseases and even than substance addictions (Hing et al., 2016; Konkolÿ Thege et al., 2015). For example, according to Brown and Russell (2019), the public perception does not see similarities between problematic gambling and substance use disorders, which leads to the belief that people could simply stop gambling. This increases the tendency to blame and blame those who suffer from this addiction, increasing stigma (Hing et al., 2015).

6.1.2 Danger Appraisal Hypothesis

On the other hand, the "danger appraisal hypothesis" holds that when a person is perceived as dangerous, they are attributed a greater responsibility for their behavior, which increases social rejection toward them (Corrigan et al., 2003). However, in behavioral addictions, the people involved do not usually show dangerous behaviors, nor is there a perception of dangerousness in relation to problematic gamblers (Hing et al., 2016) nor to video game addiction and problematic Internet use (Casale et al., 2023). In short, the danger appraisal of people with a behavioral addiction does not seem to be involved in a relevant way in the development of stigma.

6.2 Stigma in Gambling and Betting

Research on stigma in non-substance addictions has focused mainly on problematic gambling, substantiating the relevance of this (Brown and Russell, 2019; Hing et al., 2015; Hing et al., 2016; Hing and Russell, 2017; Quigley et al., 2019; Rolando et al., 2023). People with gambling problems report that this behavior negatively affects their work and family life (Hing et al., 2015) and that they often feel judged by their environment, being perceived as weak or without self-control, which generates social rejection and complicates close relationships (Rolando et al., 2023; Hing et al., 2016). This external stigmatization can be internalized, increasing the risk of self-stigma, where people feel shame and see their problem as a personal failure (Baxter et al., 2016; Hing et al., 2016). As a result, many people choose to hide their addiction, avoiding seeking help and perpetuating the problematic behavior (Hing et al., 2016; Hing et al., 2011). This fact is configured as a barrier to access to treatment.

Concealment often leads to social isolation and seeking company in other players, where they do not feel judged (Hing et al., 2015; Russell et al., 2018), perpetuating the stigma (Eldredge et al., 2016). This suggests an underestimation of secrecy and that increasing public awareness about its signs could help detect the problem before it worsens (Hing et al., 2015). However, the evidence indicates that not all forms of awareness are effective, and they can even have iatrogenic effects, increasing the stigma of the affected people. "Responsible gambling" campaigns, promoted by governments and industry to reduce the harm associated with gambling, can increase stigma by reinforcing the stereotype of the irresponsible gambler (Miller et al., 2016; Miller and Thomas, 2017). These campaigns present gambling as something controllable for the majority, attributing the problem to the lack of self-control of a minority that, it is assumed, could avoid it if they acted "responsibly" (Brown and Russell, 2019). Thus, a division is created between "responsible" and "irresponsible" players, emphasizing individual responsibility and generating guilt in those who fail to control their addiction (Thomas et al., 2016).

This approach, based on attribution theory, fosters the stigma toward problematic gambling and diverts the responsibility of government policies and the industry toward the individual (Miller et al., 2014). In fact, some affected people see these narratives as especially stigmatizing, suggesting that they are directly to blame for their situation (Miller and Thomas, 2017). It is suggested, therefore, to review or abandon the concept of "responsible gambling" to prevent this discourse from reinforcing the stigma and underlining the individual responsibility, shifting the attention from the structural factors that contribute to the problem (Miller et al., 2016; Miller and Thomas, 2017).

6.3 Stigma in Video Game Addiction

In recent years, the literature has pointed out the addictive potential of certain video games, which led to the inclusion of Internet Gaming Disorder in the DSM-5 (APA, 2013). Subsequently, the WHO (2022) incorporated the Video Game Use Disorder in the ICD-11, covering both online and offline gaming behaviors. However, according to some experts, the inclusion of video game use disorder in diagnostic manuals may have promoted an exaggerated view of the risks posed by games and generated uncertainty among the boundaries that differentiate very committed players from those for whom it poses a problem (Aarseth et al., 2017; Ferguson and Colwell, 2020).

Galanis et al. (2021) warn about the possible misclassification of regular, but non-problematic, players with a pathological label that could generate stigma. However, it is also argued that the advantages of these labels outweigh the disadvantages, as they favor the development of better treatment protocols and facilitate prevention campaigns (Pontes et al., 2022). In this respect, Galanis et al. (2023) pointed out that it is unlikely that the concept of "game addiction" is a determining factor in public stigma.

The behavior of problematic video game use is perceived as controllable, generating anger and guilt in observers (Casale et al., 2023). Although less stigmatizing than problematic gambling (Peter et al., 2018), video games often include microtransactions, such as loot boxes, power-ups, and coins, which can disrupt the player's spending. This suggests a growing convergence between video games and gambling, which could increase the stigma toward video game addiction. Thus, more research is needed to understand possible stigmatization processes similar to those observed in problematic gambling.

6.4 Vulnerability to Stigma in Behavioral Addictions

Stigma in problematic gambling particularly affects vulnerable groups, with women being one of the most affected. Women players tend to choose games in discreet places to avoid being seen and judged and avoid betting houses due to derogatory comments they receive, even from other players (Estévez et al., 2023). This stigma implies a double penalty: being a woman and a player (Estévez et al., 2023). This occurs because they do not conform to traditional gender roles (Martínez-Redondo and Arostegui-Santamaría, 2021), facing prejudices that label them as bad mothers or workers, negligent, irresponsible, incompetent, and selfish, generating rejection in their environment (Estévez et al., 2023; Casey, 2006; Holdsworth et al., 2012).

This transgression of gender expectations leads to feelings of guilt and shame, making it difficult to seek support (Hing et al., 2016) and increasing self-stigma in women to a greater extent than in men (Hing and Russell, 2017). This represents a significant barrier to access to treatment, especially considering the frequent comorbidity with disorders such as depression, anxiety, and substance use (Desai and Potenza, 2008). In fact, suicide is the main cause of death in women players (Althaus et al., 2021).

Family support for women is limited and often comes from other women (Rius-Buitrago et al., 2021), while partners may despise or mistreat them (Lamas et al., 2018). In contrast, men receive more family support and social justification (Martínez-Redondo and Luján-Acevedo, 2020). Although women are more likely to contact help centers, men are more likely to attend the appointment for an evaluation (Weinstock et al., 2011).

Other vulnerable groups include people with low incomes and minorities, who face greater stigmatization compared to individuals with higher incomes, who usually have more access to treatment, possibly due to higher education and less stigmatizing attitudes (Holdsworth et al., 2015; Horch and Hodgins, 2015).

6.5 Addressing Stigma in Behavioral Addictions

6.5.1 *Interventions to Reduce Stigma*

Strategies to reduce stigma in behavioral addictions are limited, but some from other areas could be adapted. Brown and Russell (2019) describe interventions for stigma in problem gambling, previously used in stigmatized conditions such as mental illness (Corrigan et al., 2012). Riordan et al. (2021), based on guidelines for alcohol treatment, recommend person-centered practices, non-stigmatizing language, and training for professionals to reduce stigma. These strategies could be applied to both problem gambling addiction and video game addiction.

6.5.2 *Contact*

Contact interventions aim to reduce stereotypes through interactions between individuals unfamiliar with a condition and affected individuals, who share their experiences and recovery processes (Arboleda-Flórez and Stuart, 2012). These interventions increase the empathy of outsiders and decrease the anxiety of affected individuals when addressing the condition (Thornicroft et al., 2016), facilitating identification and reducing the perception of loneliness (Corrigan et al., 2012). However, these interventions can foster compassion and affect the feeling of autonomy (Corrigan and Fong, 2014). Their effectiveness depends on awareness of the gambling disorder (Corrigan et al., 2012; Hing et al., 2016; Holmes et al., 1999).

6.5.3 *Education*

Educational interventions aim to counteract stereotypes and negative attitudes through truthful information about the gambling disorder (Arboleda-Flórez and Stuart, 2012), addressing how it develops and questioning erroneous beliefs (Eldredge et al., 2016). However, the presentation of data can increase social distancing if it highlights differences between the public and the stigmatized group (Palmer et al., 2018). The effectiveness of these interventions depends on the level of awareness of the problem (Holmes et al., 1999).

6.5.4 Use of Language

The use of language in public campaigns is crucial, as emphasizing personal responsibility can generate negative attitudes toward those suffering from gambling problems (Miller & Thomas, 2017). Inclusive and person-centered language is recommended, avoiding pejorative terms, labels, and expressions that attribute blame (Healy et al., 2022).

6.5.5 Advocacy

Advocacy interventions focus on the gambling disorder as a social justice issue, rejecting the associated negative stereotypes (Arboleda-Flórez and Stuart 2012), pointing out the interests of the gaming industry and the responsibility of the government, reducing the player's responsibility (Hancock and Smith, 2017; Miller and Thomas, 2017; Thomas et al., 2016). Increasing community awareness and reducing stigma facilitates family and friends' support, essential for help-seeking behavior in reducing barriers to treatment (Itäpuisto 2019; Wieczorek and Dąbrowska, 2018).

6.5.6 Person-Centered Practice

Person-centered practice, which fosters compassion, respect, and patient participation, is key in the treatment of mental disorders (Sharma et al., 2015). In behavioral addictions, it is necessary to involve the family, as parental behavior influences the evolution of the disorder (Bonnaire et al., 2019; Li et al., 2019).

Brown and Russell (2019) suggest that it is necessary to employ all intervention modalities to address stigma comprehensively. Depending on a single style of intervention may not address all aspects of stigma, which could be counterproductive. In addition to the proposed interventions, according to Brown and Russell (2019), "advocacy actions" are crucial. These are interventions aimed at reframing the problem, shifting the focus of attention from the individual to the collective. Such actions will necessarily involve multiple recipients, including not only players and their families but also communities, services, stakeholders, and policymakers.

6.6 Prevention of Structural and Provider Stigma

The place where treatment is offered can influence stigmatization (Rolando et al., 2023). Satel (2007) warned that sometimes medical and mental health professionals endorse stigmatizing attitudes toward mental illness, which could also apply to these behaviors. There are also studies that point to a lack of willingness to provide treatment by health professionals, considering that, for example, video game disorder should not be considered a mental health problem (Dullur and Hay, 2017). This fact not only interferes with access to treatment but could also interfere with future searches for it and the development of self-stigma.

Therefore, explicitly addressing stigma from the beginning of treatment can improve adherence to it and recovery (Hing and Russell, 2017). In addition, including outreach services or online counseling would help attract people who, for many reasons, do not want to access face-to-face services (Rodda et al., 2013).

6.7 Promoting Coping with Self-Stigma

Self-stigma in behavioral addictions occurs when a person internalizes negative stereotypes associated with their disorder and applies them to their identity (Corrigan et al., 2009). A common coping mechanism is to hide the problematic behavior (Hing and Russell, 2017), which, although it reduces shame, prevents the recognition of the problem and the search for help, hindering recovery (Nuske and Hing, 2013). Shame, fear of rejection, and social judgment about treatment discourage help-seeking (Hing et al., 2014), while the effort to hide the problem generates anxiety and stress (Corrigan et al., 2013).

Revealing the problematic behavior can result in social disapproval, but it also reduces stress and facilitates family support, reducing self-stigma and improving quality of life (Corrigan et al., 2010). Admitting the problem is effective in combating self-stigma and reducing isolation. Moreover, when a person agrees with stereotyped beliefs, they are less likely to seek help, as they try to distance themselves from the stigmatized group. On the other hand, people who attend treatment perceive fewer stereotypes, although it is not clear whether this is a result of the treatment or facilitated the search for help (Hing and Russell, 2017).

6.8 Stigma Associated with Clinical Diagnosis

Corrigan (2000) has pointed out that diagnostic labels and other indicators of mental illnesses can act as foundations for the creation of stereotypes and prejudices. This type of prejudice tends to manifest in negative behaviors, including hostility, discrimination in areas such as housing, employment, or access to treatments, and, especially, in avoidance behaviors toward the affected people (Corrigan, 2000). Thus, diagnostic labels can be particularly prone to generating stigmatizing perceptions in relation to people with behavioral addictions, providing a basis for the emergence of stereotypes (Corrigan, Markowitz et al., 2003). In line with this, Peter et al. (2018) observe that the diagnostic label of gaming or video game disorder increases stigma compared to control conditions without diagnosis. However, other studies (Palmer et al., 2018; Quigley et al., 2019) support the conclusion that the label used to describe the gaming disorder does not affect attitudes and stigma toward the disease. These results suggest that the more recent term "gaming disorder," introduced in the DSM-5 (APA, 2013), does not provoke more stigma than its predecessor "pathological gambling" in the DSM-IV (APA, 1994). Similarly, the terminology used to describe video game addiction seems to have little impact on the stigma toward gamers (Galanis et al., 2023). In short, further research is needed to clarify this key issue in relation to stigma in people with behavioral addictions.

The stigmatization of gaming disorder cannot be reduced with a simple change of terminology (Quigley et al., 2019). In the case of substance addictions, it has been proposed to reconceptualize substance use disorders as prolonged excessive use (Rehm et al., 2013; Rehm et al., 2014). This way of considering them is less stigmatizing than the label of "addiction," as it presents the consumption behavior as a continuum in which problematic consumptions are at one end (Rehm et al., 2013). In non-substance addictions, since most people perform some of these behaviors regularly, they could be located at different points on the continuum. This perspective would help to reduce stigma, focusing efforts on reducing it and thus freeing the behavior from the moral and disease connotations associated with the label of "addiction" (Hing et al., 2016).

6.9 Stigma and Overpathologization

In the last decade, a worrying trend has emerged in the field of mental health and addictions, which consists of overpathologizing certain disruptive behaviors, usually derived from frequent and intensive use of digital devices, video games, the Internet, or social networks, from the moment it generates some type of interference in daily life. According to experts, it is possible that, in an attempt to categorize and better understand human behavior, we have fallen into the temptation to pathologize the everyday, simply because at some point it may become problematic, dysfunctional, or maladaptive (Kardefelt-Winther et al., 2017). Using criteria typical of substance addictions, such as tolerance or withdrawal syndrome, health professionals have begun to label daily activities, ranging from video game use to physical exercise, also as "addictions." But what part of the epidemiology that we are building today is really a true addiction in clinical terms? What could simply be an excessive passion or enthusiasm can become a cause for concern and clumsily labeled as a pathology (Billieux et al., 2019). This could trigger an alarm cycle leading to unnecessary therapeutic interventions, a saturation of health devices, and a loss of confidence in the behavioral sciences themselves. We are at risk of treating as sick people who are not, thus weakening the credibility of our discipline and causing the stigmatization of those we are supposed to be helping.

Recognizing the problem and avoiding its trivialization does not mean overdimensioning it, a risk that could lead us to overpathologize it and confer a clinical character when it may not have it (Nogueira-López et al., 2023). In this sense, an analysis and reflection must be carried out to adequately define and quantify the problem. It is necessary for the field of mental health to be able to timely redefine addictive behaviors, focusing on symptoms that truly reflect a significant and persistent clinical dysfunction. Faced with the initial risk of trivializing the problem that the emergence of new addictions (especially in adolescence) can pose, the risk also grows of positioning ourselves on the opposite side, which reinforces the need to be especially rigorous in this field, using good diagnostic criteria and appropriate instruments. In short, an accurate diagnosis enables both professionals and affected individuals to better understand and contextualize the issue, facilitating more effective intervention and reducing the stereotypes and beliefs that fuel stigma, often stemming from the inappropriate use of diagnostic terms.

6.10 Final Considerations: Proposals for the Design of Public Policies Aimed at Reducing the Stigma Associated with Problem Gambling and Video Game Addiction

When addressing the stigma associated with problem gambling and the addiction to video games, public policies should consider several key implications:

(a) *Integration of mental health:* Public policies should recognize these behaviors as mental health problems and integrate treatment for them within broader mental health services. This approach can destigmatize these conditions and encourage people to seek help without fear of being judged (Gainsbury et al., 2014).
(b) *Awareness and education campaigns:* It is essential to raise awareness about the nature of addiction to gambling and video games. Educational programs aimed at the public and health professionals should highlight the behavioral and psychological foundations of these addictions to reduce public stigma.
(c) *Policy reforms:* Policies should reflect the most recent scientific understanding of these issues. For example, their diagnostic classification in the DSM and ICD recognizes their legitimacy as a mental health condition, which potentially reduces stigma. Public policies that align with such classifications are essential to promote non-discriminatory treatment frameworks.
(d) *Support and access to treatment:* Stigma often prevents people from seeking help. It is essential to ensure accessible and unbiased treatment options. Policies that expand access to support systems, such as anonymous telephone lines,

online counseling, and peer support groups, can mitigate the fear of stigmatization (Kuss and Griffiths, 2017).

(e) *Regulation and advertising:* It is necessary to tighten advertising regulations for gambling and online games, especially with regard to their exposure to minors. Similarly, it is necessary to regulate the incorporation of elements of gambling and betting into video games, such as loot boxes. Policies that regulate how these activities are promoted can reduce normalization and help manage public perceptions, which otherwise could contribute to stigma.

The incorporation of these considerations into public policies will help reduce stigma and create a more favorable environment for people affected by problem gambling and video game addiction.

References

Aarseth, E., Bean, A. M., Boonen, H., Colder Carras, M., Coulson, M., Das, D., Deleuze, J., Dunkels, E., Edman, J. M., Ferguson, C. J., Haagsma, M. C., Bergmark, K. H. M., Hussain, Z., Janszm, J., Kardefelt-Winther, D., Kutner, L., Markey, P., Lundenal Nielsen, R. K., Prause, N., et al. (2017). Scholars' open debate paper on the World Health Organization ICD-11 gaming disorder proposal. *Journal of Behavioral Addictions, 6*(3), 267–270. https://doi.org/10.1556/2006.5.2016.088

Althaus, J., Zendle, D., & Bowden-Jones, H. (2021). Gambling and gaming addictions in women. In G. Carrà, M. Galanter, & A. M. Baldacchino (Eds.), *Textbook of addiction treatment*. Springer.

American Psychiatric Association. (1994). *Diagnostic and statistical manual of mental disorders* (4th ed.).

American Psychiatric Association. (2013). *Diagnostic and statistical manual of mental disorders* (5th ed.). https://doi.org/10.1176/appi.books.9780890425596.

Arboleda-Flórez, J., & Stuart, H. (2012). From sin to science: Fighting the stigmatization of mental illnesses. *Canadian Journal of Psychiatry, 57*(8), 457–463. https://doi.org/10.1177/07067437120570080

Baxter, A., Salmon, C., Dufresne, K., Carasco-Lee, A., & Matheson, F. I. (2016). Gender differences in felt stigma and barriers to help-seeking for problem gambling. *Addictive Behaviors Reports, 3*, 1–8. https://doi.org/10.1016/j.abrep.2015.10.001

Billieux, J., Flayelle, M., Rumpf, H. J., & Stein, D. J. (2019). High involvement versus pathological involvement in video games: A crucial distinction for ensuring the validity and utility of gaming disorder. *Current Addiction Reports, 6*(3), 323–330. https://doi.org/10.1007/s40429-019-00259-x

Bonnaire, C., Liddle, H. A., Har, A., Nielsen, P., & Phan, O. (2019). Why and how to include parents in the treatment of adolescents presenting internet gaming disorder? *Journal of Behavioral Addictions, 8*(2), 201–212. https://doi.org/10.1556/2006.8.2019.27

Brown, K. L., & Russell, A. M. (2019). Exploration of intervention strategies to reduce public stigma associated with gambling disorder. *Journal of Gambling Studies, 36*(2), 713–733. https://doi.org/10.1007/s10899-019-09888-3

Casale, S., Boursier, V., Musicò, A., Ghinassi, S., Cigolini, G., Petrucci, E., & Gioia, F. (2023). Stigmatizing attitudes toward internet gaming disorder, problematic smartphone use and problematic social networking site use: An experimental vignette study. *Addictive Behaviors, 141*, 107665. https://doi.org/10.1016/j.addbeh.2023.107665

Casey, E. (2006). Domesticating gambling: Gender, caring and the UK National Lottery. *Leisure Studies, 25*(1), 3–16. https://doi.org/10.1080/02614360500150695

Corrigan, P. W. (2000). Mental health stigma as social attribution: Implications for research methods and attitude change. *Clinical Psychology: Science and Practice, 7*(1), 48.

Corrigan, P. W., & Fong, M. W. M. (2014). Competing perspectives on erasing the stigma of illness: What says the dodo bird? *Social Science and Medicine, 103*, 110–117. https://doi.org/10.1016/j.socscimed.2013.05.027

Corrigan, P. W., Kosyluk, K. A., & Rüsch, N. (2013). Reducing self-stigma by coming out proud. *American Journal of Public Health, 103*(5), 794–800. https://doi.org/10.2105/AJPH.2012.301037

Corrigan, P. W., Larson, J. E., & Ruesch, N. (2009). Self-stigma and the "why try" effect: Impact on life goals and evidence-based practices. *World Psychiatry, 8*(2), 75–81. https://doi.org/10.1002/j.2051-5545.2009.tb00218.x

Corrigan, P., Markowitz, F. E., Watson, A., Rowan, D., & Kubiak, M. A. (2003). An attribution model of public discrimination towards persons with mental illness. *Journal of Health and Social Behavior.* https://doi.org/10.2307/1519806

Corrigan, P. W., Morris, S., Larson, J., Rafacz, J., Wassel, A., Michaels, P., Wilkniss, S., Batia, K., & Rüsch, N. (2010). Selfstigma and coming out about one's mental illness. *Journal of Community Psychology, 38*(3), 259–275. https://doi.org/10.1002/jcop.20363

Corrigan, P. W., Morris, S. B., Michaels, P. J., Rafacz, J. D., & Rüsch, N. (2012). Challenging the public stigma of mental illness: A meta-analysis of outcome studies. *Psychiatric Services, 63*(10), 963–973. https://doi.org/10.1176/appi.ps.201100529

Desai, R. A., & Potenza, M. N. (2008). Gender differences in the associations between past-year gambling problems and psychiatric disorders. *Social Psychiatry and Psychiatric Epidemiology, 43*, 173–183. https://doi.org/10.1007/s00127-007-0283-z

Dullur, P., & Hay, P. (2017). Problem internet use and internet gaming disorder: A survey of health literacy among psychiatrists from Australia and New Zealand. *Australasian Psychiatry, 25*(2), 140–145. https://doi.org/10.1177/1039856216684714

Eldredge, L. K. B., Markham, C. M., Ruiter, R. A. C., Kok, G., Fernandez, M. E., & Parcel, G. S. (2016). *Planning health promotion programs: An intervention mapping approach.* Wiley.

Estévez, A., Macía, L., Ontalvilla, A., & Aurrekoetxea, M. (2023). Exploring the psychosocial characteristics of women with gambling disorder through a qualitative study. *Frontiers in Psychology, 14*, 1294149. https://doi.org/10.3389/fpsyg.2023.1294149

Ferguson, C. J., & Colwell, J. (2020). Lack of consensus among scholars on the issue of video game "addiction". *Psychology of Popular Media, 9*(3), 359–366. https://doi.org/10.1037/ppm0000243

Gainsbury, S., Hing, N., & Suhonen, N. (2014). Professional help-seeking for gambling problems: Awareness, barriers and motivators for treatment. *Journal of Gambling Studies, 30*(2), 503–519. https://doi.org/10.1007/s10899-013-9373-x

Galanis, C. R., Delfabbro, P. H., & King, D. L. (2021). Stigma-related arguments against gaming disorder: A call for research. *Addiction, 116*(10), 2921–2922.

Galanis, C. R., Weber, N., Delfabbro, P. H., Billieux, K., & King, D. L. (2023). Gaming disorder and stigma-related judgements of gaming individuals: An online randomized controlled trial. *Addiction, 118*, 1687–1698. https://doi.org/10.1111/add.16211

Hancock, L., & Smith, G. (2017). Critiquing the Reno Model I-IV international influence on regulators and governments (2004–2015)—The distorted reality of "responsible gambling". *International Journal of Mental Health and Addiction, 15*(6), 1151–1176.

Healy, M., Richard, A., & Kidia, K. (2022). How to reduce stigma and bias in clinical communication: A narrative review. *Journal of General Internal Medicine, 37*(10), 2533–2540. https://doi.org/10.1007/s11606-022-07609-y

Hing, N., Holdsworth, L., Tiyce, M., & Breen, H. (2014). Stigma and problem gambling: Current knowledge and future research directions. *International Gambling Studies, 14*(1), 64–81. https://doi.org/10.1080/14459795.2013.841722

Hing, N., Nuske, E., & Gainsbury, S. (2011). *Gamblers at risk and their help seeking behaviour*. Centre for Gambling Education & Research.

Hing, N., Nuske, E., Gainsbury, S. M., & Russell, A. M. T. (2016). Perceived stigma and self-stigma of problem gambling: Perspectives of people with gambling problems. *International Gambling Studies, 16*(1), 31–48. https://doi.org/10.1080/14459795.2015.1092566

Hing, N., Nuske, E., Gainsbury, S. M., Russell, A. M. T., & Breen, H. (2016). How does the stigma of problem gambling influence help-seeking, treatment and recovery? A view from the counselling sector. *International Gambling Studies, 16*(2), 263–280. https://doi.org/10.1080/14459795.2016.1171888

Hing, N., & Russell, A. M. T. (2017). Psychological factors, sociodemographic characteristics, and coping mechanisms associated with the self-stigma of problem gambling. *Journal of Behavioral Addictions, 6*(3), 416–424. https://doi.org/10.1556/2006.6.2017.056

Hing, N., Russell, A. M. T., & Gainsbury, S. M. (2016). Unpacking the public stigma of problem gambling: The process of stigma creation and predictors of social distancing. *Journal of Behavioral Addictions, 5*(3), 448–456. https://doi.org/10.1556/2006.5.2016.057

Hing, N., Russell, A. M. T., Gainsbury, S. M., & Nuske, E. (2016). The public stigma of problem gambling: Its nature and relative intensity compared to other health conditions. *Journal of Gambling Studies, 32*(3), 847–864. https://doi.org/10.1007/s10899-015-9580-8

Hing, N., Russell, A., Nuske, E., & Gainsbury, S. (2015). *The stigma of problem gambling: Causes, characteristics and consequences*. Centre for Gambling Education & Research, Southern Cross University. Victorian Responsible Gambling Foundation.

Holdsworth, L., Hing, N., & Breen, H. (2012). Exploring women's problem gambling: A review of the literature. *International Gambling Studies, 12*(2), 199–213. https://doi.org/10.1080/14459795.2012.656317

Holdsworth, L., Nuske, E., & Hing, N. (2015). A grounded theory of the influence of significant live events, psychological co-morbidities and related social factors on gambling involvement. *International Journal of Mental Health & Addiction, 13*(2), 257–273. https://doi.org/10.1007/s10899-015-9580-8

Holmes, E. P., Corrigan, P. W., Williams, P., Canar, J., & Kubiak, M. A. (1999). Changing attitudes about schizophrenia. *Schizophrenia Bulletin, 25*, 447–456. https://doi.org/10.1093/oxfordjournals.schbul.a033392

Horch, J. D., & Hodgins, D. C. (2015). Self-stigma coping and treatment-seeking in problem gambling. *International Gambling Studies, 15*(3), 470–488. https://doi.org/10.1080/14459795.2015.1078392

Itäpuisto, M. (2019). Problem gambler help-seeker types: Barriers to treatment and help-seeking processes. *Journal of Gambling Studies, 35*(3), 1035–1045. https://doi.org/10.1007/s10899-019-09846-z

Kardefelt-Winther, D., Heeren, A., Schimmenti, A., van Rooij, A., Maurage, P., Carras, M., Edman, J., Blaszczynski, A., Khazaal, Y., & Billieux, J. (2017). How can we conceptualize behavioural addiction without pathologizing common behaviours? *Addiction, 112*(10), 1709–1715. https://doi.org/10.1111/add.13763

Kilian, C., Manthey, J., Carr, S., Hanschmidt, F., Rehm, J., Speerforck, S., & Schomerus, G. (2021). Stigmatization of people with alcohol use disorders: An updated systematic review of population studies. *Alcoholism: Clinical and Experimental Research, 45*(5), 899–911. https://doi.org/10.1111/acer.14598

Konkolÿ Thege, B., Colman, I., el-Guebaly, N., Hodgins, D. C., Patten, S. B., Schopflocher, D., Wolfe, J., & Wild, T. C. (2015). Social judgments of behavioral versus substance-related addictions: A population-based study. *Addictive Behaviors, 42*, 24–31. https://doi.org/10.1016/j.addbeh.2014.10.025

Kuss, D. J., & Griffiths, M. D. (2017). Social networking sites and addiction: Ten lessons learned. *International Journal of Environmental Research and Public Health, 14*(3), 311. https://doi.org/10.3390/ijerph14030311

Lamas, J. L., Santolaria, R., Estévez, A., & Jauregui, P. (2018). *Guía clínica específica "Mujer y juego" [Specific clinical guideline "Women and gambling"]*. Delegación del Plan Nacional Sobre Drogas.

Li, A. Y. L., Chau, C. L., & Cheng, C. (2019). Development and validation of a parent-based program for preventing gaming disorder: The game over intervention. *International Journal of Environmental Research and Public Health, 16*(11), 1984. https://doi.org/10.3390/ijerph16111984

Martínez-Redondo, P., & Arostegui-Santamaría, E. (2021). *Situación en España de la Violencia de Género y el abuso de sustancias [The situation of gender violence and substance abuse in Spain]*. Ministerio de Sanidad.

Martínez-Redondo, P., & Luján-Acevedo, F. (2020). *Hombres y adicciones. Intervención desde perspectiva de género [Men and addictions. Intervention from a gender perspective]*. UNAD.

Miller, H. E., & Thomas, S. L. (2017). The problem with 'responsible gambling': Impact of government and industry discourses on feelings of felt and enacted stigma in people who experience problems with gambling. *Addiction Research & Theory, 26*(2), 85–94. https://doi.org/10.1080/16066359.2017.1332182

Miller, H. E., Thomas, S. L., Robinson, P., & Daube, M. (2014). How the causes, consequences and solutions for problem gambling are reported in Australian newspapers: A qualitative content analysis. *Australian and New Zealand Journal of Public Health, 38*, 529–535. https://doi.org/10.1111/1753-6405.12251

Miller, H. E., Thomas, S. L., Smith, K. M., & Robinson, P. (2016). Surveillance, responsibility and control: An analysis of government and industry discourses about problem and responsible gambling. *Addiction Research & Theory, 24*, 163–176. https://doi.org/10.3109/16066359.2015.1094060

Nogueira-López, A., Rial-Boubeta, A., Guadix-García, I., Villanueva-Blasco, V. J., & Billieux, J. (2023). Prevalence of problematic internet use and problematic gaming in Spanish adolescents. *Psychiatry Research, 326*, 115317. https://doi.org/10.1016/j.psychres.2023.115317

Nuske, E., & Hing, N. (2013). A narrative analysis of help-seeking behaviour and critical change points for recovering problema gamblers: The power of storytelling. *Australian Social Work, 66*(1), 39–55. https://doi.org/10.1080/0312407X.2012.715656

Organización Mundial de la Salud. (1992). *CIE-10 Clasificación Internacional de Enfermedades, 10ª revisión.*

Organización Mundial de la Salud. (2022). *CIE-11 Clasificación Internacional de Enfermedades, 11ª revisión*. https://icd.who.int/es

Palmer, B. A., Richardson, E. J., Heesacker, M., & DePue, M. K. (2018). Public stigma and the label of gambling disorder: Does it make a difference? *Journal of Gambling Studies, 34*(4), 1281–1291. https://doi.org/10.1007/s10899-017-9735-x

Peter, S. C., Li, Q., Pfund, R. A., Whelan, J. P., & Meyers, A. W. (2018). Public stigma across addictive behaviors: Casino gambling, eSports gambling, and internet gaming. *Journal of Gambling Studies, 35*, 247–259. https://doi.org/10.1007/s10899-018-9775-x

Pontes, H. M., Montag, C., Elhal, J. D., Monteiro, A. V., Evren, C., Throuvala, M. A., Macur, M., McDowall, A., Rumpf, H., Carbonell, X., Kuss, D., López-Fernámdez, O., & Griffiths, M. (2022). *Stigma and gaming disorder: Should we take a 'glass half full' or 'glass half empty' perspective?* Society for the Study of Addiction. https://doi.org/10.1111/add.15831

Quigley, L., Prentice, J., Warren, J. T., Quilty, L. C., Dobson, K. S., & Hodgins, D. C. (2019). What's in a name? Evaluating the public stigma of gambling disorder. *Journal of Gambling Studies, 36*, 1205–1228. https://doi.org/10.1007/s10899-019-09924-2

Rehm, J., Marmet, S., Anderson, P., Gual, A., Kraus, L., Nutt, D. J., Room, R., Samokhvalov, A., Scafato, E., Trapencieris, M., Wiers, R. W., & Gmel, G. (2013). Defining substance use disorders: Do we really need more than heavy use? *Alcohol and Alcoholism, 48*(6), 633–640. https://doi.org/10.1093/alcalc/agt127

Rehm, J., Probst, C., Kraus, L., & Lev-Ran, S. (2014). The addiction concept revisited. In P. Anderson, G. Bühringer, & J. Colom (Eds.), *Reframing addiction: Policies, processes and pressures* (pp. 103–117). ALICE RAP Project.

Riordan, B. C., Winter, D. T., Barrett, L., Ritter, A., Lancaster, K., Seear, K., Butler, K., & Haber, P. S. (2021). Guidelines for the treatment of alcohol problems: An introduction. In P. S. Haber & B. C. Riordan (Eds.), *New Australian guidelines for the treatment of alcohol problems: An overview of recommendations* (pp. S3–S5). Medical Journal of Australia.

Rius-Buitrago, A., Soriano-Villarroel, I., & López-González, H. (2021). "Yo sabía que nadie me iba a juzgar": La adicción al juego online desde la perspectiva de género ["I knew no one would judge me": Online gambling addiction from a gender perspective]. *Musas, 6*, 138–155. https://doi.org/10.1344/musas2021.vol6.num1.8

Rodda, S., Lubman, D. I., Dowling, N. A., Bough, A., & Jackson, A. C. (2013). Web-based counseling for problem gambling: Exploring motivations and recommendations. *Journal of Medical Internet Research, 15*(5), e99. https://doi.org/10.2196/jmir.2474

Rolando, S., Ferrari, C., & Beccaria, F. (2023). "To me, it was just a vice". Stigma and other barriers to gambling treatment in Piedmont, Italy. *Journal of Gambling Studies, 39*(4), 1909–1925. https://doi.org/10.1007/s10899-023-10214-1

Russell, A. M. T., Langham, E., & Hing, N. (2018). Social influences normalize gambling-related harm among higher risk gamblers. *Journal of Behavioral Addictions, 7*(4), 1100–1111. https://doi.org/10.1556/2006.7.2018.139

Satel, S. (2007). In praise of stigma. In J. E. Henningfield, P. B. Santora, & W. K. Bickel (Eds.), *Addiction treatment: Science and policy for the twenty-first century* (pp. 147–151). Johns Hopkins University Press.

Sharma, T., Bamford, M., & Dodman, D. (2015). Person-centred care: An overview of reviews. *Contemporary Nurse, 51*(2–3), 107–120. https://doi.org/10.1080/10376178.2016.1150192

Thomas, S. L., Bestman, A., Pitt, H., David, J., & Thomas, S. (2016). *Lessons for the development of initiatives to tackle the stigma associated with problem gambling*. Victorian Responsible Gambling Foundation.

Thornicroft, G., Mehta, N., Clement, S., Evans-Lacko, S., Doherty, M., Rose, D., Koschorke, M., Shidhaye, R., O'Reilly, C., & Henderson, C. (2016). Evidence for effective interventions to reduce mental-health-related stigma and discrimination. *The Lancet, 387*(10023), 1123–1132. https://doi.org/10.1016/S0140-6736(15)00298-6

Weiner, B. (1986). *An attributional theory of motivation and emotion*. Springer.

Weiner, B. (1995). *Judgments of responsibility: A foundation for a theory of social conduct*. Guilford Press.

Weiner, B., Perry, R. P., & Magnusson, J. (1988). An attributional analysis of reactions to stigmas. *Journal of Personality and Social Psychology, 55*(5), 738. https://doi.org/10.1037/0022-3514.55.5.738

Weinstock, J., Burton, S., Rash, C. J., Moran, S., Biller, W., Krudelbach, N., Phoenix, N., & Morasco, B. J. (2011). Predictors of engaging in problem gambling treatment: Data from the West Virginia problem gamblers help network. *Psychology of Addictive Behaviors, 25*, 372–379. https://doi.org/10.1037/a0023240

Wieczorek, Ł., & Dąbrowska, K. (2018). What makes people with gambling disorder undergo treatment? Patient and professional perspectives. *Nordic Studies on Alcohol and Drugs, 35*(3), 196–214. https://doi.org/10.1177/1455072518772397

Chapter 7
Evaluation of an Online Intervention to Reduce Stigma Among Healthcare Workers in Latin America

Jazmín Mora-Rios, Hugo Noel Valdivia Ramos, Jimena Kalawaski, and José Luis Vázquez

7.1 Introduction

It is recognized throughout the world that stigma represents one of the major barriers to the care of people with mental health problems, including substance use. From highly industrialized to less developed countries, stigma related to mental illness affects the emotional well-being of those suffering from mental disorders and also of their families. Stigma causes isolation and shame, which discourages people from seeking help.

In his classic study on stigma, Goffman (1963) defined the concept as a negative and degrading personal attribute that differentiates a person from others, placing them in an undesirable or inferior category, which leads to feelings of guilt, shame, and humiliation.

Society attributes a series of negative traits to people who suffer from mental health problems, especially those with severe conditions such as schizophrenia and addiction (Sordi et al., 2021; Monteiro et al., 2013; Mora-Ríos et al., 2017). These people are often criticized and discredited, assumed to be unpredictable and dangerous, perceived as having no control over their lives, and blamed along with their

J. Mora-Rios (✉)
Direction of Epidemiological and Psychosocial Research. Ramón de la Fuente Muñiz National Institute of Psychiatry, Mexico City, Mexico
e-mail: morarj@inprfm.gob.mx

H. N. Valdivia Ramos
National Autonomous University of Mexico, Mexico City, Mexico

J. Kalawaski · J. L. Vázquez
Demand Reduction Unit, Executive Secretariat of the Inter-American Drug Abuse Control Commission (CICAD), Organization of American States (OAS), Santiago, Chile
e-mail: JKalawski@oas.org; JVazquez@oas.org

T. Mota Ronzani (ed.), *Social Stigma and Drug Use*,
https://doi.org/10.1007/978-3-031-94813-8_7

families for their condition. Mental illness generates fear, rejection, pity, and mistrust. These ideas are promoted in the social imaginary through the family, media, political figures, and opinion leaders.

These negative beliefs are held both by the general population and by healthcare workers. Some studies have reported that healthcare workers have a fatalistic perception of mental health problems (Schulze, 2007), believing that it makes no sense to invest in treatment because they affect people who "cannot be cured"; they think the only possible forms of care are confinement and control through medication, especially in the case of disorders such as schizophrenia and substance abuse (Murney et al., 2020). Rojas Vistorte et al. (2018) found greater stigmatization by older and more experienced healthcare workers. Negative attitudes were found more in medical personnel than in those in other fields, especially concerning disorders such as schizophrenia and depression. There was also a directly proportional relationship: the greater the degree of stigmatizing attitudes, the greater the tendency to express rejection and create social distance from people with these problems. Among the reasons that could explain this stigmatization by healthcare workers, it has been suggested that mental health is emphasized less than physical health in their training as students, which could lead to a limited and fragmented approach to health, with less humanized care.

Studies have shown attitudes of rejection even in mental health specialists (Arvaniti et al., 2009; Lauber et al., 2006). However, direct contact with people with mental illness seems to reduce stigma in the attitudes of health professionals more than scientific knowledge (Clement et al., 2012; Couture & Penn, 2003; Knaak et al., 2014; Smith & Cashwell, 2011).

This study is part of a global comparative and cross-cultural research network since 2004. The overall goal of the network is to achieve multidisciplinary advances in research on stigma and the dynamics of structural discrimination and social exclusion in mental illness. Mexico joined this initiative in 2007. Funding was obtained from the Sectoral Funds for Health and Social Security Research (FOSSSIS-CONACYT) to carry out a broad-based study on stigma and discrimination in mental illness in different parts of the population, including people with a psychiatric diagnosis, families, healthcare workers, and the general population. The goal was to develop a community intervention model based on the needs of the main actors involved in the treatment and rehabilitation of people with a mental disorder, with a gender and human rights approach, to generate action strategies in this sector. The Mexico study found that participants with a psychiatric diagnosis identified the family as the primary source of stigma and discrimination and health care workers as secondary. These findings prompted our interest in developing the proposal for the online course (Mora-Rios et al., 2017).

The objective of the course is to sensitize those who work in health institutions, as they are key to transforming the conditions of care and improving the quality of life and inclusion of people affected by mental health problems. We seek to provide resources and undertake actions that expand knowledge on these topics and make them accessible to people who provide health care. The course is aimed at professionals from health teams in first-level care institutions in Latin America, although it may also interest auxiliary healthcare workers.

The objective of this study was to evaluate the effect of this online intervention for healthcare workers aimed at reducing stigmatizing attitudes toward mental illness and to identify whether such intervention constitutes a valuable resource for healthcare workers of 13 Latin American countries, 2017.

7.2 Development

The methodology of the broader research project, from which the online course was devised, has already been published (Mora-Ríos et al., 2013; Mora-Ríos & Bautista, 2014). The project was approved by the Ethics Committee of the Ramón de la Fuente Muñiz National Institute of Psychiatry. Written informed consent was obtained through the process, guaranteeing the anonymity and confidentiality of the information. The online course is called "Stigma and Mental Health: Challenges in Constructing Quality Health Care." It was implemented with the support of the Sectoral Funds for Health and Social Security Research (Mora-Ríos et al., 2017). The first course was given in 2018 to 107 healthcare workers.

This study analyzes the course results from 1 September to 26 November 2021, administered with the support of the Education Department of the Ramón de la Fuente Muñiz National Institute of Psychiatry. The course was offered remotely using the MOODLE platform.

7.3 Course Description

The contents of the course are divided into five modules: (1) What do we know about mental health?, (2) Stigma and its consequences for health, (3) Expressions of stigma and discrimination in clinical practice, (4) What can we do?, and (5) Recommendations. To provide dynamic content, infographics, audio, and videos were included, presenting the testimonies of people with lived experience of mental health disorders; these used professional actors to protect the identities of the informants on whose participation they were based. Testimonies from family members and others with lived experience and from healthcare workers were also included. The course had 16 individual activities and nine group activities (participation in forums).

In response to an announcement by the Demand Reduction Unit of the Executive Secretariat of the Inter-American Commission for the Control of Drug Abuse (CICAD), 75 participants from 12 different countries in Latin America (Argentina, Brazil, Chile, Costa Rica, Colombia, Ecuador, Guatemala, Mexico, Nicaragua, Panama, Peru, and Uruguay) enrolled and were sent usernames and passwords. Of these, 9% never signed into the platform, and 11% of those who signed in performed no activities in the course. The course was offered free of charge, and participants were asked to consent to use their answers for research purposes. They were asked to perform all activities to receive a certificate at the end of the course.

7.4 Sociodemographic Characteristics of Participants

Table 7.1 shows data for those who completed the course. The majority were women (76%), and the rest (24%) were men from 12 countries, mainly from Mexico (20%), Peru (12.7%), and Panama (10.9%). Their ages were 24–65, with an average age of 39; 60% were aged 31–44, so they were generally young. The disciplines represented were psychology (65%), medicine (13%), nursing (12%), social work (5%), and others (e.g., sociology). The most common level of studies was a master's degree (40%), followed by bachelor's and specialty degrees (33% and 22%, respectively). One participant from the nursing area with a high school diploma works in an addiction center in Mexico. Approximately 76% of participants reported working in the care of people with mental health problems.

7.5 Measurements

The following measurements were used to assess attitudes toward mental illness:

1. Six items from the Mental Health Knowledge Schedule (MAKS-10; Evans Lako, et al., 2010) were used. The original version consists of 12 items measuring general mental health knowledge. For this study, we used a five-point agreement-disagreement response format on a Likert scale. The questionnaire measures six areas of knowledge related to stigma based on six items: help-seeking, recognition, support, employment, treatment, and recovery. A higher score corresponds to a greater understanding of the stigma of mental illness.
2. Reported and Intended Behavior Scale (RIBS; Evans-Lacko et al., 2011). This scale originated from the Star Social Distance Scale (Evans-Lacko et al., 2011) and measures intended behavior. It consists of eight items, of which the first four have a three-point response range (yes, no, and don't know). The remaining four items measure the intention of behavior and are answered on a five-point Likert scale indicating the level of agreement and disagreement. The highest score indicates less stigmatizing behavior. In this study, only the last four items were considered, maintaining the original contexts, and a new one was added, the willingness to have a relationship.
3. The Opinions Toward Mental Illness (OMI) questionnaire was initially developed by Cohen and Struening (1962). It consists of 51 items that evaluate five dimensions: authoritarianism, benevolence, mental health ideology, social restrictiveness, and interpersonal etiology of mental illness. The overall reliabil-

Table 7.1 Sociodemographic characteristics of participants who completed the course

	Women		Men		Total	
	n	%	*n*	%	*n*	%
Age (years)						
24–30	5	9.1	1	*1.8*	*6*	*10.9*
31–37	*11*	20	6	*11*	*17*	*30.9*
38–44	*11*	20	5	9.1	*16*	29.1
45–51	11	20	–	–	*11*	*20*
52–65	*4*	7.3	1	1.8	*5*	*9.1*
Nationality						
Argentina	*1*	1.8	–	–	*1*	*1.8*
Chile	*5*	9.1	–	–	*5*	*9.1*
Colombia	*2*	3.6	1	1.8	*3*	5.5
Costa Rica	2	*3.6*	–	–	*2*	3.6
Ecuador	2	*3.6*	*3*	*5.5*	*5*	9.1
Guatemala	*4*	6.7	1	1.8	*5*	*9.1*
Honduras	*2*	3.6	–	–	*2*	3.6
Mexico	*9*	15.0	*2*	3.6	*11*	20.0
Nicaragua	*2*	*3.6*	1	1.8	*3*	5.5
Panama	*6*	10.9	–	–	*6*	10.9
Peru	*4*	7.3	*3*	5.5	*7*	12.7
Uruguay	*4*	*7.3*	–	–	*4*	7.3
Profession						
Psychology	*29*	*69.0*	7	*12.7*	*36*	65.5
Medicine	*4*	*7.3*	3	*5.5*	*7*	12.8
Nursing	*5*	*9.1*	2	*3.3*	*7*	11.7
Social work	*2*	*3.6*	1	*1.8*	*3*	5.5
Other	*2*	*3.6*	–	–	2	3.6
Level of education						
High school	–	–	1	*1.8*	*1*	1.8
Bachelor's degree	*16*	*29.1*	2	*3.6*	*18*	32.7
Specialty	*5*	*9.1*	7	*12.7*	*12*	21.8
Master's degree	*19*	*34.5*	3		*22*	40.0
Doctorate	2	*3.6*	–	–	2	3.6
Works in care						
Yes	*32*	*58.2*	10	*18.2*	*42*	76.4
No	*10*	*18.2*	3	*5.5*	*13*	23.6
Total	*42*	*76.4*	13	*23.6*	*55*	100

ity was 0.83. The response format is a four-point Likert scale: 0 = totally disagree, 1 = disagree, 2 = agree, and 3 = totally agree. The overall internal consistency is adequate (alpha = 0.90). For this study, we used a modified version based on the version validated in Mexico by Altamirano (2012), which was previously adapted to the context of the Mexican population (Mora-Ríos et al., 2013).

The participants completed all the questionnaires before the first training session of the intervention group (August 2021) and after the completion of the last training session (October 2021). Five instructors, three women and two men, reviewed the activities and provided support and guidance. Participants met with the team in two online sessions, the first at the beginning of the course to provide information about the platform and activities to be developed and the second to give feedback to the participants regarding doubts about the activities or platform.

7.6 Data Analysis

The t-test for related samples was used to compare the means between the pre-test and post-test phases for hypothesis testing. The magnitude of the differences was evaluated using the effect size (Cohen's *d*), interpreted according to the reference values small = 0.2, moderate = 0.5, and large = 0.8 (Lakens, 2013). This analysis included the MAKS, the RIBS, and the OMI scores. The assumption of normality was verified using the Shapiro-Wilk test. The data were analyzed using the statistical programs JASP version 0.19.1 (JASP Team, 2024) and G*Power version 3.1.9.7 (Erdfelder et al., 1996).

7.7 Results

The majority of the participants evaluated the course favorably (60%). All showed interest in the course topics. In addition to reading, each participant carried out activities. There were forums where participants could share their reflections and experiences about how stigma and discrimination were expressed in their respective countries.

Table 7.2 shows the comparison of the means of the total scores of the questionnaires on mental health stigma: the MAKS, the RIBS, and the OMI. These were administered in the pre-test and post-test phases. Significant differences were found between the means of the pre-test and post-test in the MAKS, with a moderate effect

Table 7.2 Comparison of the means of the stigma questionnaires in the pre-test and post-test

	Pre-test		Post-test					
Scale	*M*	*SD*	*M*	*SD*	*t (df)*	*p*-value	*SE*	1-β
Mental health knowledge schedule	24.25	2.24	25.81	2.42	−4.318 (54)	<0.001	−0.58	0.99
Reported and intended behavior scale	21.01	2.64	22.30	2.57	−3.830 (54)	<0.001	−0.51	0.97
Opinions toward Mental Illness (OMI) questionnaire	171.56	14.42	182.52	11.58	−6.526 (54)	<0.001	−0.88	0.99

Note: Student's *t*-test. Cohen's *d* effect size

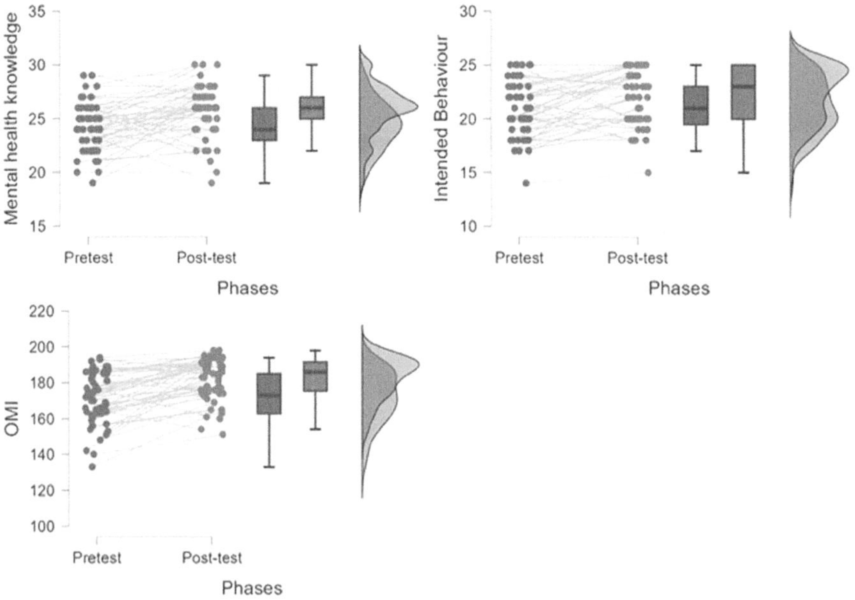

Fig. 7.1 Distribution and density of the results of the stigma questionnaires between phases. Note: This figure shows the distribution and density of the scores of the Mental Health Knowledge Scale (MAKS), Reported and Intended Behavior Scale (RIBS), and the Opinions toward Mental Illness (OMI) questionnaire in the pre-test and post-test phases. The box and whisker plots show an increase in the medians of the scores after the intervention. The density graphs indicate a shift toward higher scores in the post-test phase, suggesting improved knowledge, behavioral intention, and a favorable change in opinions about mental illness

size, $t(54) = -4.318$, $p < 0.001$, 95% CI [−2.290, −0.838], $d = -0.58$, and statistical power $(1 - \beta) = 0.99$. As shown in Fig. 7.1, most participants had increased scores after the intervention, suggesting greater knowledge about mental health stigma at the course's end.

Significant differences were also observed for the RIBS, with a moderate effect size, $t(54) = -3.830$, $p < 0.001$, 95% CI [−1.967, −0.615], $d = -0.51$, and statistical power $(1—\beta) = 0.97$. Figure 7.1 shows an increase in the mean scores for intended behavior in the post-test, as indicated by the upward-trending lines in the connected dot graph and the increase in the post-test medians, reflected in the box plots.

Finally, there was a significant increase in the post-test scores of the OMI questionnaire, with a large effect size, $t(54) = -6.526$, $p < 0.001$, 95% CI [−14.332, −7.596], $d = -0.88$, and statistical power $(1–\beta) = 0.99$. Figure 7.1 shows an increase in the post-test scores for most participants, suggesting that favorable attitudes toward mental illnesses increased after the intervention.

Participants were asked if the course could be a resource to reduce the stigmatizing attitudes of healthcare staff in their countries. As seen in Fig. 7.2, 95% of participants said it had helped them greatly, and three said it had helped somewhat. More than a specific change in attitudes, what was achieved was a strengthening of the

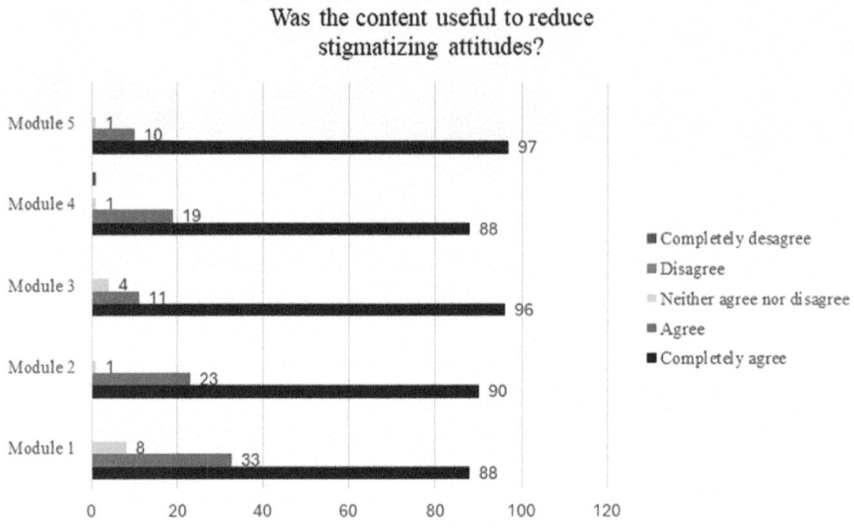

Fig. 7.2 Evaluation of the online course Stigma and Mental Health

positioning of the participants and a reflection on their experiences with other participants in the forums included in the course.

Note: This figure shows the evaluation of the usefulness of the intervention for modifying discriminatory attitudes and practices in health care workers. The bars indicate that most participants rated the five modules positively, with the last two being the best rated.

In addition, participants were asked open-ended questions. One question asked whether they would recommend the course to others, and nearly all replied that they would. They also said that the course was helpful in their professional and personal training and enabled them to expand their knowledge on stigma and discrimination and consider how to apply them. They said that the course sensitized them by encouraging them to identify and reflect on their beliefs and strengthening their competencies, resources, and possible strategies. By contrasting the testimonies with their reality, they said, the course helped them to analyze the situations they had experienced and to sensitize them to their own stigmatizing attitudes and discriminatory actions in the past. One example is given related to benevolent stigma, or treating with pity the person with mental health problems or addiction, which could underestimate their abilities. In comments about the activities, most said that they liked being able to put the material reviewed into practice. Below are some examples of reasons given as to why they would recommend the course:

> I would recommend it because it helped me expand my perception of the topic and make changes. Anyone taking this course will at least have to reflect on their attitudes.
>
> Yes, because one has to be sensitized. It also helps us grow as people since when we have a relative or someone close to us, we have the tools to provide the help they need.
>
> Yes, because it incorporates up-to-date practical and theoretical information that is valuable and applicable to Latin American reality.
>
> The feedback from our coordinator also made me reflect and think. It is very complete.

Participants also recommended including examples of community interventions to combat stigma from different parts of Latin America, mainly related to substance use; providing more material on inequality, interculturality, human rights, and public policy; adding more detailed information on people in vulnerable groups; such as migrants, people living on the streets, and the LGTTTBIQ+ community; expanding on topics related to employment and structural discrimination; and including strategies to involve communications and social media. These are all complex and interesting topics, and they demonstrate the interest in Latin America in understanding the forms and manifestations of stigma in the local context.

The aspects of the course most valued by participants were the videos, video animations, and testimonials (of healthcare workers, family members, and substance users), as they allowed them to identify expressions of stigma in their work environments and their effects on people and to learn more about people's needs. One participant emphasized that it was good to know that all the testimonials were based on real cases. Participants also criticized the format of two activities suggested by the platform (nos. 11 and 16) and suggested carrying the activity out freely. These suggestions helped improve the course.

7.8 Final Considerations

This study found that this online course is helpful in reducing stigmatizing attitudes in healthcare workers. The course content is culturally relevant for healthcare workers in Mexico and other parts of Latin America. Stigma and discrimination in health care are widespread problems in different regions of Latin America (Semrau, et al., 2015, Sordi et al., 2021). Participants showed interest in the course and highlighted the importance of training healthcare workers on these issues, especially in primary care.

These findings coincide with those of Valdivia (2024), who demonstrated the effect of this course in modifying the attitudes of healthcare students at the end of and 1 month after completing the course. In this work, we evaluate only the effect of the intervention after the course has ended. One of the future tasks suggested by this experience is a follow-up study over a more extended period, at 1 month, 6 months, and a year after the intervention, to evaluate whether the favorable attitudes are maintained over time, as has been done in other studies (Clement et al., 2012; Knaak et al., 2014). This intervention and its effectiveness constitute important contributions specially considering that in recent years, efforts to address stigma in, Latin America through anti-stigma iniciatives have increasingly been recognized (Thornicroft et al., 2022).

Our findings on the effectiveness of this course highlight the importance of providing quality comprehensive training to healthcare workers, with collaboration between the health team and others who participate in care in such fields as medicine, psychology, nursing, and social work. The training information should be up-to-date, based on scientific evidence, and use non-stigmatizing language. The use and problematic consumption of substances requires specific training that emphasizes health teams in contact with different population groups, such as infants, adolescents, women, and young people, and that develops particular strategies for the care of people who experience multiple discrimination.

Finally, an approach based on human rights and social inclusion is essential. It is necessary to promote care, voluntary treatment, and interventions adapted to the cultural contexts of different Latin American countries to provide quality care that is dignified and inclusive and that is sensitive to issues of stigmatization in attitudes, skills, and knowledge.

Quality research must be carried out on the barriers to seeking and finding treatment by health professionals, as well as self-stigma, the consequences of stigmatizing attitudes, and actions that promote dignified treatment focused on human rights. It is also necessary to encourage evaluation of the effectiveness of programs aimed at reducing stigma and discrimination (Thomas et al., 2015) to implement effective practices based on evidence.

References

Altamirano, C. (2012). *Validación factorial del cuestionario de opiniones hacia la enfermedad mental (OMI) en personal de salud.* Tesis de maestría, Universidad Nacional Autónoma de México.

Arvaniti, A., Samakouri, M., Kalamara, E., Bochtsou, V., Bikos, C., & Livaditis, M. (2009). Health service staff's attitudes towards patients with mental illness. *Social Psychiatry and Psychiatric Epidemiology, 44*(8), 658–665. https://doi.org/10.1007/s00127-008-0481-3

Clement, S., van Nieuwenhuizen, A., Kassam, A., et al. (2012). Filmed v. live social contact interventions to reduce stigma: Randomised controlled trial. *British Journal of Psychiatry, 201*(1), 57–64. https://doi.org/10.1192/bjp.bp.111.093120

Cohen, J., & Struening, E. L. (1962). Opinions about mental illness in the personnel of two large mental hospitals. *Journal of Abnormal and Social Psychology, 64*, 349–360.

Couture, S., & Penn, D. (2003). Interpersonal contact and the stigma of mental illness: A review of the literature. *Journal of Mental Health, 12*(3), 291–305. https://doi.org/10.1080/0963823100118276

Erdfelder, E., Faul, F., & Buchner, A. (1996). GPOWER: A general power analysis program. *Behavior Research Methods, 28*(1), 1–11.

Evans-Lacko, S., Rose, D., Little, K., Flach, C., Rhydderch, D., Henderson, C., & Thornicroft, G. (2011). Development and psychometric properties of the reported and intended behaviour scale (RIBS): A stigma-related behaviour measure. *Epidemiology and Psychiatric Sciences, 20*(3), 263–271. https://doi.org/10.1017/s2045796011000308

Evans-Lacko, S., Little, K., Meltzer, H., Rose, D., Rhydderch, D., Henderson, C. (2010a). Development and psychometric properties of the Mental Health Knowledge Schedule. *Canadian Journal of Psychiatry, 55*: 440–448. https://doi.org/10.1177/070674371005500707

Goffman, E. (1963). *Stigma: Notes on the management of spoiled identity*. Prentice Hall.

JASP Team. (2024). JASP (Version 0.19.1) [Computer software].

Knaak, S., Modgill, G., & Patten, S. B. (2014). Key ingredients of anti-stigma programs for health care providers: A data synthesis of evaluative studies. *Canadian Journal of Psychiatry, 59*(10 Suppl 1), S19–S26. https://doi.org/10.1177/070674371405901s06

Lakens, D. (2013). Calculating and reporting effect sizes to facilitate cumulative science: A practical primer for t-tests and ANOVAs. *Frontiers in Psychology, 4*, 863.

Lauber, C., Nordt, C., Braunschweig, C., & Rössler, W. (2006). Do mental health professionals stigmatize their patients? *Acta Psychiatrica Scandinavica, 429*, 51–59.

Monteiro, S. S., Villela, W. V., & Soares, P. S. (2013). The interaction between axes of inequality in studies on discrimination, stigma and HIV/AIDS: Contributions to the recent international literature. *Global Public Health, 28*(5), 519–533. https://doi.org/10.1080/17441692.2013.779738

Mora-Ríos, J., & Bautista, A. (2014). Estigma estructural, género e interseccionalidad: Implicaciones en la atención a la salud mental. *Revista Salud Mental, 37*(4), 303–312.

Mora-Ríos, J., Bautista, N., & Natera, G. (2013). Adaptación cultural de tres instrumentos de investigación sobre estigma y enfermedad mental en México. *Salud Mental, 36*(1), 9–18.

Mora-Ríos, J., Ortega-Ortega, M., & Medina-Mora, M. E. (2017). Addiction-related stigma and discrimination: A qualitative study in treatment centers in Mexico City. *Substance Use & Misuse, 52*(5), 594–603. https://doi.org/10.1080/10826084.2016.1245744

Murney, M. A., Sapag, J. C., Bobbili, S. J., & Khenti, A. (2020). Stigma and discrimination related to mental health and substance use issues in primary health care in Toronto, Canada: A qualitative study. *International Journal of Qualitative Studies on Health and Well-Being, 15*(1), 1744926. https://doi.org/10.1080/17482631.2020.1744926

Rojas Vistorte, A. O., Silva Ribeiro, W., Jaen, D., Jorge, M. R., Evans-Lacko, S., & Mari, J. d. J. (2018). Stigmatizing attitudes of primary care professionals towards people with mental disorders: A systematic review. *International Journal of Psychiatry in Medicine, 53*(4), 317–338. https://doi.org/10.1177/0091217418778620

Schulze, B. (2007). Stigma and mental health professionals: A review of the evidence on an intricate relationship. *International Review of Psychiatry, 19*, 137–155.

Semrau, M., Evans-Lacko, M., Koschorke, L., Ashenafi, L., & Thornicroft, G. (2015). Stigma and discrimination related to mental illness in low and middle-income countries. *Epidemiology and Psychiatric Sciences, 24*, 382–394.

Smith, A. L., & Cashwell, C. S. (2011). Social distance and mental illness: Attitudes to mental health and substance use issues in primary health care in Toronto, Canada: A qualitative study. *International Journal of Qualitative Studies on Health and Well-being.*

Sordi, B., Hernandez, R, Bobbili, S. & Arena, C. (2021). Health care providers and people with mental illness. An integrative review on antistigma interventions. *International Journal of Social Psychiatry, 67*,7: 840–853. https://doi.org/10.1177/0020764020985891.

Thomas, N., McLeod, B., Jones, N., & Abbott, J. (2015). Developing internet intervention to target the individual impact of stigma and health conditions. *Internet Interventions*, 351–358.

Thornicroft, G., Sunkel, C., Alikhon, A., Baker, S., Brohan, E., El Chammay, R., Davie, K., Demissie, M., Duncan, J., Fckadu, W., Gronholm, P., Guerrero, Z., Gurung, D., Habtamu, K., Hanlon, C., Heim, E., Henderson, C., Hijazi, Z., Hoffman, C....& Winkler, P. (2022). The Lancet Commission on ending stigma and discrimination in mental health. *The Lancet, 4009*, (10361)? 1438-1480. https://doi.org/10.1016/s0140-6736(22)01470-2

Valdivia, H. (2024). *Evaluación de una intervención en línea para reducir el estigma de la enfermedad mental en estudiantes de la salud.* Tesis doctoral, Universidad Nacional Autónoma de México.

Chapter 8
Extreme Experiences: Social Exclusion of Young Users of Inhalants, Crack, and Heroin in Mexico

Mario Joaquín Domínguez and Hugo César Moreno

8.1 Introduction

To analyze negative images of substance users, we turn to the production of subjectivities described by Michel Foucault (2002) and Roberto Esposito (2005, 2006a, 2007) because this concept provides a useful theoretical-methodological toolbox for the definition, characterization, and analytical construction of subjects based on their experience with substance use. In this way, we can identify stigma and exclusion in a context where the use of psychoactive substances is almost always assumed to be a problem of pathology and punishment of antisocial behavior, one that must be addressed through prohibition. In addition, to better understand the experience of young substance users, it is necessary to understand how the production of subjectivity occurs in the contemporary world, within the framework of neoliberal capitalism.

This approach allows us to understand the construction of young substance users as subjects and the way in which they relate to the apparatuses (structures and institutions) that define them. This theoretical approach is indispensable to the location and positioning of the discussion that identifies subjects in the dual condition of being young and drug users. This dual condition promotes stigma and exclusion, discriminatory processes that, in addition to excluding and marginalizing, lead to processes of criminalization and decitizenship. In this regard, Sepúlveda's (1997) observation about young people who use coca paste is of interest:

M. J. Domínguez (✉)
Department of Social Sciences in Health, Ramón de la Fuente Muñiz National Institute of Psychiatry, Mexico City, Mexico
e-mail: mariodom@inprf.gob.mx

H. C. Moreno
Institute of Social Sciences and Humanities, Benemérita Universidad Autónoma de Puebla, Puebla, Mexico

T. Mota Ronzani (ed.), *Social Stigma and Drug Use*,
https://doi.org/10.1007/978-3-031-94813-8_8

> The issue of a particular type of youth (urban/working-class) and its connection to the phenomenon of coca paste leads us to a problem characterized by prejudice and stereotype, where stigmatization sanctions and penalizes subjects and thought, and marginalizes lives, imposing negative and contradictory signs of identity. It leaves painful marks that coincide more with official speech and discourse than with those thoughts and feelings that tell us about the complex forms of subjectivation that develop on the very edges of society. (p. 103)

To this extent, discussion about substance use and users makes a kind of sense in its perception of the problem as pathological, in its adoption of the perspectives of health and punishment to combat antisocial behavior with prohibition and, in the best of cases, with prevention and treatment programs. This perspective has recently begun to be displaced, with consideration of the human rights of subjects in terms of sophisticated formulations that seek to reconfigure the cartographies in which users are located, that is, to include consideration of class, racialization, gender, age, and other social conditions and situations. These include the theoretical reflections of Esposito and Foucault on the production of subjectivities as juridical subjects, characterized as free, but who are nonetheless domesticated, subjected, and classified by institutions, by knowledge, and by scientific rationalism. That is, modern freedom is incorporated into the subject as a freedom that will lead to the possibility of being (acting as) oneself and not something else. It is therefore necessary to understand how substance use operates in the relationships between subjects and social institutions such as the family, school, work, and health care.

Given these assumptions, we must recognize that it is not enough to identify users as juridical subjects, since this "embodied freedom" of their subjectivity will take possession of their will (Esposito, 2006a), although this does not imply a complete lack of resistance or opposition. In other words, by integrating the institutional parameters, they will be defined as social subjects and legally accepted within the system that imposes the law. However, these codes of freedom will be under the protection of a legality that includes and excludes individuals by guaranteeing their political rights, which makes them free subjects, insofar as they are juridical subjects, but also subjects of interests. This results, as Esposito notes, in a collective immunity, a nationality of interests and rights: that is, the liberal rights of the sovereign citizen (Moreno, 2013). In this regard, the apparatus of the school excels in producing the subjectivity necessary to a society relying on the production of subjects who are civically and technically equipped to participate "freely" by being good citizens and good workers.

The transformations introduced by the neoliberal moment of capitalism thus affect in various ways the apparatuses of public education, public health, labor rights, and so forth, directly affecting individual life, reorganizing and disrupting time and space in everyday life (Bauman, 2000; Giddens, 1993; Han, 2012). The rationalization of labor is intensified within the framework of production mobilized by consumption, so that contemporary capitalism can be thought of as a consumer capitalism (Bauman, 2000; Han, 2012), deregulating the capital-labor relationship and leading to other forms of productive organization, increasing the use of flexible hiring and precarious employment, as well as processes of self-exploitation under the neoliberal principle of self-entrepreneurship (Foucault, 2007; Han, 2012). The deterioration of labor forms plays an essential role in contemporary forms of social exclusion, what Castells (1999) calls "disaffiliation."

In neoliberal capitalist society, labor is no longer defined by production but by consumption: that is, the workforce is detached from political processes, as technological advances in production, logistics, and organization allow for flexibility in production, reducing the bargaining power of labor against capital. Labor is subsumed into the production process, which is mobilized by consumption, which in turn mobilizes market economies demanding political arrangements that allow for the commodification of everything, including health, safety, and education. This process is accompanied by the exacerbation of what Esposito (2007) calls "immunization," the process of the separation of subjects through the breaking of community ties, of what is common. Their social character is broken, affecting the notion of community that represents a danger for capitalist society. The subject is immunized, stripped of social bonds and common life, leaving a notion of the common based on biological traits, that is, a biopolitics that drives apparatuses of control anchored in biological characteristics (Esposito, 2007).

It is pertinent, then, to ask how contemporary subjectivities are generated, how social apparatuses are articulated to produce subjectivities for the current social system, and how they produce disposable subjects. In the case of young people, Rossana Reguillo observes how these articulations of apparatuses create "accelerated youth disaffiliations," the process in which young people are rapidly disconnected from the system and left as individuals to resolve their own lives (Reguillo, 2010).

The ways of assuming one's own subjectivity have changed, and we believe that young people who consume psychoactive substances form contradictory youth subjectivities, using apparatuses that respond to processes of exclusion and marginalization, often exacerbating them, but also exercising them as forms of resistance and production of subjectivity contrary to the principles of the "good working citizen." They forge divergent paths that are not necessarily gambling with death, but whose extreme nature is something like death.

8.2 Drugs and Limit Experiences as Devices of Discontrol

Substance use is not exclusive to a particular class or social group, age group, or gender. However, there are differences in practices determined by the subject, type of substance, and contexts of use. New drug markets, social inequalities, and precarity affect the spread of new substances and the ways of experiencing substance use. For example, one person living on the street, asked what drugs he had used, replied:

> *Activo*, mushrooms, peyote, marijuana, cocaine, crack, heroin, nubain, but you know why I stopped shooting up? Because it was messing up my veins. (30-year-old male, heroin user)

Apart from the question of whether the habitual and problematic use of drugs led this man to the street or whether the situation of living on the streets led him to daily serious drug use, the interesting thing about his answer is his awareness of the consequences of repeated use of a type of substance and its administration—in this case, the injection of heroin. Access to substances is easy or difficult according to the context, and a change in substance is both a question of access and of a user's wanting to reduce risks. There is a user's awareness of what they consume and its relationship to their health or the risk of death, where substance use becomes a social apparatus, where the center of operations is the user and the way they regulate, increase, or end the use of a substance. Another example relative to the question of access is offered by another person living on the street, a regular user of inhalants, who was asked how he obtained other types of drugs:

> No, well, they invite me because… the truth, well, coke is very expensive, dude, so I don't have enough to be buying that shit. Instead, when I run into one of my buddies… when he has some, he just tells me, here goes your line. (18-year-old male, inhalant user)

The use of psychoactive substances differs according to the context and what the user is looking for. Using marijuana is not the same as using heroin, using inhalants is not the same as using cocaine. Their chemical composition, effects, costs, availability, paraphernalia, risks, and consequences are all different. A crack user shared the following:

> I don't like it in a can or in a Yakul [small plastic container for a brand of probiotic drink]. I'm pipe only, if I don't have a pipe… I'll give you fifty [pesos] for your pipe, dude, even if it's really burnt, I'll give you fifty for your pipe, better in a pipe. Because the hit gets to you more, more direct. But yes, when you inhale it, it's not the same… like there's nowhere for the smoke to escape. After I've put in about five or six rocks so that the hit gets to me more, more badass… the damn grease is already built up, I give it a rebound and my ears even go *zzzzz*. Recently I'm using more… my sight goes and my mind goes blank, I start to see white… (21-year-old male, crack user)

These differences are also found in the perception of society and among the users themselves. There is an unwritten hierarchy according to which it is more degrading to use some drugs than others. In general, the perception of the substance user is negative, but there are substances, such as heroin, inhalants, and crack (also known as "piedra") used by poorer people that are perceived as more degrading. In colloquial terms, it is worse to be a "tecato" (heroin user), "piedroso" (crack user) or *monoso* (an inhalant user) than a "marihuano" or a "pacheco" (marijuana user).

In a study of crack use that we conducted from 2011 to 2013, we identified and developed four typologies that serve as categories of analysis to distinguish the conditions of crack or rock smokers: (1) amateurs, (2) stable users, (3) "piedroso," and (4) veterans (Valdez et al., 2015). Other studies (De Oliveira & Nappo, 2008; German & Sterk, 2002) have constructed similar typologies that have proven useful.

Amateur users are in the initial phases of crack use; their use is not yet frequent, and they still hold a job or stay in school. They usually associate mainly with people who do not use crack or other drugs, their use represents a small part of their daily life, and they do not identify as "piedrosos" a pejorative expression employed by users themselves. For example, Reka,[1] who studied engineering and works as a photographer and had been using rock for a few months, says:

> Just... it's variable, because suddenly I have to pay something and then I say no... and the whole week goes by and I don't smoke any, but if I've paid all my things... well then I do smoke it, but not every day. With a crackhead it's almost every day; they live to smoke it. (34-year-old female, crack user)

Stable users try to control their crack use; these are people with intermittent use and more or less structured lives that help them reduce the consequences of use, and their use is mainly in private spaces. Edu, 30 years old, studied communication, currently works as a reporter, and smokes rock on weekends, on the street or on the roof of his house:

> I don't consider myself so addicted... I have always controlled myself a little more, like I have been a little more thoughtful ... in a way knowledge also heals you a little and you can find... many answers... most of the gang... doesn't study that kind of thing, and well, they are less aware of the consequences... (30-year-old male, crack user)

The *piedroso* relate more to other users and drug dealers; they spend most of their time trying to obtain resources to continue their use and often become involved in criminal activities. They themselves often identify as "crackheads," a derogatory term, and often exchange sex for drugs. Mike says that "they are not well seen, those who have not burned out, well, there is no problem... but if you see a guy like that crackhead, you know he is a rat or a fucking bum." Serafín is an example. At 17, he smoked rock for the first time and throughout his history of use, he has been involved in crime. At the time of the interview, he worked for a dealer and considered himself a "crackhead."

> I have known drugs since I was a child, because my father is, or was, a drug addict... then I started working with my uncle, and my uncle smoked every day. We didn't even work anymore, we just smoked all day. I smoked everything. The guys in my class, some of them become athletes, some just smoked weed, and I became a crackhead, and a crackhead in that group is total rejection. Since I'm a crackhead, the gang... with a crackhead it's always going to be shitty. Because the crackhead is going to give it all away for one more *piedra*. (23-year-old male, crack user)

Veteran users have prolonged use of crack but have managed to keep their lives relatively stable. They are able to gather resources for their use with minor temporary jobs. They socialize more with people who use alcohol. They try to control their use of crack by using other substances, such as marijuana, which allows them to use crack sporadically. An older man says:

> Marijuana... to this day, yes there are times when I roll a cigarette... before it was daily... and at all hours... when I was young, yes, yes I smoked it all day... yes, yes I smoke it [*piedra*], but I decide when I'm going to smoke it, not when you tell me... I can go buy it and smoke it, but I only smoke one and that's it... I don't have enough money to get addicted... (59-year-old male, crack user)

---

[1] All interviewees quoted in this article are identified with pseudonyms to protect their privacy.

On the other hand, there are the users of *activo*, an industrial solvent that is inhaled as a drug in Mexico City neighborhoods, especially among the homeless population. Some young users are devotees of Saint Jude, and every 28th of the month, thousands of faithful arrive at his church, especially on October 28 (Ortiz et al., 2015). Not all are homeless and not all inhale *activo*, but there is a stereotypical image of the young *vicioso* ("addict") or *monoso* (active user).

> I have heard some comments about some guys who are *monosos*, they inhale *activo* and then they run around like bad guys, stealing, but they don't steal from the people in the neighborhood, they rob taxis or something… and they're not from here, but these are things that I have heard. (39-year-old male, crack user)

> Well, these days I don't like to be at home … because there are only problems at home, well, only getting yelled at, I mean, since I don't work and then since I'm an addict [inhales *activo*]… I don't like to be yelled at… I like to be free… (19-year-old male, inhalant user)

Activo is a very cheap and readily available substance, so it is associated with people who live on the street (Ortiz et al., 2017). However, for these same reasons, it is also used by junior high (12–15 years old) and high school students (15–19 years old). Its use in any quantity causes serious physical and mental health problems that configure the dirty character and are totally detached from citizen qualities. But some users, depending on their social origin, manage to live with its use without reaching the most intense moments of consumption and despise the direct association between inhalant use and contempt for people living on the streets and human waste condition:

> I don't like it when they say, oh, those from the street!, well what happened, like from the street, many say that we are from the street, but we are not from the street, we are from our mom and our dad (34-year-old male, inhalant user).

Another group of people who are discriminated against for their substance use are heroin users, or *tecatos*. These are poor people who have lost social position by prioritizing the search for resources to buy drugs. They are found primarily on the border with the United States, living in contexts of social inequality, with little or no care and a lack of opportunities for effective rehabilitation, surrounded by violence and the risks of HIV, hepatitis C, or death by overdose (Fleiz et al., 2019).

> People look down on us, I mean, a *tecato*, a *cristalon*, the *tecato* is the worst, the truth, they see us as if we are less people, that we are worth less and I feel that in reality it should not be like that, but people see us like that. Well we ourselves may be all dirty or so, but well we don't look at ourselves for the physical, it's like a bond that exists between all the tecatos. (34-year-old woman, heroin user)

For many young people, substance use is guided by a more complex cultural plot, where leisure and activities, whether at work, at school, or in social life, enable relationships between the substance and their social apparatuses, functioning as measures of control (keeping a job, staying in school) or as catalysts for problematic use where losing a job can lead to an increased intensity of use or immediate social relationships of family or neighborhood. Sources of income serve as social apparatuses in contrast to school or work.

Family relationships and substance use configure a subjectification apparatus that feeds stigma and generates complex environments where violence and survival put the substance at the center of social relationships, from serving as the foundation of illegal family businesses (Zamudio & Carlos, 2009) to opening the door to problematic use, which in turn allows many young people to become workers for drug-dealing enterprises such as *narco-tienditas*, or small-scale dealers. There are different social relationships through which young people relate to drugs, either through trafficking, where they are recruited by a gang offering payment in money or drugs (Domínguez et al., 2019), or because their family or neighbors deal drugs and they take it on like any other casual job.

For this reason, it is not useful simply to assume that a person's relationship with substances, as a worker, is only a matter of income: the income is often barely enough to survive. In poor neighborhoods, where there is a lack of opportunities in employment, education, or recreation, and where there are few outlets for political, social, or cultural participation, substance use and dealing go beyond achieving a certain avoidance of reality or confrontation with authority; they function as a social apparatus that respond to the precariousness with which apparatuses of civic education, social control, and staying healthy in order to work are exercised.

It is necessary here to explain precisely what we mean by "social apparatus." Briefly, we have in mind the concept of Foucault as defined by Gilles Deleuze (1989) and Giorgio Agamben (2014) that imagines lines or series connecting and organizing a machine producing subjectivity. These lines are linguistic, textual, visual, and tactile, and they form mandates, orientations, regulations, laws, and orders. Skeins, grids, or maps—any such image serves to describe an apparatus structured through a fabric made up of sequences that connect territories, where bodies are simultaneously territories and agents of intervention.

The school, for example, is a social apparatus structured by its space and the way its elements are arranged: classrooms, courtyards, benches, blackboards, as well as bodies according to their reason to be there, be they principals, administrators, teachers, security guards, janitors, or students. All of these respond to regulations and curricular criteria, which in turn are defined by legislation. The school as a social apparatus serves for the civic and technical education of students, to equip them with the qualities necessary to be good citizens and workers. The intent is to create a certain subjectivity, that is, a subject with certain characteristics. But there are always other lines: escape routes, hidden paths, and other elements that complicate the skein.

Such lines emerge from all subjects in processes of subjectivation. Following Foucault and Agamben, the subject is always under the influence of social apparatuses whose function is to subjectify, that is, to create subjects. The subject is that which is always in process by being subjected to connections of institutional knowledge from medicine, psychiatry, and law—but also from sociology and economics—that perform this subjectivation: knowledge subjects individuals or groups among which discourses circulate that form identity, and the subjects are subjected. Thus, the question of social apparatuses is the question of subject formation.

Foucault observes the modes of subjectivation as forms of objectification of the subject by social apparatuses that seek to produce a subject according to the needs of its mandate: healthy, strong, civil, and honest. But, as we will show, there are always subjective lines that emerge from a subject as a product of other apparatuses (family, religion, neighborhood), that is, other sources of knowledge that align with or interfere with the social apparatus of the school, exploding some forms, promoting others, and bringing higher levels of knowledge into conflict with subjected forms. The extensive territory in which the physical space of the school is located has already initiated a process of subjectivation, and so there are conflicts and new lines reconfiguring relationships within the apparatus, including acts that run contrary to the law but are said to improve relationships, such as backpack and other searches that violate children's rights.

With respect to substance use, we can discern how it articulates with social apparatuses, for example, biopolitical ones, understanding these as processes that seek to guide the production of subjectivity toward strong, healthy citizens prepared to work and able to avoid distractions that would affect their physical and mental health. Substance use is out there and if we consider the social apparatuses of public health, we find that substance use is a line of subjectivation that thwarts the generation of healthy subjects. It is no coincidence that this apparatus considers any substance use to be problematic, even if it is only recreational and occasional. The same is true for schools, where more than a mere distraction, substance use becomes a barrier to learning and discipline, as well as a knowledge that hinders the performance of the social apparatus in collective terms. Thus, the assumption that all substance use has a negative effect on health and free physical development leads to discriminatory processes against users that serve as mechanisms of social isolation, stripping these subjects of social, political, cultural, and economic attributes. Discrimination is at the level of action; that is, it is the behavior that produces stereotypes and prejudices and translates into hostile and exclusionary treatment of a person or group, invalidating their practices and knowledge, in addition to ignoring the complexity and social productions of substance use.

Clearly, substance use can lead to social problems and destroyed lives. It is not our intent here to deny that reality but to consider that the universe of substance users is much more complex than the images in a government anti-drug ad. It is necessary to understand how a social apparatus is woven outside the hegemonic apparatuses from the threads of problematic use, survival, and resistance, where users stay on the edges of the extreme experience, between caring for themselves and an awareness of substance use as an extreme experience that leads to resistances, infrapolitics, and subjectivations in opposition to the capitalist societal system.

The claim by one of the interviewees that he stopped injecting because "I was already messing up my veins" reveals a relationship of knowledge about the substance and his own body, as well as his ability to avoid the abyss. Deleuze and Guattari's (2004) notion of the body without organs may be useful in understanding this. A body without organs is, for these authors, a form of desubjectivation that implies the death of a living entity. In order not to die, the body without organs is always shaping itself. It is the play between subject and subjectivation, a constant tension that allows the subject to endure the exercise of social apparatuses. The interviewee who said "Recently I'm using more… my sight goes and my mind goes blank, I start to see white" illustrates the notion of the body without organs as a process of desubjectivation, where the eyes and memory are lost, but these organs resume their function before death comes, and the body makes its way back from the extreme experience.

Understanding substance use as more than purely a public health situation implies closing our eyes to infrapolitical realities (Scott, 2004); that is, substance use also includes a dimension of resistance to hegemonic social apparatuses that do not achieve their promised results among the poorest of the population. When one of our informants says "I don't like being scolded… I like to be free," referring to his substance use, he is standing on the border of social exclusion and the institutional inclusion of confinement, which ranges from the rehabilitation center to the hospital and psychiatric hospital, to the prison. But he also expresses the possibility of creating street apparatuses, where the collective allows for survival and the management of use. There is undoubtedly a relationship between problematic use and life on the street, but it would be very risky to assume that one defines the other, especially without observing that street life generates collectives of help, care, and survival: "Well, we may be all dirty and such, but, well, we don't see each other for our appearance, it's like a bond that exists among *tecatos*."

The user's relationship with the substance is also defined by their ability to get it. "I don't have enough to be buying that shit," declares one. "I do smoke it," says another, "but not every day. With a crackhead it's almost every day; they live to smoke it." "I have always controlled myself a little more, like I have been a little more thoughtful," says a third, exemplifying how the relationship with the substance involves a class situation and defines the management of use. Among those who are not quite as poor, the pleasure of substance use is managed according to how it is felt in the body and issues of access are used as a management tool: "I can go buy it and smoke it, but I only smoke one and that's it… I don't have enough money to get addicted."

8.3 Drugs and Abandonment as a Subjectivation Apparatus at the Extreme: "Fucking Society Has Already Puked Me Up"

Reguillo (2010) warns that his category of "overflowing modernity" is not a process of homogenization, as societies have different ways of appropriating the materials of modernity. However, contemporary biopolitics, according to Esposito, is a negative, a biopolitics of life, has the mandate to "make live" one particular way and "let die" other forms of life (Moreno, 2020a, 2020b).

It is social apparatuses like the legal and health systems that decide which lives are "worthy of being lived." In this precarized narrative of life itself, guilt and responsibility are laid on the individual subject, displacing the responsibility of the institutions in such a way that individuals feel responsible for their "inability" to fit into the system.

> Already at the time of addiction and all, well, what you prefer is to be alone and keep on, so to speak, getting high, you no longer worry… the responsibility, your job and all, again at that moment I threw everything away, I lost everything, the job, my obligation, I lost the respect of society, I lost my parents, I lost everything because I isolated myself, I isolated myself from all people…" (36-year-old male, crack user)

As we have been arguing here, we have arrived at an analysis of the biopolitics and biopower of substance use (Foucault, 2002), mediating between the structures and logic of capital and cultural interpretation. We understand that biopolitics as a technology of power does not mean the suppression of other technologies (such as discipline, the panopticon, and sovereignty) but is constructed to take life as the center of domination; that is, public policy proposals, laws, orders, and a variety of other strategies are carried out based on the quality of being alive and link political power with other social agencies to exercise a governmentality that has life as its object, according to the principles of "making live" and rejection unto the death (Foucault, 2007).

We also understand that contemporary biopolitics is a biopolitics of life (Esposito, 2006b), which means that it designs policies seeking to promote a single form of life, and is exacerbated by the current neoliberal impulse in capitalism that presents itself as capable of turning anything, even life, into a commodity. Neoliberal biopolitics, if the trope is allowed, insofar as it appeals to rationality, knowledge, and science as an instrument of domination, is based on economics as the fundamental science.

The power-knowledge that emerges from this relationship is at the service of regularization and control that is exercised over individuals, or to be more precise, over the bodies that must be disciplined (Foucault, 2002). In this sense, if the scientific knowledge of medicine is responsible for treating or curing sick subjects, in a system that includes and excludes them at the same time, in both the scientific and the political sense (Esposito, 2006a), the power-knowledge of economic science amplifies the functions of exclusion and, at the same time, of inclusion in isolating institutions that turn untamed lives into pure life (Agamben, 2003), generating economic benefits: life as a bare commodity. Here, discipline is not simply an art of distributing bodies but the use of techniques and tactics to combine forces and obtain an effective apparatus of control and extraction of profit (Foucault, 2002).

Rights, both human and political, and in equal measure the process of subjectivation, are the analytical subject of contemporary biopolitics, because this biopolitics presents the dilemma between the inclusion of the citizen and the exclusion of those without rights, of the non-citizens, who are assumed to be subjects without "a life worthy of being lived," a "bare life" (Agamben, 2003; Esposito, 2006a). That this life, in Foucauldian terms, is simply biological and serves purposes of exclusion and extermination: colonization, war, crime, madness, and mental illness, among other phenomena (Foucault, 2002). It is inscribed even more in the negative form of biopower, which uses elimination through euthanasia, eugenics, and genocide as a form of domination and of generation of profit (Esposito, 2006a). Biopolitics is incorporated in the subject, and it penetrates and objectifies bodies in order to tell them politically who they are.

> All the *tecatos* [junkies], all of us *tecatos* are a fucking disease... a plague, a thing that isn't normal, we're like those guys in the movie... the living dead, I mean the fucking zombies... I even say so about myself, I discriminate against myself... fucking addict. (38-year-old male, heroin user)

The disciplines in charge of enforcing the law, based on the principles of fields such as criminal, civil, and labor law, sanction the practices of these subjects, which are linked to delinquency, crime, idleness, and violence. Scientific power-knowledge treats them as useless lives, "lives not worthy of being lived," in the eyes both of the law and of medicine. These lives, as Foucault explains in his work on madness and the prison, are subject to the dominion of biopower, controlled through confinement in clinics and prisons (Foucault, 2002).

With the term "biopolitics," we refer to institutional care for the biological lives of individuals through the implementation of disciplinary apparatuses that render the subject an object of (political) care. "Life must be separated and enclosed in spaces of progressive desocialization that immunize it from any drift toward community" (Esposito, 2005, p. 199), because "to insure a common life, the law is forced to introduce into it something that holds it back behind itself, to render it less common, immune" (Esposito, 2005, p. 43).

The immunization in the link between young people and drugs has placed the young subject in a condition overloaded with valuations and labels that often result in de facto criminalization, and that, with substance use, reaffirms the intervention of the state and its institutions. Because of their practices and behaviors, they are said, without analysis and regardless of whether they actually have a problem with substance use, to need control and care. However, even given the notion of disease, not everyone ends up having an addiction.

It may be that problematic use of psychoactive substances (Sepúlveda et al., 2008) causes the labels to be applied in a generalized way to all users, so that they themselves are convinced that they are what they are said to be. However, not all users see themselves in that way; on the contrary, some question the political discourse that tries to define them.

> We are "addicts," we are "street kids," the *monosos* of the street. I like vice, I like vice. (22-year-old male, inhalant user)
>
> They see us as sick and say no way, why would I invest in someone who's killing himself? (26-year-old male, crack user)
>
> You'll never get cured... but it would be interesting... okay, they're sick, but the root of the disease, what is it? (25-year-old woman, crack user)

It is necessary to recognize that in the construction of the subjectivity of young substance users in contemporary societies, most subjects are controlled by their own use: they monitor themselves and are docile (Esposito, 2005). However, the apparatuses and technologies used to control, measure, and channel individuals and turn them into docile and useful subjects are found in hospitals, schools, the military, families, and churches—in the spaces where bodies are subjected, manipulated, and disciplined (Foucault, 2002).

There is no pharmaco-biological apparatus meant to turn citizens into useless subjects; it is, rather, the articulation of the pharmaco-biological relations of the subjects with other apparatuses that promote the designation of "lives not worthy of being lived." Because although substance use is just one of many forms of consumption created by modernity, in that sense consumer subjects are also consumers of drugs. We use the word "drug" here to associate a set of senses and meanings. Contemporary neoliberal societies have built a complex pharmaceutical industry to support public and private health systems.

Drugs are just another element inserted into social apparatuses to control rambunctious children, to improve the abilities of neurodivergents, to alleviate ills, and to reduce the pain of workers. But those same drugs promote problematic use. This is not the place to detail how the opioid crisis in the United States was constructed, but it is a product of the public health-medicine-pharmaceutical industrial complex, a crisis that is characteristic of capitalism in its neoliberal stage (Suárez, 2020).

According to Derrida, "*Pharmacia* (*Pharmakeia*) is also a common noun signifying the administration of the *pharmakon*, the drug: the medicine and/or poison" (1981, p. 70). In the drug or *pharmakon,* there is a dual power: relief or poisoning; the same substance heals or kills. In this sense, substance use is not a desire to narcotize the population; nor is there a conscious interest in producing mentally ill people or criminals. The interest is to separate these "disposable subjects" from the rest of the population because the interest of biopower is that healthy subjects not be contaminated (Foucault, 2002). But if the *pharmakon* is used to improve health, to "make live," one is facing the possibility of divergences in use. Derrida notes that the *pharmakon* contains both pleasure and pain: "This type of painful pleasure, linked as much to the malady as to its treatment, is a *pharmakon* in itself. It partakes of both good and ill, of the agreeable and the disagreeable. Or rather, it is within its mass that these oppositions are able to sketch themselves out" (1981, p. 99). Relieving pain means offering relief that, in turn, provides pleasure. The analysis of substance use should include the right to relief and pleasure, even the right to painful pleasure.

Although not everyone perceives themselves with exclusionary labels or discriminates against themselves, they know that others do label them as contaminating subjects, and they resist, in the attempt to accomplish what Foucault calls making one's own life a work of art, by appealing to a political stance based on culture, elaborating oppositional forms of power both within and outside the political, on the border, in the interstices that remain between culture and civilization, in the impolitic (Esposito, 2006b). There, the subject produces oppositional values, in what Foucault calls an affirmative biopolitics, which makes no distinction between animal life and the human life that constitutes the subject: the "animalization of man" flows into the aesthetics of existence (Esposito, 2006b, quoted in Moreno, 2014, p. 80).

> They don't stop calling me a thief, a drug addict... they look at you funny... everyone stares at me, as if I were a fucking Martian. What they think of me is the worst, dude, that I'm a fucking drug addict and that guy is never going to get ahead, fucking failure... society doesn't accept you, it's never going to accept you, that's why among ourselves we understand each other... No way, fucking society has already puked me up, the truth is it has already puked me up... and people are always going to be pointing at you, people have already labeled you, for them you'll always be a drug addict. (32-year-old male, crack user)

When Michel Foucault says in his interview with Paul Rabinow, "I believe that from the idea that the self is not given to us, we can only extract a practical consequence: we must constitute ourselves, manufacture ourselves, order ourselves as a work of art" (Rabinow, 1984), he puts into play the idea of apparatuses producing subjectivity (the self is not given to us), to the extent that the subject is always in the process of subjectivation and is therefore always in a position to give itself a lifestyle, a unique form of life, as a work of art (we must constitute ourselves, manufacture ourselves, order ourselves as a work of art). In art, the form is not necessarily beautiful, but in the uncanny (Freud, 1990), there is an aesthetics that opposes the idea of a unique form of life. The use of the *pharmakon* carries the possibility of living that extreme experience between pain and pleasure, and perhaps it is time to think about substance use from the perspective of the right to pleasure and allowing oneself a unique form of life.

8.4 Final Considerations

We reiterate that our intention is not to analyze substance use as a desirable situation, but we distance ourselves from the idea of thinking about it from the perspective of disease, criminalization, and decitizenship. We seek to understand substance use as a constant of human development that fosters diverse forms of life, linking social, cultural, and economic productions at a distance from the violence and death that today embodies the global economy of drugs, both licit and illicit. The testimonies presented here are from people who have been stigmatized, excluded to the extent that they do not feel they "fit into society," who say: "I do not feel accepted, I feel rejected." Their relationships with substances are diverse, and there are care and management processes that allow them the "painful pleasure" involved in the use of the *pharmakon*.

We hear the voices of people in extreme situations, nomads on the edge implied by the extreme experience of problematic substance use and the social exclusion into which they are thrown: "I lost the respect of the society, I lost my parents, I lost everything because I isolated myself, I isolated myself from everyone." But it is impossible to ignore the awareness regarding their situation and the acceptance of the relationships they establish with their peers and the rest of society ("all of us *tecatos* are a fucking disease... a plague, a thing that isn't normal"), but from that position there is also the creation of other forms of life ("that's why we understand each other"), forms of life that must be treated from a position of inclusion (medical and psychiatric), and that treats them with dignity and respect for their rights.

When we talk about a way of life, we are thinking about the idea of a biopolitics for life like that of Roberto Esposito, a biopolitics that, rather than defining how life should be, contributes to the proliferation of ways of life, that promotes human diversity and confers dignity on divergences, even on those ways of life that are supposedly deviant. In this way, we assume that substance use must be understood from the dichotomy of its *pharmakon* etymology. That is, it entails the double meanings of relief and damage, cure and death, pain and pleasure. Thinking about substance use with the idea that there is a right to pleasure would allow effective treatments that avoid death and violence.

References

Agamben, G. (2003). *Homo sacer. El poder soberano y la nuda vida*. Edit. Pre-Textos.

Agamben, G. (2014). *Qué es un dispositivo. Seguido de El amigo y La Iglesia y el Reino*. Adriana Hidalgo editora.

Bauman, Z. (2000). *Trabajo, consumismo y nuevos pobres*. Gedisa.

Castells, M. (1999). *Fin de Milenio*. México.

De Oliveira, L. G., & Nappo, S. A. (2008). Characterization of the crack cocaine culture in the city of São Paulo: A controlled pattern of use. *Revista de Saude Publica, 42*(4), 664–671.

Deleuze, G. (1989). ¿Qué es un dispositivo? In *Michel Foucault, filósofo* (pp. 155–163). Gedisa.

Deleuze, G., & Guattari, F. (2004). *Mil mesetas. Capitalismo y esquizofrenia*. Pre-Textos.

Derrida, J. (1981). Plato's pharmacy. In *Dissemination*. University of Chicago Press.

Domínguez, M. J., Ortiz, A., Ramírez, I., & Palomares, G. (2019). Monas, charcos y mamilas: de la inhalación a la venta del activo en "niños de la calle". In H. C. Moreno & M. Urteaga (Eds.), *Juventud, Trabajo y Narcotráfico. Inserción laboral de los jóvenes en organizaciones delincuenciales* (pp. 227–246). Benemerita Universidad Autonoma De Puebla.

Esposito, R. (2005). *Immunitas. Protección y negación de la vida*. Amorrortu.

Esposito, R. (2006a). *Bíos. Biopolítica y filosofía*. Amorrortu.

Esposito, R. (2006b). *Categorías de lo impolítico*. Buenos Aires.

Esposito, R. (2007). *Communitas. Origen y destino de la comunidad*. Amorrortu.

Fleiz, C., Domínguez, M., Villatoro, J. A., Vazquez, F., Zafra, E., Sánchez, R., Resendiz, E., Bustos, M., & Medina, M. E. (2019). *Cuqueando la chiva: contextos del consumo de heroína en la frontera norte de México*. INPRFM.

Foucault, M. (2007). *Historia de la sexualidad. 1 La voluntad de saber, México*. Siglo XXI Editores.

Foucault, M. (2002). *Vigilar y castigar*. México.

Freud, S. (1990). Lo ominoso. In *Obras Completas* (Vol. XVII). Amorrortu.

German, D., & Sterk, C. E. (2002). Looking beyond stereotypes: Exploring variations among crack smokers. *Journal of Psychoactive Drugs, 34*(4), 383–392.

Giddens, A. (1993). *Consecuencias de la modernidad*. 1a. edición en Alianza.

Han, B.-C. (2012). *La sociedad del cansancio*. Herder.

Moreno, H. (2013). Sociedad y comunidad, vida e inmunidad. *La sociedad política en Roberto Esposito, Metapolítica*, núm. 80, enero- marzo: 38–49. www.metapolitica.com.mx

Moreno, H. (2014). Vida común o vida en común. La biopolítica y el sujeto. *Roberto Esposito, Metapolítica*. núm. 86, julio-septiembre: 77–86. www.metapolitica.com.mx

Moreno, H. (2020a). Entre la tanatopolítica y la necropolítica. In A. Fuentes Díaz & F. J. Cortazar Rodríguez (Eds.), *Vidas en vilo. Marcos necropolíticos para pensar las violencias actuales* (pp. 63–94). Universidad de Guadalajara, Centro Universitario De Los Lagos.

Moreno, H. (2020b). Biopolítica, tanatopolítica y necropolítica. In I. Covarrubias (Ed.), *Democracia, derecho y biopolítica. Problemas y desafíos de la vida en común* (pp. 233–276). Gedisa/Universidad Autónoma de Querétaro.

Rabinow, P. (1984). Michel Foucault: "El sexo es aburrido". En el Pais. https://elpais.com/diario/1984/06/27/cultura/457135204_850215.html?event=go&event_log=go&prod=REGCRARTMX&o=cerradomx

Ortiz, A., Domínguez, M. J., & Palomares, G. (2015). El consumo de disolventes inhalables en la festividad de San Judas Tadeo. *Salud Mental, 38*(6), 433–439.

Ortiz, A., Domínguez, M., Palomares, G., & Medina-Mora, M. E. (2017). Activo distribution and paraphernalia among "street children". *Salud Mental, 40*(4), 165–170.

Reguillo, R. (2010). Los jóvenes en México. (Coord.), Fondo de Cultura Económica, Consejo Nacional para la Cultura y las Artes. México. 2012 *Formas políticas del desencanto*. Siglo XXI editores.

Sepúlveda, M. (1997). El silencio de los angusitados. In M. Hopenhayn (Ed.), *La grieta de las drogas: desintegración social y políticas públicas en América Latina* (pp. 103–112). Naciones Unidas. Comisión Económica para América Latina y el Caribe. CEPAL.

Sepúlveda, M., Báez, F., & Montenegro, M. (2008). *No en la puerta de mi casa* (Implantación no conflictiva de dispositivos de drogodependencias). Grup Igia.

Scott, J. (2004). *Los dominados y el arte de la resistencia*. Discursos ocultos. Ediciones Era.

Suárez, S. (2020). *Crisis de opioides en Estados Unidos*. Universidad de La Laguna.

Valdez, A., Kaplan, C., Nowotny, K. M., Natera-Rey, G., & Cepeda, A. (2015). Emerging patterns of crack use in Mexico City. *International Journal of Drug Policy, 26*(8), 739–745.

Zamudio, A., & Carlos, A. (2009). Los Perico: un ejemplo de cómo las familias se vinculan al negocio del comercio de drogas al menudeo. In *Revista Sociedad y Economía, núm. 16, enero, 2009* (pp. 123–137). Universidad del Valle Cali.

Chapter 9
Stigma, Discrimination, and Substance Use: An Intersectionality-Based Approach

Jazmín Mora-Rios, Marcela Tiburcio, and Adán Aranda

9.1 Introduction

The aim of this study is to draw on the theoretical approach based on intersectionality to achieve a greater understanding of the complexity of addiction in low- and middle-income regions. Mexico, like Latin American countries such as Brazil, Colombia, Argentina, and Peru, is characterized by deep social inequalities. To this end, we provide a review of the research that has adopted intersectionality in the approach to addiction and refer to our own research findings as part of a previously published mixed methods study (Mora-Rios et al., 2017) on stigma and discrimination in different groups (users, relatives, health personnel, and the general population). For the purposes of this study, we refer only to persons with lived experience in addiction, as well as health personnel working in this field.

Addictions are a growing problem globally and have increased the global burden of mental and addictive disorders associated with high levels of mortality and chronic disease. It is estimated that around 284 million people aged 15–64 used drugs worldwide in 2020, a 26% increase over the previous decade (UNODC, 2022).

J. Mora-Rios (✉)
Direction of Epidemiological and Psychosocial Research. Ramón de la Fuente Muñiz National Institute of Psychiatry, Mexico City, Mexico
e-mail: morarj@inprf.gob.mx

M. Tiburcio
Department of Social Sciences in Health, Ramón de la Fuente Muñiz National Institute of Psychiatry, Mexico City, Mexico
e-mail: tibsam@inprf.gob.mx

A. Aranda
Faculty of Psychology, National Autonomous University of Mexico, UNAM, Mexico City, Mexico

T. Mota Ronzani (ed.), *Social Stigma and Drug Use*,
https://doi.org/10.1007/978-3-031-94813-8_9

The stigma associated with substance use interferes with the timely search for care. Kohn et al. (2018) revealed that the gap for the treatment of substance use disorders is greater in Latin America (83.7%) than in North America (69.1%). Moreover, it is possible that in low-and middle-income countries, the magnitude of this problem is underestimated due to the limited research on stigma (Rehm & Shields, 2019).

Stigma is a concept proposed by sociologist Erving Goffman (1963) to designate the social rejection a person experiences because of a condition that discredits them socially. The process of stigmatization, according to sociologists Link and Phelan (2001), has to do with an asymmetric power process from which an anomalous identity is constructed from the interaction between stigmatizers and stigmatized. This process includes labeling, attributing beliefs and assigning stereotypes, and a separation between subjects into "them" versus "us," which implies a loss of status of the stigmatized subject and can contribute to discrimination. For the purposes of this analysis, we consider the definition of stigma proposed by Medina-Perucha et al. (2019): the "social process that involves the segregation of groups and social individuals based on socially valued attributes, and that result in inequities based on social, political, or economic power" (p. 316).

Research on stigma and addiction has gained great interest in recent years (Commission on Narcotic Drugs, 2022; UNODC, 2022). In a comprehensive review, Yang et al. (2017) identified 2,386 articles on stigma and addiction published through August 2016, originating from the United States and various European countries, including the United Kingdom. However, despite advances in the field, myths and stereotypes persist related to irresponsibility, lack of control, and criminality attributed to people who use substances. These are deeply rooted in the general population and are expressed in fear, rejection, avoidance, denial of rights, discrimination, loss of opportunities and timely access to adequate care, which has additional negative effects on the stigmatized person, limiting their activities and restricting their participation in social life.

This persistence was shown in one study that was carried out in different European countries in the 1990s and 2020s, which found that stigmatizing attitudes toward people who use substances continued to predominate (Kilian et al., 2021). In Latin America, addiction tends to generate greater social rejection from the general population than other mental health-related problems, as has been documented in countries such as Brazil, Chile, and Mexico (Mora-Rios et al., 2017; Sapag et al., 2022).

In Mexico, data generated in national surveys on substance use identified an increase in the negative attitudes of the general population toward those who used drugs in 2016 than in those who used them in 2011 (Bustos-Gamiño et al., 2022). There was an estimated 26% increase in substance use in 2010–20, mainly of cannabis and amphetamines, with only one in 11 users requiring treatment. Of those who seek treatment, it is estimated that 85% are men. The average age of onset of use of any psychoactive substance is 13.6 years, and there is an approximate delay of 11.5 years from the beginning of experimentation to seeking help related to use (CONADIC, 2021).

Within this complex reality, the social stigma faced by people with substance use disorders intersects with other manifestations of discrimination and inequality. This stigma, seen from the perspective of intersectionality, could reveal patterns of exclusion and discrimination that are essential to understand and address the problem.

9.2 Concept of Intersectionality

Intersectionality has a long history, but it has been popularized by the work of Crenshaw (1989). Its origins come from Black feminist thought and the activism of women of color. Hankivsky (2012) took up the concept to account for its scope in understanding different social phenomena, as it allows for the analysis of the simultaneous interaction of various social factors at different levels.

Intersectionality is an analytical tool that refers to the interconnection of sociopolitical categories that contribute to discrimination in different areas, including ethnicity, gender, migration status, social class, and age. These categories overlap and generate a synergistic effect. For Grzanka (2020), intersectionality "is the study and critique of how multiple social systems intersect in producing and sustaining complex inequities" (p. 453), with an emphasis on the role of justice. In this sense, the approach is useful for addressing addiction, as it is a public health problem closely linked to processes of globalization, with production and marketing networks at a global level, that involve other social determinants based on social inequality, power structures, and gender, as well as ideological, political, and cultural aspects of drugs.

From the perspective of intersectionality, it is essential to include structural and institutional discrimination in the analysis, which refers to the set of norms, policies, and procedures of public and private entities that deliberately restrict the rights and opportunities of people with mental disorders, legitimize power differences, and reproduce inequities and social exclusion (Link & Phelan, 2001). It is also vital to include the dimension of power. Mental health care has been marginalized from public policy and is reproduced in institutions, including health care institutions. An example of this marginalization is the lack of resources and care strategies allocated to the care for people with mental health problems and addictions. According to national and international estimates, resources for mental health, in addition to being insufficient, are distributed inequitably and are used inefficiently; despite the availability of treatments, only a minority of people with substance use problems receive attention.

In an interesting review of these topics, Meyers et al. (2021) argue that intersectional stigma is multidimensional, as it involves various forms of oppression, including racism, xenophobia, and stigmatization of substance use. It is also multilevel, as it operates on individual, interpersonal, and community levels, and it is multidirectional, because it involves reciprocal influence among these levels. This approach allows for the highlighting of qualitative differences within the stigmatized group at the interpersonal level that generate unique experiences. The relational

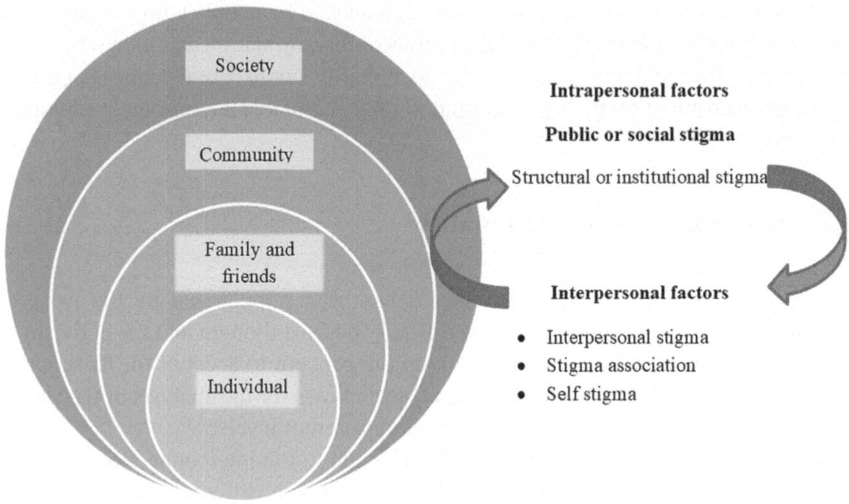

Fig. 9.1 Influence between the interpersonal and individual levels of stigma

conceptualization approach incorporates mutual influence, gender diversity, and individual and contextual conditions that participate in exclusion processes. It also takes into account significant aspects of culture in Latin America that cannot be isolated from the health conditions of the population.

Figure 9.1 illustrates the process of stigmatization. The norms, values, stereotypes, and prejudices that are expressed through discriminatory behaviors are part of a shared knowledge that is learned and legitimized by different social institutions. This requires consideration of the mutual influence between individual and macro-social factors that shape the exclusion processes directed at different social groups. However, this knowledge is not static, so interpersonal contact and the active participation of people, groups, and institutions are fundamental to the generation of new forms of knowledge and the approach to social phenomena.

9.3 Intersectionality and the Social Stigma of People Who Use Substances

From an intersectional perspective, it is possible to understand how social stigmatization of people who use substances interacts with phenomena such as racism and sexism. Various studies have documented that people who use substances who belong to specific sexual diversity and ethnic groups tend to be treated inequitably (Kulesza et al., 2016; Lipperman-Kreda et al., 2020; Nelson, 2021). For example, it is more likely that an Indigenous, Black, or Hispanic person with addictions will be sent to jail rather than to a health care institution for treatment.

Various social groups participate in the stigmatization of people who use substances. For example, the media often present more sympathetic narratives of opioid use in the white population, in contrast to the criminalization of people of color, who are described as transgressors, irresponsible, and immoral. This leads to difficulties in entering the labor market except with precarious jobs and low wages, and it promotes hatred and rejection of these people (Kulesza et al., 2016).

Gunn et al. (2018) explore the impact of stigma on drug users, particularly from family and partners, and find that women with a history of substance use, imprisonment, or behaviors associated with addiction are subject to multiple forms of discrimination. These authors address the intersection of various stigmatizing factors in the lives of women who have been incarcerated and have a history of substance use.

English et al. (2018) examine a group of Black. Latino, and multiracial men of diverse sexual identities, who have historically been the object of stigma and discrimination. Their interest was to explore the intersection of race, sexual orientation, and stigma and its relationship to substance use in these men. A principal finding was that racial discrimination was associated with difficulties for emotional regulation in those who had been victims of attacks and hate crimes.

In a systematic review of qualitative studies on the subject, Meyers et al. (2021) suggest that a qualitative intersectional approach considering stigmatized identities is most appropriate for the analysis of complex issues such as substance use and gender, and that these identities affect the health and well-being of people who use substances. However, quantitative studies found no evidence of the impact of gender on stigmatization, so the measurements used to address these issues may not account for the complexity of stigmatization processes. However, qualitative studies have documented that women using substances report double or triple conditions of exclusion, due to cultural expectations that are linked to their gender expectation as caregivers. Women who use drugs are considered transgressors, evil, selfish, and promiscuous (Meyers et al., 2021; Walters et al., 2023). The physical, emotional, economic, and sexual violence to which these women are subjected could be naturalized, seen as a kind of punishment or consequence for not fulfilling their assigned role (Lozano-Verduzco et al., 2016, Mora-Ríos et al., 2017: Gunn et al., 2018). In addition to the social and cultural difficulties they face, these women also experience discrimination within the health care system. Health care providers reproduce these stereotypes, giving priority to their other health problems, which negatively affects their health and well-being (Meyers et al., 2021).

Along the same lines, Kelly et al. (2021) found a marked relationship between substance use disorder and suicide risk in people with diverse sexual orientations and in specific ethnic groups (Hispanics, Blacks), in comparison with white heterosexual adults. The suicide risk was higher in Black and Hispanic women. Finally, a qualitative study (Ghasemi et al., 2021) found that stigmatization and discrimination against Afghan immigrants were related to the gender and migratory status of the informants, which accentuated the inequality experienced by people who use substances and prevented them from accessing treatment.

9.4 Intersectionality, Stigma, and Substance Abuse in Latin America

In Mexico, a number of authors have proposed intersectional analyses of addiction. Núñez (2019) critiques regulatory and prohibitionist frameworks that have criminalized drug use and advocates instead for public policies that consider intersectionality and a perspective of gender and other identities. In a narrative review, Torres-Lorenzo et al. (2022) highlight the importance of including intersectionality and a gender perspective in addressing violence and substance use in women.

In a mixed methods study we carried out in Mexico City (Mora-Rios et al., 2017), we inquired about the experiences of stigma and discrimination related to the use and abuse of substances from the perspective of people with substance use disorder, family members, and health providers. All informants diagnosed with substance abuse disorder reported being the object of stigma and discriminatory practices as a result of their use at some point in their lives, primarily by their families and health personnel, and consisting mainly of criticism, hostile attitudes, and blame for their use. Discriminatory practices were described in unregulated self-help groups (AA), mainly physical and verbal aggression. Family members expressed feelings of guilt, shame, anger, helplessness, and hopelessness, so they preferred to isolate themselves or avoid meetings, anticipating rejection. Health care providers, in addition to recognizing stigma as a problem present in all types of care services, mentioned providers' lack of training in addiction and mental health issues and the apathy of mental health institutions, as well as the lack of recognition of health care personnel working in this area.

9.5 Social Context, Vulnerability, and Emerging Problems

Migrants as a group face particular conditions of vulnerability is. Mexico has a significant flow of migrants, both of citizens and foreigners traveling to the United States in search of better living conditions. Substance use is an additional problem among this population during its journey to the United States. Migrants also face unemployment, discrimination, insecurity, poverty, social isolation, separation from family networks, and exploitation, which further complicate their situation.

Opioid use is an emerging problem in the states close to Mexico's border with the United States. Many of the people affected are Central American and African migrants deported by the United States, some of them born with withdrawal syndrome because their mothers used drugs during pregnancy. These people, in their conditions of vulnerability, are captured by groups dedicated to trafficking in substances including opioids, methamphetamine, and fentanyl. They lack resources, are in poor health conditions, and lack access to care services. Other no less important challenges are faced by older adults, victims of violence by crime, and terrorism and forced displacements by drug traffickers.

As part of the effort to eradicate stigma and discrimination with respect to addiction, it is necessary to implement a different paradigm, one that is dialogical, due to the complexity of the phenomenon. It must involve different social groups, people who use substances, family members, health personnel, decision makers, and civil society, all of whose testimonies and experiences are key to modifying attitudes toward people who use substances.

While in the traditional paradigm efforts are focused on reducing stigma by improving accessibility to care services, a new paradigm should be oriented toward recovery, agency, and inclusion. It should fight for access to minimum supports, such as housing, employment, and care services. This is one of the main challenges in reducing stigma toward people who use substances: to have clean, adequate facilities, so as not to perpetuate the idea that these facilities are designed for punishment. In Latin America, community interventions are increasingly being carried out to address stigma, using participatory strategies which have given good results, but it is necessary to evaluate the impact of these interventions, and such evaluation remains a challenge.

As for health care professionals, it is necessary to provide additional training and support, as they are limited in their work by a lack of resources and a burden of administrative activities that interfere with patient care. It is essential to establish a commitment with the main actors involved in the health care process. Political will is required, adopting a more comprehensive vision that includes mental health and addiction as a key focus of the well-being of the population, to face the complexity of the problems linked to the care process. It must be part of a broader social commitment, with an inclusive and open view of the sociocultural diversity of the population and a more human approach.

9.6 Final Considerations

In this study, an intersectionality paradigm allows us to understand in a more complete and nuanced way the experiences of people who use substances. Intersectionality refers to the dynamic relationship between social determinants, the subject, and their context. In this sense, it alludes to the presence of multiple conditions that seriously affect people, generating their social exclusion, and that are part of their social context.

Stigma is a significant source of stress and social disadvantage for people who use substances, and it has a significant effect on their well-being. It represents an additional burden that intersects with other conditions, creating double and triple disadvantages. Studies show that there are certain vulnerable groups, especially women, who are exposed to violence when they transgress the gender expectation that they be caregivers. However, it is essential to investigate more fully the resources of this population in facing adversity, and to assume a more reflective and critical positioning to address the questions of stigma and discrimination in the defense of their rights. It is necessary to go beyond centering the problem on blaming people who use substances and their families, who are the ones who suffer directly the consequences of substance abuse (Orford et al., 2005).

In low- and middle-income countries, it is essential to expand research on addictions from an intersectional perspective to influence the development of public policy that assumes a greater commitment to the care of the most vulnerable parts of the population, to make their needs visible, and to implement specific culturally relevant actions that contribute to social inclusion.

References

Bustos-Gamiño, M., Mora-Ríos, J., Villatoro-Velázquez, J. A., Fleiz-Bautista, C., Molina-López, A., & Medina-Mora, M. E. (2022). Changes in attitudes toward people with substance use disorder: A comparative study of the general population in Mexico. *International Journal of Environmental Research and Public Health, 19*(14), 8538. https://doi.org/10.3390/ijerph19148538

Comisión Nacional Contra las Adicciones (CONADIC). (2021). *Informe sobre la salud mental y el consumo de sustancias psicoactivas en México*. México.

Commission on Narcotic Drugs. (2022, March 14–18). *Summary of the discussions of the informal technical consultation on promoting non-stigmatizing attitudes to ensure the availability of, access to and delivery of health, care and social services for drug users, 14–16 January 2020, Vienna, Austria. Sixty-fifth session*. Vienna.

Crenshaw, K. (1989). Demarginalizing the intersection of race and sex: A black feminist critique of antidiscrimination doctrine, feminist theory and antiracist politics. *University of Chicago Legal Forum, 1989*(1), 139–167.

English, D., Rendina, H. J., & Parsons, J. T. (2018). The effects of intersecting stigma: A longitudinal examination of minority stress, mental health, and substance use among Black, Latino, and multiracial gay and bisexual men. *Psychology of Violence, 8*(6), 669–679. https://doi.org/10.1037/vio0000218

Ghasemi, E., Rajabi, F., Negarandeh, R., Vedadhir, A., & Majdzadeh, R. (2021). HIV, migration, gender, and drug addiction: A qualitative study of intersectional stigma towards Afghan immigrants in Iran. *Health & Social Care in the Community, 30*(5). https://doi.org/10.1111/hsc.13622

Goffman, E. (1963). *Stigma: Notes on the management of spoiled identity*. Prentice-Hall.

Grzanka, P. R., Flores, M. J., VanDaalen, R. A., & Velez, G. (2020). Intersectionality in psychology: Translational science for social justice. *Translational Issues in Psychological Science, 6*(4), 304–313. https://doi.org/10.1037/tps0000276

Gunn, A. J., Sacks, T. K., & Jemal, A. (2018). "That's not me anymore": Resistance strategies for managing intersectional stigmas for women with substance use and incarceration histories. *Qualitative Social Work, 17*(4), 490–508. https://doi.org/10.1177/1473325016680282

Hankivsky, O. (2012). Women's health, men's health, and gender and health: Implications of intersectionality. *Social Science & Medicine, 74*(11), 1712–1720. https://doi.org/10.1016/j.socscimed.2011.11.029

Kelly, L. M., Shepherd, B. R., & Becker, S. J. (2021). Elevated risk of substance use disorder and suicidal ideation among Black and Hispanic lesbian, gay, and bisexual adults. *Drug and Alcohol Dependence, 226*, 108848. https://doi.org/10.1016/j.drugalcdep.2021.108848

Kilian, C., Manthey, J., Carr, S., Hanschmidt, F., Rehm, J., Speerforck, S., & Schomerus, G. (2021). Stigmatization of people with alcohol use disorders: An updated systematic review of population studies. *Alcoholism: Clinical and Experimental Research, 45*(5), 899–911. https://doi.org/10.1111/acer.14598

Kohn, R., Ali, A. A., Puac-Polanco, V., Figueroa, C., Lopez-Soto, V. A., Morgan, K., Saldivia, S., & Vicente, B. (2018). Mental health in the Americas: An overview of the treatment gap. *Revista Panamericana de Salud Pública, 42*. https://doi.org/10.26633/rpsp.2018.165

Kulesza, M., Matsuda, M., Ramirez, J. J., Werntz, A. J., Teachman, B. A., & Lindgren, K. P. (2016). Towards greater understanding of addiction stigma: Intersectionality with race/ethnicity and gender. *Drug and Alcohol Dependence, 169*, 85–91. https://doi.org/10.1016/j.drugalcdep.2016.10.020

Link, B. G., & Phelan, J. C. (2001). Conceptualizing stigma. *Annual Review of Sociology, 27*, 363–385. https://doi.org/10.1146/annurev.soc.27.1.363

Lipperman-Kreda, S., Wilson, A. F., Hunt, G., Annechino, R., & Antin, T. M. J. (2020). Substance use among sexual and gender minorities: Association with police discrimination and police mistrust. *Sexuality, Gender & Policy, 3*(2), 92–104. https://doi.org/10.1002/sgp2.12019

Lozano-Verduzco, I., Romero-Mendoza, M., & Marín-Navarrete, R. (2016). Violence narratives of Mexican women treated in mutual-aid residential centers for addiction treatment. *Substance Abuse Treatment, Prevention, and Policy, 11*(1). https://doi.org/10.1186/s13011-016-0083-0

Medina-Perucha, L., Scott, J., Chapman, S., Barnett, J., & Dack, C. (2019). A qualitative study on intersectional stigma and sexual health among women on opioid substitution treatment in England: Implications for research, policy, and practice. *Social Science & Medicine, 222*, 315–322. https://doi.org/10.1016/j.socscimed.2019.01.022

Meyers, S. A., Earnshaw, V. A., D'Ambrosio, B., Courchesne, N. S., Werb, D., & Smith, L. C. (2021). The intersection of gender and drug use-related stigma: A mixed methods systematic review and synthesis of the literature. *Drug and Alcohol Dependence, 223*, 108706. https://doi.org/10.1016/j.drugalcdep.2021.108706

Mora-Ríos, J., Ortega-Ortega, M., & Medina-Mora, M. E. (2017). Addiction-related stigma and discrimination: A qualitative study in treatment centers in Mexico City. *Substance Use & Misuse, 52*(5), 594–603. https://doi.org/10.1080/10826084.2016.1245744

Nelson, E. E. (2021). Intersectional analysis of cannabis use, stigma, and health among marginalized Nigerian women. *Sociology of Health & Illness, 43*(3), 660–677. https://doi.org/10.1111/1467-9566.13244

Nuñez, C. (2019). Género y toxicodependencia. Una mirada interseccional. *Tareas, 162*, 107–126. Recuperado de https://www.redalyc.org/journal/5350/535059263010/

Orford, J., Natera, G., Copello, A., Atkinson, C., Mora, J., Velleman, R., Crundall, I., Tiburcio, M., Templeton, L., & Walley, G. (2005). *Coping with alcohol and drug problems: The experiences of family members in three contrasting cultures*. Routledge.

Rehm, J., & Shield, K. D. (2019). Global burden of disease and the impact of mental and addictive disorders. *Current Psychiatry Reports, 21*(2). https://doi.org/10.1007/s11920-019-0997-0

Sapag, J., Traub, C., Velasco, P. M., Arratia, T., Alvarado, R., Aracena, M., Poblete, F., Villarroel, L., Bravo, P., Álvarez-Huenchulaf, C., Escalona, A. J., Vargas-Malebrán, N., Bobbili, S. J., Bustamante, I., Khenti, A., & Corrigan, P. W. (2022). Reducing stigma toward mental illness and substance use issues in primary health care in Chile: Protocol of a cluster controlled trial study. *Frontiers in Psychiatry, 13*, 1083042.

Torres-Lorenzo, A., Ayala-Ramos, G. E., Morales-Vargas, P. V., Aldwen-Cruz, K. M., Ríos-Rivera, G. D., & Rodríguez-Caraballo, D. J. (2022). Uso de sustancias en mujeres y violencia de género: Desde una perspectiva feminista e interseccional. *Sección Especial: Violencia De Género, 33*(2), 352–364. https://doi.org/10.55611/reps.3302.11

United Nations Office on Drugs and Crime. (2022). *Drug World Report 2022*. Disponible en: https://www.unodc.org/unodc/en/data-and-analysis/world-drug-report-2022.html

Walters, S. M., Kerr, J., Cano, M., Earnshaw, V., & Link, B. (2023). Intersectional stigma as a fundamental cause of health disparities: A case study of how drug use stigma intersecting with racism and xenophobia creates health inequities for Black and Hispanic persons who use drugs over time. *Stigma and Health*. Advance online publication. https://doi.org/10.1037/sah0000426

Yang, L. H., Wong, L. J., Grivel, M. M., & Hasin, D. S. (2017). Stigma and substance use disorders. *Current Opinion in Psychiatry, 30*(5), 378–388. https://doi.org/10.1097/yco.0000000000000351

Part II
Social Stigma, Gender, Family Contexts and Drug Use

Chapter 10
Stigma, Prejudice, and Media: Impact on the Care of Relatives of People Who Use Drugs

Joanna Gonçalves de Andrade Tostes-Bianchetti, Telmo Mota Ronzani, Rodrigo Goycolea Martinic, and Pollyanna Santos da Silveira

10.1 Stigma and Dependence: The Conceptual and Cultural Bases of This Relationship

The process of stigmatization has been extensively studied, both theoretically and empirically, and is commonly defined as the interplay of labeling, stereotype attribution, social separation, status loss, and discrimination, reinforced through power dynamics (Hatzenbuehler et al., 2013; Link & Phelan, 2001). In this process, individuals or groups are devalued and socially excluded due to characteristics perceived as deviant (Corrigan & Watson, 2002).

The relationship between stigma and dependence is complex and deeply rooted in conceptual frameworks and cultural perceptions. Stigma constitutes a form of social disqualification that significantly impacts identity and access to treatment (Gnanapragasam et al., 2023). Cultural perceptions shape stigma, as societal disapproval often leads to self-stigmatization among individuals with substance

J. G. de Andrade Tostes-Bianchetti
Postgraduate Program in Psychology, Universidade Federal de Juiz de Fora, Juiz de Fora, Brazil
e-mail: joanna@tostes.org

T. M. Ronzani (✉)
Department of Psychology, Universidade Federal de Juiz de Fora, Juiz de Fora, Brazil
e-mail: telmo.ronzani@ufjf.br

R. G. Martinic
Escuela de Terapia Ocupacional, Facultad de Odontología y Ciencias de la Rehabilitación, Universidad San Sebastián, Santiago, Chile
e-mail: rodrigo.goycolea@uss.cl

P. S. da Silveira
Faculty of Psychology, Universidade Católica de Petrópolis, Petrópolis, Brazil

T. Mota Ronzani (ed.), *Social Stigma and Drug Use*,
https://doi.org/10.1007/978-3-031-94813-8_10

dependence (Nearchou et al., 2024). Such cultural factors contribute to negative portrayals of people who use drugs, reinforcing stigma and hindering social reintegration (De Shalit et al., 2024; Gnanapragasam et al., 2023).

Different models of dependence influence public stigma. For example, biological explanations can attenuate stigma by framing dependence as a medical problem rather than a moral failure (Siddiqui & Rutherford, 2023). Some direct consequences of stigmatization are the development of social exclusion strategies with punishment systems or social barriers, hindering access to basic human rights. Classic examples include prejudices related to class and race, as well as the exclusion of marginalized groups, such as people labeled as "mad" or "addicts" (De Shalit et al., 2024; Ronzani et al., 2016).

Stigma in healthcare settings exacerbates global health inequities, crossing economic, social, and cultural borders (Monteiro & Villela, 2013). In this field, many individuals who would benefit from available treatments, improving symptoms and disabilities, refrain from seeking help or discontinue treatment prematurely due to the anticipated social consequences (Ronzani, 2018). Among the elements that can explain this low participation in mental health programs, perhaps the most important are the effects on the social environment (Ronzani, 2018). Thus, if on the one hand the condition of deviant social status of drug users can serve to discourage use, on the other hand, stigmatization can affect the health of those who use illicit drugs. Chronic exposure to stigma-related stress can worsen health outcomes or decrease the quality of care received (Ahern et al., 2007).

The consequences of stigma in its interface with health become even more worrying, considering that they are not limited to the attribution of negative characteristics to certain individuals, but rather reduce opportunities for access to information and services that offer health care, enabling a more dignified life, and end up further increasing health disparities (Ferreira et al., 2014; Ronzani & Furtado, 2010). In addition, studies have identified among those who internalize stigma, feelings of guilt, hopelessness, distress, self-reproach, and depression. These variables, in turn, are pointed out as associated with a more restricted social network, anticipation of rejection in social situations and the resulting social isolation, including unemployment (Tsang et al., 2010; Vauth et al., 2007).

10.2 Social Determinants, Stigma, and Drug Use

The interaction between social determinants, stigma, and drug use is complex and multifaceted. Social determinants, such as socioeconomic status, education, and mental health significantly influence drug use behavior and attitudes toward dependence. Stigma exacerbates these challenges, leading to discrimination and restricted access to treatment. Fundamental factors such as housing, employment, and education shape individuals' mental health and substance use patterns (Gnanapragasam et al., 2023).

Health disparities are defined as the differences between the health profiles of subgroups of the population, encompassing outcomes on physical and mental health. These disparities range from self-perceived health status to mortality rates, from psychological well-being to severe mental disorders (Hatzenbuehler et al., 2013). However, there needs to be a deeper understanding to overcome descriptive and depoliticized discourses, considering that the differences between these health profiles may not have any relation to social injustice, but they can also highlight it in a pronounced way (Ronzani et al., 2023). The hegemonic medical model often reinforces medicalization as a universal solution while obscuring the ideological and social control mechanisms that regulate behaviors and disorders (Delgado & Imedio, 2011).

It is undeniable that changing the macrosocial structures in health in short periods of time is unfeasible, especially when it needs to be carried out in conjunction with actions from various other sectors. However, incremental strategies must be developed to facilitate communication between healthcare providers and users, as well as to create spaces to sensitize and train health professionals. It is necessary to discuss stigma and its impact on production, maintenance, and confrontation of social inequalities and health inequities (Massignam et al., 2015).

Monteiro and Villela (2013) suggest that the specific contexts in which stigma operates are linked to its greater or lesser success. When more egalitarian interpersonal relationships are established in these contexts, there is a tendency for the production and diffusion of stigma to be less expressive and, therefore, significant improvements can be obtained in health promotion strategies and in reducing disparities. Implicit biases show that people who inject drugs, especially those from ethnic minority origins, are more likely to be associated as deserving of punishment and not help, indicating the presence of implicit beliefs related to the stigma of dependence (Kulesza et al., 2016).

From this understanding, the sphere of care should include understanding the history of substance use and the relationship between individuals and groups inserted in a certain sociocultural context. Drug use is analyzed within an interaction between drug–individual–environment, capable of giving real meaning to the problems related to this consumption (Ronzani, 2018). Although drug use is present in various social classes and in different contexts, some determinants increase the social or disease burden in relation to this use. That is, there is not a simple and direct cause and effect relationship. Some of these social determinants already related to drug use in the literature are poverty, race, gender, unemployment, housing, education, malnutrition, among others (Ronzani et al., 2023). Understanding these determinants allows us to glimpse the social vulnerability of substance consumption, in order to optimize the planning of actions and care for users (McCormack et al., 2015; Ronzani et al., 2023).

Although social determinants play a fundamental role in influencing drug use, stigma remains a significant barrier to effective treatment and support. Addressing these interrelated issues requires comprehensive public health and education strategies to reduce stigma and improve access to care.

10.3 Stigma and Health Care

Studies conducted around the world have pointed out that the stigma related to substance use disorders is intense, but it is still necessary to know more about its underlying processes. To minimize the impacts of stigma, a deeper view from different perspectives on the problem must be achieved, including the general population, general health professionals and specialized services, and drug users in treatment (van Boekel, 2015; Tostes et al., 2020b).

Regarding specifically the social reintegration of people with mental disorders, in general, the community surrounding mental health services plays a fundamental role in its success or failure. The stigma toward users of these services, especially when it comes from neighborhood residents, hinders users' adherence to treatment and compromises the resumption of daily activities, important for their clinical improvement and social reintegration (Thornicroft et al., 2016; Tostes et al., 2020a).

According to the literature review conducted by van Boekel (2015), more conservative doctors and nurses expressed more negative attitudes toward their patients who use injectable drugs, because they believe in the controllability of use by users. Another study, conducted with nurses, psychologists, counselors, and doctors, pointed out that there was not a collaborative relationship with drug users in treatment. The results also pointed out that beliefs and prejudices could be imposed on users, even unintentionally, ending up disempowering precisely those they should empower (Curtis & Harrison, 2001).

Despite the lack of knowledge about mental disorders being pointed out by the literature as a variable that is related to the presence of stigma, in the study by Serra et al. (2013) conducted with a large sample of university students, peculiar results were found. Having a reasonable knowledge about these disorders and being able to distinguish them contrasts with the fact that these students were skeptical about the possibility of recovery and the effectiveness of a treatment for people with these disorders. Negative attitudes of students related to mental disorders, in general, were also found in the studies by Pedrão et al. (2002) with nursing students. Specifically regarding drug addicts, the study by Sungu (2015) conducted with university students showed that attitudes were considerably negative, mainly in relation to social and family interactions.

Although some progress can be observed in relation to the fight for the health and human rights of drug users, mainly obtained by organizations in favor of these users, it is still necessary to establish and consolidate various partnerships. Some points of alliance are considered priorities, such as the improvement of the treatment offered by health professionals and the police approach, the expansion of housing alternatives, and the implementation of services aimed at harm reduction (Crabtree et al., 2016). The findings of the presence of stigma among health professionals and the need to minimize its impact gained prominence among researchers and on political agendas in recent decades, as pointed out by a recent systematic review, although low funding and the implementation of interventions lack considerable advances (Tostes et al., 2020b).

10.4 The Role of the Media in the Process of Stigmatization

The media plays a pivotal role in perpetuating and reinforcing stigma related to substance use. In Brazil, for instance, crack users are frequently depicted as dangerous, aggressive, and morally culpable for their condition (Silveira et al., 2018). Predominantly, media narratives employ moralizing and sensationalist discourses, further deepening social exclusion and stigmatization.

According to the "Agenda-Setting" theory, the media significantly influences the political agenda. Topics that receive widespread media coverage become priority in public opinion, shaping government actions. This phenomenon happens recursively, as the media influences public opinion, and public opinion influences the media. That is, to ensure its consumer market, the press is inclined to address topics considered of greater interest to the population. In addition, journalism tends to address taboo topics such as drugs avoiding the confrontation of prevailing cultural values (Brooks et al., 2023).

Studies that analyzed journalistic articles about drugs in Brazil confirmed the pattern of biased, alarmist journalistic coverage. For illegal drugs, the studies indicated that the articles analyzed highlighted the increase in consumption and the problems resulting from use and trafficking. There were a few contextual articles that addressed the different psychosocial perspectives necessary for understanding such a complex topic (Ronzani et al., 2009a, b; Felix & Vianna, 2015). On the other hand, regarding alcoholic beverages, the content of the media presents itself paradoxically. The glamorization of trade and consumption, stimulated in marketing actions, coexists with the process of stigmatization of alcohol dependence addressed by means of communication, such as journalism. The person who develops dependence then becomes a deviant who failed in their ability to control over alcohol (Ronzani et al., 2009a, b).

Regarding the problems reported in the press, proactive approaches are rarely presented or therapeutic options discussed. Often, the problems are seen as cases like "without solution" or "failed". Hospitalization is mentioned as the main form of treatment, without questioning its limitations and inadequacies for most cases. The study conducted by Mastroianni (2006), with journalists, pointed out that they admitted the low quality of the content published on the topic, presenting as justification the need for speed in writing (high productivity) and competition among communication vehicles (preference for "sensationalist" topics). In addition, some journalists considered it risky to question prevailing social values, preferring to construct their articles anchored in more accepted cultural conceptions, even if they did not find them accurate.

Despite these challenges, the media is often considered a reference for truth in Brazil. The media has a strong influence on professional practice and, consequently, on the quality of services for users, drug addicts and their families. It is essential that professionals in the field act critically towards journalism. Based on the example of the National Agency for Children's Rights—ANDI (2005), which for many years worked actively to improve journalistic coverage, similar initiatives may drive the improvement of the published material. The media can be a great ally of health and human rights, gradually minimizing the process of stigmatization, when aligned with ethical information and evidence-based health communication strategies (Silveira et al., 2018).

10.5 Stigma, Drugs, Media, and Gender Perspectives: The Impact on Family Members

The stigma around substance use and mental health significantly affects family members of users, often leading to feelings of shame, isolation, and decreased quality of life. This is an associated or courtesy stigma, which involves the way families are perceived and treated by society. The interaction between stigma, substance use, media, and gender perspectives significantly compromise the family members of individuals with substance use disorders (Jackson, 2023).

In the context of courtesy stigma, people are judged based on their association with individuals with substance use disorders or mental illness. There is a decrease in communication and an increase in shame, especially among parents of adolescents with chronic mental disorders, increasing shame and reluctance to seek treatment (Jackson, 2023). Discrimination by society exacerbates the emotional suffering faced by families, as they deal with negative perceptions and lack of understanding about mental health problems (Maldonado et al., 2023).

Similarly, gender roles can exacerbate stigma, considering that mothers are generally blamed for their children's substance use, reinforcing negative stereotypes about motherhood. Fathers can also suffer stigma, but usually in different contexts, such as social expectations of masculinity (Wilkens & Foote, 2018). Gender roles often dictate the type of support available, with mothers frequently bearing the weight of care responsibilities and facing unique challenges in accessing mental health resources (Khan et al., 2022).

Gender also proved to be a prominent variable in the systematic review conducted by Meyers et al. (2021), which explored how some factors interact to influence the experiences and treatment outcomes of individuals who use drugs. The studies showed diverse results: some found higher levels of stigma among women who used drugs compared to men (Meyers et al., 2021); others showed that there were no significant gender differences in the level of stigma. In addition, women tended to report stigma as a barrier more than men (Stringer & Baker, 2018). Possibly, this is due to facing additional barriers related to family responsibilities and mental health (Agterberg et al., 2020). Regarding drug use, for men, family support reduced the frequency of use; but daily contact increased the frequency of drug use, due to stress and demands. On the other hand, for women, the feeling of trust in the family was a hindrance to continued involvement with drug use (Zhang & Demant, 2021).

Added to this complex scenario is the existence of gender violence and depressive symptoms, which proved to be significant risk factors for substance use among transgender women, highlighting the combined effects of stigma and mental health problems (Nuttbrock et al., 2014). Social support and affirmation policies are protective factors against substance use, especially for young people from sexual and gender minorities, although they are studied less frequently (Kidd et al., 2018).

Despite the challenges in this context, there is growing recognition of the need for interventions that meet the needs of both people with drug addiction and their families, promoting resilience and recovery (Shanmugam, 2021) and understanding the role of media in this process. Stereotypical representations can perpetuate courtesy stigma, influencing public perceptions negatively and further isolating families from support networks (Khan et al., 2022; Ricci & Dixon, 2015).

Campaigns aimed at reducing stigma, such as the initiatives of the National Alliance on Mental Illness (NAMI) in the United States, highlight the importance of changing public perceptions to better support families (Ricci & Dixon, 2015). Although stigma has profound negative effects on families, some studies suggest that increasing awareness and education can mitigate these impacts by promoting resilience and support networks among affected families (Jackson, 2023; Ricci & Dixon, 2015).

10.6 Final Considerations

The literature has been showing that understanding the stigmatization process related to drug users can be of fundamental importance for political direction and the implementation of intervention strategies. If, on the one hand, people face health conditions associated with social disabilities that prevent them from performing many social roles and achieving life goals, on the other hand, social reactions to the severe forms of some conditions can be equally devastating (Pescosolido et al., 2021; Silveira et al., 2015).

Stigmatizing drug users can serve as a means of imposing social norms to establish boundaries and socially acceptable behaviors. Seen from this perspective, stigmatization could be considered a successful strategy to reduce such behaviors (Ronzani, 2018). However, moralizing strategies associated with repressive perspectives have been considered ineffective. By focusing only on the negative characteristics of the user, they end up restricting the possibilities of welcoming and accessing health services (Tostes et al., 2020b).

Stigmatizing views on drug users legitimize ineffective approaches that attribute to users the responsibility for the problems not only that they themselves face, but blame users for social problems, such as violence and social inequality. They are clear barriers to seeking treatment and work, fundamental dimensions for recovery and social reintegration. Minimizing the impact of stigma is necessary to ensure the proposition and implementation of prevention, treatment, and social reintegration strategies. Users need to be involved in the decision-making process of the treatment so that individuals' demands are considered.

The intersection between drug use, stigma, gender issues, and family dynamics is a complex area of study. Family dynamics play a crucial role, with different impacts according to gender. The language used to describe drug use and the context of initiation to drug use by the media also affect levels of stigma. Intersectionality with race/ethnicity and gender further exacerbate the stigma experienced by individuals. Addressing these issues requires a critical and gender and culture sensitive view to reduce stigma and improve treatment outcomes.

Therefore, it is essential to consider culture, contexts, and intersectionalities to develop strategies for reducing stigma in specific groups, decreasing various barriers to healthcare access, and promoting more prevention initiatives. In this sense, the way the media in general disseminates and describes drug users is strategic so that the consequences of stigma are minimized.

References

Agência Nacional dos Direitos da Infância (ANDI). (2005). *Mídia e drogas*. Cortez.

Agterberg, S., Schubert, N., Overington, L., & Corace, K. (2020). Treatment barriers among individuals with co-occurring substance use and mental health problems: Examining gender differences. *Journal of Substance Abuse Treatment, 112*, 29–35. https://doi.org/10.1016/j.jsat.2020.01.005

Ahern, J., Stuber, J., & Galea, S. (2007). Stigma, discrimination and the health of illicit drug users. *Drug and Alcohol Dependence, 88*, 188–196.

Brooks, C., Mirzoev, T., Chowdhury, D., Deuri, S. P., & Madill, A. (2023). Using evidence in mental health policy agenda-setting in low- and middle-income countries: A conceptual meta-framework from a scoping umbrella review. *Health Policy and Planning, 38*(7), 876–893. https://doi.org/10.1093/heapol/czad038

Corrigan, P. W., & Watson, A. C. (2002). The paradox of self-stigma and mental illness. *Clinical Psychology: Science and Practice, 9*, 35–53.

Crabtree, A., Latham, N., Bird, L., & Buxton, J. (2016). Results of a participatory needs assessment demonstrate an opportunity to involve people who use alcohol in drug user activism and harm reduction. *Harm Reduction Journal, 13*(37). https://doi.org/10.1186/s12954-016-0140-3

Curtis, J., & Harrison, L. (2001). Beneath the surface: Collaboration in alcohol and other drug treatment. *Journal of Advanced Nursing, 34*, 737–744. https://doi.org/10.1046/j.1365-2648.2001.01711.x

De Shalit, A., van der Meulen, E., Chu, S. K. H., & Thomas, R. (2024). Drug use stigma and reprisal: Barriers to prison needle exchange in Canada. *The Prison Journal, 104*(3), 344–364. https://doi.org/10.1177/00328855241240142

Delgado, M. J. R., & Imedio, L. R. (2011). La menopausia un ciclo de vida: Análisis comparativo de la percepción que las mulheres urbanas y rurales de la provincia de Granada tienen de su propia menopausia. In R. F. Alves (Ed.), *Psicologia da Saúde: Teoria, intervenção e pesquisa* (pp. 121–141). EDUEPB.

Felix, C. B., & Vianna, A. C. F. (2015). O preconceito e o estigma na cobertura midiática sobre drogas no Rio de Janeiro. *Contemporanea: Revista de Comunicação e Cultura (UFBA), 13*(3), 566–581. Dossiê Temático Comunicação e Direitos Humanos: políticas e cidadania no contexto. https://doi.org/10.9771/contemporanea.v13i3.14399

Ferreira, G. C. L., Silveira, P. S., Noto, A. R., & Ronzani, T. M. (2014). Implicações da relação entre estigma internalizado e suporte social para a saúde: Uma revisão sistemática da literatura. *Estudos de Psicologia, 19*(1), 1–88.

Gnanapragasam, S. N., Astill Wright, L., Pemberton, M., & Bhugra, D. (2023). Outside/inside: Social determinants of mental health. *Irish Journal of Psychological Medicine, 40*(1), 63–73. https://doi.org/10.1017/ipm.2021.49

Hatzenbuehler, M. L., Phelan, J. C., & Link, B. G. (2013). Stigma as a fundamental cause of population health inequalities. *American Journal of Public Health, 103*, 813–821.

Jackson, P. R. (2023). *7.2 The multigenerational impact of substance use disorder–related stigma and how to address it with families*. https://doi.org/10.1016/j.jaac.2023.07.166

Khan, F., Lynn, M., Porter, K., Kongnetiman, L., & Rebecca, H.-S. (2022). "There's no supports for people in addiction, but there's no supports for everyone else around them as well": A qualitative study with parents and other family members supporting youth and young adults. *The Canadian Journal of Addiction, 13*, S72–S82. https://doi.org/10.1097/CXA.0000000000000149

Kidd, J., Jackman, K., Wolff, M., Veldhuis, C., & Hughes, T. (2018). Risk and protective factors for substance use among sexual and gender minority youth: A scoping review. *Current Addiction Reports, 5*, 158–173. https://doi.org/10.1007/s40429-018-0196-9

Kulesza, M., Matsuda, M., Ramirez, J., Werntz, A., Teachman, B., & Lindgren, K. (2016). Towards greater understanding of addiction stigma: Intersectionality with race/ethnicity and gender. *Drug and Alcohol Dependence, 169*, 85–91. https://doi.org/10.1016/j.drugalcdep.2016.10.020

Link, B. G., & Phelan, J. C. (2001). Conceptualizing stigma. *Annual Review of Sociology, 27*, 363–385.

Maldonado, D. A. C., Martins, L. F., & Ronzani, T. M. (2023). Estigma de Cortesia e condições de saúde: revisão sistemática de literatura. *Psicologia em Estudo, 28*, e52111. https://doi.org/10.4025/psicolestud.v28i0.52111

Massignam, F. M., Bastos, J. L. D., & Nedel, F. B. (2015). Discriminação e saúde: Um problema de acesso. *Epidemiologia e Serviços de Saúde, 24*(3), 541–544. https://doi.org/10.5123/S1679-49742015000300009

Mastroianni, F. C. (2006). *As drogas psicotrópicas e a imprensa brasileira: Análise do material publicado e do discurso dos profissionais da área de jornalismo* (Dissertação de Mestrado). Universidade Federal de São Paulo, São Paulo, SP, Brasil.

McCormack, R. P., Hoffman, L. F., Norman, M., Goldfrank, L. R., & Norman, E. M. (2015). Voices of homeless alcoholics who frequent Bellevue Hospital: A qualitative study. *Annals of Emergency Medicine, 65*(2), 178–186. https://doi.org/10.1016/j.annemergmed.2014.07.029

Meyers, S. A., Earnshaw, V. A., D'Ambrosio, B., Courchesne, N., Werb, D., & Smith, L. R. (2021). The intersection of gender and drug use-related stigma: A mixed methods systematic review and synthesis of the literature. *Drug and Alcohol Dependence, 223*, 108706. https://doi.org/10.1016/j.drugalcdep.2021.108706

Monteiro, S., & Villela, W. (2013). Estigma E Saúde: Uma Relação Vital Em Debate (Resenha). *Cadernos de Saúde Pública, 30*(2), 439–441.

Nearchou, F., French, A., Buckley, A., Koretsidou, C., O'Gara, C., & Watchorn, A. (2024). Stigma and Alcohol Use Disorder: Insights from a qualitative study in patients, family members and health care providers. https://doi.org/10.31234/osf.io/dm7gv

Nuttbrock, L., Bockting, W., Rosenblum, A., Hwahng, S., Mason, M., Macrì, M., & Becker, J. (2014). Gender abuse, depressive symptoms, and substance use among transgender women: A 3-year prospective study. *American Journal of Public Health, 104*(11), 2199–2206.

Pedrão, L. J., Avanci, R. C., & Malaguti, S. E. (2002). Perfil das atitudes de alunos do curso de enfermagem frente à doença mental, antes da influência da instrução acadêmica, proveniente de disciplinas de área específica. *Revista Latino-Americana de Enfermagem, 10*(6), 794–799. https://doi.org/10.1590/S0104-11692002000060000

Pescosolido, B. A., Halpern-Manners, A., Luo, L., & Perry, B. (2021). Trends in Public Stigma of Mental Illness in the US, 1996-2018. *JAMA network open, 4*(12), e2140202. https://doi.org/10.1001/jamanetworkopen.2021.40202

Ricci, B., & Dixon, L. (2015). What can we do about stigma. *Psychiatric Services, 66*(10), 1009–1009. https://doi.org/10.1176/APPI.PS.661004

Ronzani, T. M. (2018). *Drugs and social context: Social perspectives on the use of alcohol and other drugs*. Springer.

Ronzani, T. M., Costa, P. H. A., Paiva, F. S., Cruvinel, É., Formagini, T. D. B., & Medeiros, A. X. (2016). A interface da vulnerabilidade abordada pela atenção básica na saúde e assistência. In Garcia F, Costa MR, Guimarães LP, Neves MCL, organizadores. *Vulnerabilidade e o Uso de Drogas* (pp. 245–262). Belo Horizonte: 3i Editora.

Ronzani, T. M., Fernandes, A. G. B., Gebara, C. F. P., Oliveira, A. S., Scoralick, N. N., & Lourenço, L. M. (2009a). Media and drugs: A documental analysis of the Brazilian writing media between 1999 and 2003. *Ciência & Saúde Coletiva, 14*(5), 1751–1761. https://doi.org/10.1590/S1413-81232009000500027

Ronzani, T. M., Furtado, E. F., & Higgins-Biddle, J. (2009b). Stigmatization of alcohol and other drug users by primary care providers in Southeast Brazil. *Social Science & Medicine, 69*(7), 1080–1084. https://doi.org/10.1016/j.socscimed.2009.07.009

Ronzani, T. M., & Furtado, E. F. (2010). Estigma social sobre o uso de álcool. *Jornal Brasileiro de Psiquiatria, 59*(4), 326–332.

Ronzani, T. M., Pereira, T. S., Castro, J. B., & Dimenstein, M. (2023). Social determinants and drug dependence: Systematic review of literature. *Psicologia: Teoria E Pesquisa, 39*, e39407. https://doi.org/10.1590/0102.3772e39407.en

Serra, M., Lai, A., Buizza, C., Pioli, R., Preti, A., Masala, C., & Petretto, D. R. (2013). Beliefs and attitudes among Italian high school students toward people with severe mental disorders. *Journal of Nervous and Mental Disease, 201*(4), 311–318. https://doi.org/10.1097/NMD.0b013e31828f1429

Shanmugam, P. K. (2021). Psychoeducation impact for family members of substance users: An evaluation the workbook "Addiction: A Family Disease". *Journal of Substance Use, 26*(2), 202–211. https://doi.org/10.1080/14659891.2020.1807632

Siddiqui, H., Rutherford, M.D. (2023). Belief that addiction is a discrete category is a stronger correlate with stigma than the belief that addiction is biologically based. *Subst Abuse Treat Prev Policy 18*, 3. https://doi.org/10.1186/s13011-022-00512-z

Silveira, P. S., Casela, A.L.M., Monteiro, E.P., Ferreira, G.C.L., Freitas, J.V.T., Machado, N.M, Costa, P. H.A., Ronzani, T.M., & Noto, A.R. (2018). Crack e Mídia: O que dizem as principais revistas jornalísticas do país?. Estudos e Pesquisas em Psicologia, 18(1), 50–71.

Silveira, P. S., Soares, R. G., Gomide, H. P., Ferreira, G. C. L., Casela, A. L. M., Martins, L. F., & Ronzani, T. M. (2015). Social distance toward people with substance dependence: A survey among health professionals. *Psicologia em Pesquisa (UFJF), 9*(2), 170–176. https://doi.org/10.5935/1678-0928.20150018

Stringer, K. L., & Baker, E. H. (2018). Stigma as a Barrier to Substance Abuse Treatment Among Those With Unmet Need: An Analysis of Parenthood and Marital Status. *Journal of family issues, 39*(1), 3–27. https://doi.org/10.1177/0192513X15581659

Sungu, H. (2015). Attitudes towards substance addiction: A study of Turkish university students. *Educational Research and Reviews, 10*(7), 1015–1022. https://doi.org/10.5897/ERR2015.2376

Thornicroft, G., Deb, T., & Henderson, C. (2016). Community mental health care worldwide: Current status and further developments. *World Psychiatry, 15*(3), 276–286. https://doi.org/10.1002/wps.20351

Tostes, J. G. A., Bandeira, M., & Oliveira, M. S. (2020a). Predictors of neighbors' attitudes toward persons with mental illness and therapeutic residential services in Brazil. *Stigma and Health, 5*(2), 138–145. https://doi.org/10.1037/sah0000178

Tostes, J. G. A., Dias, R. T., Reis, A. A. S., da Silveira, P. S., & Ronzani, T. M. (2020b). Interventions to reduce stigma related to people who use drugs: Systematic review. *Paidéia (Ribeirão Preto), 30*, e3022. https://doi.org/10.1590/1982-4327e3022

Tsang, H. W., Fung, K. M., & Chung, R. C. (2010). Self-stigma and stages of change as predictors of treatment adherence of individuals with schizophrenia. *Psychiatry Research, 180*(1), 10–15. https://doi.org/10.1016/j.psychres.2009.09.013

van Boekel, L. C. (2015). *Stigmatization of people with substance use disorders: Attitudes and perceptions of clients, healthcare professionals, and the general public.* Ipskamp Drukkers.

Vauth, R., Kleim, B., Wirtz, M., & Corrigan, P. W. (2007). Self-efficacy and empowerment as outcomes of self-stigmatizing and coping in schizophrenia. *Psychiatry Research, 150*(1), 71–80. https://doi.org/10.1016/j.psychres.2006.01.020

Wilkens, C. &, Foote, J. (2018). "Bad Parents," "Codependents," and other stigmatizing myths about substance use disorder in the family. 33–53. https://doi.org/10.1007/978-3-030-02580-9_3

Zhang, S. Y., & Demant, J. (2021). Effects of self-control, drug-use peers and family attachment on drug use among Chinese users: A gender-specific analysis. *Drug and alcohol review, 40*(7), 1369–1376. https://doi.org/10.1111/dar.13295

Chapter 11
An Analysis of Bibliographic Productions About the Use of Substances by LGBTQIA+ Youth in Brazil: Debating Stigma and Prejudice

Juliana Perucchi, Caroline Nazar Machado Cândido, Fernanda Zeloschi, Arthur de Paula Ribeiro, and Thamiris Ribeiro

11.1 Introduction

In recent international research (Evans-Polce et al., 2020) there came evidence that people from the so-called sexual and gender minorities are at greater risk of abusing alcohol and other drugs and, from this perspective, would be more exposed to developing disorders in health related to substance intake, compared to heterosexual and cisgender individuals. For at least two decades, studies have shown the discrepancy in mental health outcomes in minority groups, concerning substance use, sexual orientation and gender identity, when compared to groups of cisgender or heterosexual people (Gilman et al., 2001; Sandfort et al., 2001). And as systematic review studies point out (Plöderl & Tremblay, 2015; Coulter et al., 2019), this discrepancy has increased in recent years. In Brazil, for quite some time, there is evidence that among lesbian women, the abusive use of drugs (mainly alcohol and tobacco) is reflected in the high rate of chronic diseases among this population (Facchini & Barbosa, 2006). The relationship between stress, stigma, and chemical dependency among lesbians, gays, bisexuals, transsexuals, *queers*, intersexuals, and asexuals (LGBTQIA+) has been the target of scientific scrutiny in some theories, such as the theory of minority stress (Paveltchuk & Borsa, 2020). In this theoretical perspective, it is affirmed that the stigmatizing and stressful social environment to which LGBTQIA+ people are subjected, in many of their social relations can trigger serious mental health problems for them (Friedman, 1999; Hendricks & Testa, 2012).

The world has advanced in issues related to the rights of people to live their sexuality freely in consonance with their life perspectives and genderidentities. However, prejudice and stigma are still quite powerful in conditioning the mental health of

J. Perucchi (✉) · C. N. M. Cândido · F. Zeloschi · A. de Paula Ribeiro · T. Ribeiro
Department of Psychology, Universidade Federal de Juiz de Fora, Juiz de Fora, Brazil
e-mail: juliana.perucchi@ufjf.br

T. Mota Ronzani (ed.), *Social Stigma and Drug Use*,
https://doi.org/10.1007/978-3-031-94813-8_11

individuals and, in this sense, there is already evidence to affirm that LGBTQIA+ people present higher rates of mental health impairment when compared to heterosexual or cisgender people (Bränström et al., 2016; Pachankis & Safren, 2019; Paveltchuk & Borsa, 2020). It is also proven that this is due, among other aspects, to the social stigma related to sexual minorities. The problem is not in the fact that the person lives a non-heterosexual orientation or is not a cisgender person, but rather, in the stigma associated with the identities of lesbians, gays, bisexuals, transsexuals, transvestites, etc., as it exposes the group to social vulnerability, not their sexual orientation or their gender identity per se (Valdiserri et al., 2018; Vargas et al., 2019).

In a successful attempt to conceptualize stigma, Bruce Link and Jo Phelan (2001) revisit the propositions of Erving Goffman (1975) as a starting point of their conceptual reflection and, once returning to this author, they attribute to him a pertinent focus, prioritizing the relationship between stereotype and attribute as sources that enable the conditions of materiality for stigma to emerge, highlighting that "human differences are socially selected" (Link & Phelan, 2001, p. 368). These authors significantly advance the original proposition by proposing that "a stigma exists when elements of labeling, stereotyping, separation, loss of status, and discrimination occur simultaneously in a power situation that allows such components to happen" (Link & Phelan, 2001, p. 377). Returning to the theory of stigma, they attribute to it the notion of power, which allows to highlight other elements of the social relationship in which stigma occurs. Thus, the particularities of socially marginalized groups—those of which, exactly due to such marginalization, constitute minorities of rights—that suffer from the effects of the abusive use of alcohol and other drugs will demand measures of protection of life and health. However, one cannot face a problem (such as drug and psychoactive substance abuse) while at the same time causing the strengthening of prejudice and stigma towards these people. And, in this sense, scientific productions that contemplate and correlate these analysis universes are relevant to understand what has been produced in research, in Brazil, on such themes: LGBTQIA+ population and use/abuse of drugs.

11.2 Method

This study aimed to ascertain the existence of the influence of hostile and stressful social environments, as a result of gender and sexuality discrimination, in creating conditions for the abusive use of alcohol and other drugs among the LGBTQIA+ population in Brazilian academic literary production. Searches were conducted in the databases *Scientific Electronic Library Online* (Scielo Brazil) and *Virtual Health Library* (BVS), from August to September 2024, in two phases. In the first, the descriptors "LGBT," "LGBTQIA+," "LGBTQIAPN+," "Alcohol," "Alcohol and other drugs," "Alcohol abuse," "Drug abuse," and "Drugs" were used with the Boolean operator *AND*. Those descriptors helped the group in recognizing the field, pointing out the need for a more detailed definition of the terms, defining the best for each axis. Regarding the theme of gender and sexuality, the descriptors "LGBT," "LGBTQI," "LGBTQIAPN," "Sexuality," "Gender," "Heterosexuals," "Lesbians," "Bisexuals," "Gays," "Transsexuals," "Transvestites," and "Trans" were used; as for the theme of alcohol and other drugs, the terms used were "Harm reduction," "drugs," "licit," "illicit," "alcohol," "alcoholism," "substance use," and "substances." Serial searches were conducted with predetermined combinations of one term from each group using the Boolean operator *AND*, in an arithmetic progression logic, resulting in a total of 192 searches (96 in each database). The file production was guided by the *Preferred Reporting Items for Systematic Reviews and Meta-Analyses* (PRISMA), whose main structure is given by the stages of (1) identification, (2) screening, and (3) selection (Galvão et al., 2015). The results of each of the described phases are presented in flow form in Fig. 11.1.

Inclusion criteria: only scientific articles, original and available electronically, of free access, in Portuguese language and addressing the theme in the Brazilian national territory, published in the specific timeframe from 2019 to 2024. Repeated results and those that did not answer the research problem were excluded. The

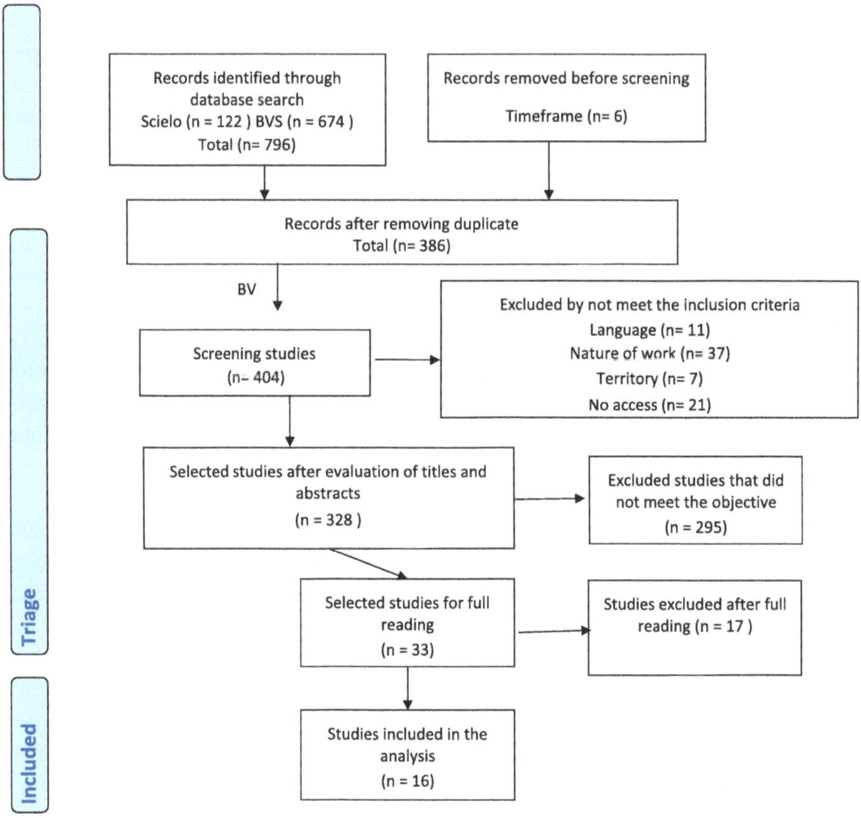

Fig. 11.1 Systematic review flow

analysis did not consider specific methods in order to avoid the rigidity of the scope. The intention to revisit the compiled knowledge reaffirms itself as an opportunity to seek new meanings and, perhaps, point out paths and possibilities for reflection (Galvão & Ricarte, 2019). During the searches and archiving of the texts, the titles were read to identify the inclusion and exclusion criteria. The works suitable for the study went through the reading of the abstracts and those that aligned with the theme—use of alcohol and other drugs, stigma and LGBTQIA+ population—were read in full (33). Of these, 17 were excluded, resulting in a total of 16 articles for analysis.

11.3 Results and Discussion

The analyzed articles consider drugs as any natural or synthetic substance, legal or illegal, capable of altering people's perception or states of consciousness. The variability of these substances is enormous: alcohol; opioids (such as heroin, codeine, and other synthetic substances); cannabinoids (marijuana, hashish, synthetic cannabinoids, spices); sedatives or hypnotics (barbiturates, benzodiazepines); cocaine; stimulants (such as amphetamines); hallucinogens (LSD; *ecstasy*), *Sex-performance-enhancing drugs* (*poppers*), to enlist some of the most cited in the studies. Considering the nature of the articles, the areas in which they were elaborated and the population cut contemplated in the content of the bibliographic materials analyzed, it is relevant to highlight that all the selected articles are scientific productions in the field of health, being five from the area of epidemiology (Leal et al., 2024; Bassichetto et al., 2024; Castoldi et al., 2021; Mota et al., 2024; Braga et al., 2022), three from public health (Sousa et al., 2020; Campos et al., 2023; Damacena et al., 2022), three from nursing (Souza et al., 2022a, b; Sousa et al., 2023; Lima et al., 2021), two from collective health (Marques et al., 2021; Ribas & Silva, 2023), two from psychology (Souza et al., 2022a); and one from mental health (Cortes et al., 2022). In addition to authors from the mentioned areas, there are also researchers from the areas of medicine (Leal et al., 2024; Sousa et al., 2023), preventive and social medicine (Braga et al., 2022) and sociology (Leal et al., 2024) signing the publications.

The analyzed articles are of different types of studies, contemplating both qualitative and quantitative methodologies. Those of a qualitative nature started from narrative reviews, integrative reviews, critical essays, and theoretical-reflective studies (Souza et al., 2022a; Marques et al., 2021; Ribas & Silva, 2023; Cortes et al., 2022; de Souza et al., 2022; Sousa et al., 2023). Cross-sectional and transversal design studies were used by authors who worked the data quantitatively (Leal et al., 2024; Bassichetto et al., 2024; Castoldi et al., 2021; Mota et al., 2024; Campos et al., 2023; Damacena et al., 2022; Sousa et al., 2020; Souza et al., 2022b; Lima et al., 2021; Braga et al., 2022). Among the instruments used for data collection were questionnaires followed by testing for Sexually Transmitted Infections (STIs), semi-structured forms, online surveys, interviews, and recruitment through

Respondent-Driven Sampling (RDS). There was also the use of scales, such as the Social Support Satisfaction Scale (ESSS) and testing through the *The Alcohol, Smoking and Substance Involvement Screening Test* (ASSIST).

The publications adopted different strategies for characterizing the participant populations. The LGBTQIA+ population, broadly, appears as the main population segment addressed in various studies (Marques et al., 2021; Ribas & Silva, 2023; Souza et al., 2022b; Braga et al., 2022); in two of these previously cited studies (Marques et al., 2021; Souza et al. 2022b), there are specifics regarding age range and self-declaration of these LGBTQIA+ identities. Gays and lesbians, exclusively, made up the population sample of only one study (Souza et al. 2022a), while trans women and transvestites appeared more frequently as the main population addressed by the articles (Leal et al., 2024; Bassichetto et al., 2024; Cortes et al., 2022; Mota et al., 2024). Similarly, men who have sex with men (MSM) also constituted a good part of the publications analyzed—noting the use of this category as a way to distinguish this population, epistemologically, from men perceived and/or self-identified as gay (Sousa et al., 2020, 2023; Souza et al. 2022a; Damacena et al., 2022). The other articles addressed groups whose characteristics did not encompass perspectives of sexuality and/or gender in a specific way, such as adult users of the Sanitary Dermatology Clinic (ADS) in Porto Alegre (Castoldi et al., 2021), undergraduate students aged 18 or older who were enrolled in health-related courses (Campos et al., 2023), and relatives of young people hospitalized for self-poisoning (Lima et al., 2021).

The so-called minority stress theory appears as a theoretical backdrop that postulates that social minorities, that is, population groups at a disadvantage compared to other normative groups, experience specific stressors—related to idiosyncrasies of the characteristics and attributes of these groups in particular. Anchored in this theoretical approach, the correlation that appears is the one established between internalized homophobia, linked to socially perceived stigma and added to social homophobia perpetuated by the groups to which the person belongs. These aspects accentuate the risk of substance abuse among the LGBTQIA+ population. The use of multiple substances is present in the daily reality of the LGBTQIA+ population, mainly alcohol and tobacco (Sousa et al., 2020). The high rates of psychological suffering of sex and gender minorities are accompanied by a high rate of vulnerability and exposure to social problems such as drug abuse (Coulter et al., 2019).

In this sense, as one of the analyzed articles asserts, Mota et al. (2024), whose scope included the discussion about the use of multiple substances among transsexual women and transvestites, the risks associated with this use include outcomes directly related to it, such as dependence and mental disorders, as well as secondary outcomes such as, for example, risk behaviors or decreased risk perception in the acquisition or transmission of the Human Immunodeficiency Virus (HIV) and other sexually transmitted infections. It is worth highlighting here, other studies (Cardoso & Ferro, 2012; Freitas, 2020) that emphasize how risk behaviors can be linked to stigma which, in turn, as Goffman (1975) asserts, provokes social exclusion. Such elements can operate as triggers of illness and provoke an increased risk of sexually transmitted infections, abusive use of alcohol and other drugs.

Transsexual and transvestite people face severe restrictions on access to resources necessary for the proper maintenance of a dignified, safe, and healthy life, as they are the target of various forms of discrimination and gender-based violence (Magno et al., 2018; Leal et al., 2024; Hughto et al., 2015; Reisner et al., 2016; Reback & Fletcher, 2014). Consequently, these people are often involved in informal activities, such as sex work, or even, in illicit activities, such as drug trafficking (Hughto et al., 2015; Reisner et al., 2016; Reback & Fletcher, 2014). In this line of reflection, another analyzed article problematized the incarceration of transsexual and transvestite women (Leal et al., 2024), highlighting that drug trafficking has been, in Brazil, the main reason for the incarceration of these women. This evidence corroborates what is evidenced by the data from the Ministry of Justice and Public Security of the country (National Council of Justice, 2021; Ministry of Justice and Public Security, 2022; Ministry of Justice and Public Security, 2023) since, such data indicate that the Brazilian female prison population is characterized by convictions related to illicit drugs, especially drug trafficking and association with trafficking, very similar to what also occurs with cisgender women in Brazil. Otherwise, female incarceration in the country is linked to indicators of social vulnerability of these women, such as misogyny and transphobia, racism, unemployment, low level of education, and, inevitably, a history of drug abuse. Among the possible explanations for the greater involvement of cisgender, transsexual, and transvestite women with drug trafficking, is their relationship with intimate partners or with family members involved in crime. The analyzed article (Freitas, 2020) highlights that stigma in transgenderism can trigger implications direct impacts on the living conditions of this population, such as low educational level, lack of housing, involvement with drug trafficking and abusive use of these substances, in addition to the difficulty of insertion in the labor market and the possibility of income generation restricted to sex work, corroborating other studies about the stigma experienced by transvestites and transgender women (Magno, 2018).

It is known that stigma affects physical and mental health, making it difficult for people to access different resources and services, accentuating health inequalities. The stigma experienced by LGBTQIA+ people promotes a hostile and stressful environment that can trigger various problems (Hatzenbuehler et al., 2013; King et al., 2008). It is worth highlighting here what the American Psychological Association (APA) guide titled *Best Practice Highlights LGBTQ* (Cabaj, 2023, p. 8) says: "*LGBTQ persons who struggle with higher rates of anxiety, affective disorder related conditions, and substance use disorders most likely have struggled with stigma and the coming out and self-acceptance process.*"

This study also points out that risk practices are frequent among LGBTQIA+ adolescents and young people who live alone, without partners or family members, among which are the use of stimulant drugs (such as cocaine, *crack* and *ecstasy*) and unprotected sexual practices accompanied by concomitant use of substances, which characterizes practices called "*chemsex*" or "*chemical sex*," which consists of the ingestion of drugs combined with sexual practices. Under these circumstances, there is evidence pointing to low proportions of risk perception among the adherents of these practices (Damacena et al., 2022). In this perspective, risk is conceptualized as any undesirable consequences resulting from some human action, this being considered a damage capable of prediction and control (Luiz & Cohn, 2006). Thus, risks emerge as capable of being targeted for management and intervention through government policies. However, once deliberated, such risk management policy ends up conditioning and tutoring people's lives and conducts, which can trigger situations of inequalities and injustices (Mendes, 2015).

Another aspect to be addressed, concerns drug use and social support (Souza et al. 2022b). Low satisfaction with available social support points to possible difficulties faced by sexual minorities in finding support in family groups, friendship, or even, in society in general. The text points out that "family support has been associated with an increase in the degree of satisfaction in various domains in the lives of LGBTQIA+ people, including lower rates of suicide, suffering, depression, hopelessness, and substance use" (Souza et al., 2022b, p. 8). Such findings accompany evidence found in research that points out that a well-structured social network, composed of social support, is associated with the reduction of risk behaviors of homosexual youth, significantly, such as the consumption or abusive use of psychoactive substances (Falleiros Braga et al., 2017).

This reflection corroborates the proposition brought by another of the analyzed articles, in order to elucidate the consequences of drug use by young people and their family context, highlighting the facilitation of violence contexts and the damage resulting from the decrease of social interaction in family by the young user. In an article that problematized antecedents of young people who attempted suicide (Lima et al., 2021), the reflection on how young people and, especially, young people from vulnerable populations, such as LGBTQIA+ people, represent a group at high risk for suicide is highlighted. Being this a significant cause of deaths by external causes at this stage of the life cycle, it seems pertinent to highlight that the suicide rate among young people, in Brazil, grew 6% per year between the years 2011 and 2022 (Alves et al., 2024). The article highlights that the nuclear family model does not necessarily protect against suicide attempts among young people, but family support, regardless of the format, is a protective factor. In Brazil, LGBTQIA+ adolescents face vulnerabilities such as prejudice, drug abuse, gender identity conflicts and mental disorders. Thus, the different bibliographic productions analyzed converge to the historical finding pointed out by the international literature (Evans-Polce et al., 2020), that the LGBTQIA+ population does, in fact, have higher rates of drug use, mainly, of tobacco and alcohol. In general, the analyzed studies also point out that lifestyles and characteristics related to prejudice and sex-gender hierarchies in this population are related to what has been highlighted in the theory of minority stress.

The impact of COVID-19 on marginalized groups also appeared as content in some of the researched articles (Marques et al., 2021; Braga et al., 2022) regarding the marginalized population and the use or abuse of alcohol and other drugs. It is stated that "there are multiple and complex relationships that can be established between uses of psychoactive substances, social vulnerability and the sanitary and social impacts of the coronavirus pandemic" (Marques et al., 2021, p. 8). In this sense, the analyzed articles highlight that, if there was already a concern about the psychosocial impacts of the pandemic on the general population—with evidence for an increase in mental health symptoms, such as worsening of anxiety and depression conditions, in addition to the significant increase in the consumption of alcohol and other drugs in the Brazilian population—they also emphasize the necessary understanding of these impacts and their developments on specific groups and the emerging need to build research approaches that contemplate their needs and specificities, as a vulnerable group. The discussion about the factors associated with the worsening of lifestyle during the pandemic of COVID-19, in the Brazilian population of lesbians, gays, bisexuals, transsexuals, transvestites, and related identities, has already been the subject of scientific scrutiny (Fontanari et al., 2019; Braga et al., 2022). Also in a study analyzed (Campos et al., 2023) on the use of psychoactive substances among health area university students before and during the COVID-19 pandemic, there is evidence that homosexual and bisexual orientation of cisgender men and women remained associated with the consumption of alcohol and illicit drugs.

One of the studies analyzed (Sousa et al., 2020) sought to investigate the factors associated with the practice of sex under the influence of drugs (*chemsex*) among MSM during the period of social isolation, in the context of the COVID-19 pandemic. Using a multicenter *online* survey, applied to the territories of Brazil and Portugal in April 2020, the research showed that—while the two countries were experiencing restrictive health measures to prevent the advancement and aggravation of the disease—the practice of *chemsex* in Brazil (69.9%) during the period surveyed was more than double that in Portugal (30.1%), with almost all of them (95%) having casual sex and a percentage of 31.4% having group sex and 47.6% having sex without a condom. The study also revealed that those who reported having group sex during the period of social distancing were twice as likely to engage in the practice of *chemsex*. Last but not least, a significant portion (95%) of the research subjects, the MSM who engaged in *chemsex* did so in an act with a casual partner during the rise of the pandemic's epidemiological curve (April 2020), in both countries surveyed (Brazil and Portugal). The study concludes that: "The occurrence of chemsex was high, especially in Brazil, where the proposed social isolation did not sensitize MSM to adherence, given the option for casual sex" (Sousa et al., 2020, p.9). The authors also highlight a perspective that deserves attention in this reflection: "It seems evident that the pursuit of pleasure proved to be more relevant in the face of the proposed COVID-19 protection measures, which makes MSM more exposed" (p. 9). However, it is worth revisiting here the relevant discussion about the challenge of identifying situations of vulnerability and greater exposure to risk without, however, reiterating or resorting to careless affirmations in the face of the polysemy that words possess. By proposing such conclusions, the text casts a shadow of interpretive possibility that allows one to infer that the "pursuit of pleasure" is "more relevant" than "protection against COVID-19" by MSM; however, it neglects the reflection that inversely, but to the same extent, one can conjecture that the strategies for preventing COVID-19 were not sufficiently adequate in achieving success in the contexts of risky sexual practices among MSM. In this sense, it seems more fruitful and relevant to concentrate analytical efforts on problematizing such contexts of "exposure"; not from a moralizing or prohibitionist perspective of what Michel Foucault (2020) called "the use of pleasures," but in a work of health risk management.

Still within the scope of the discussion about health risk management, it is known that the population of alcohol and/or other drug users is one of those recommended as key populations by the Ministry of Health of Brazil (2017) for access to post-exposure prophylaxis to HIV (PEP), in public services and, in the wake of this cut, the file of the present bibliographic review included an article (Castoldi et al., 2021), reporting on a research that sought to describe the profile of users who started prophylaxis (PEP) in a public service in southern Brazil, evaluating the use of this technology by such populations. It was "a retrospective longitudinal study in an outpatient clinic of the Unified Health System (SUS) that found evidence that, among the key populations of the study, there was a higher frequency of alcohol and/or other drug users (49.6%) and of men who have sex with men (38.1%) in the search for PEP." (Castoldi et al., 2021, p.1) Pertinent the successful attempt of this text analyzed in articulating the elements of gender, social class, and education, revealing in its research results, the high education of PEP users; which may be an indication of access to information, suggesting—still according to the text—that "people with fewer years of schooling are in a situation of greater vulnerability, including for the prevention of HIV infection" (Castoldi et al., 2021, p.6).

The articles analyzed corroborate evidence from studies with the LGBTQIA+ population (King et al., 2008; Plöderl & Tremblay, 2015; Fontanari et al., 2019), indicating the need for affirmative public policies that effectively contemplate this population, especially, transvestites and transsexual women. The consideration of high rates of vulnerability indicators, such as school dropout, low education, and problematic use of alcohol and drugs, due to stigma and prejudice, are factors that amplify discrimination, marginalization, and violence, hindering important spheres of life such as their insertion in the job market and the promotion of their quality of life (Jesus, 2012). Another integrative review study analyzed (Ribas & Silva, 2023), which deals with harm reduction (RD) for the population of transsexual women and transvestites, highlights that "constructed with a lot of dynamics, RD practices seek to look not only at the substance, but also at the subject, in a macro way, for their relationship with the drug and with the world"; further stating that, in this sense, "it is necessary to expand their actions with a view to other objectives, such as those of guaranteeing citizenship and the "human rights" (Ribas & Silva, 2023, p. 7). The emphasis seems relevant, pointed out by the analyzed text, on the importance of continuous education and training of professionals working in SUS equipment. Beyond the training of professionals, it is essential their articulation with the specific needs and vulnerabilities of this population.

Focusing on the mental health of transgender women, an integrative review analyzed in the present review (Cortes et al., 2022) highlights that, in addition to public services ensuring the execution of the right to health by minority populations, it is fundamental that governments develop, above all, health and mental health interventions that reach these people. Since there are health demands that are peculiar to these groups, as is the case, for example, of the transsexualizing process. The intention, according to the analyzed text, would be to minimize problems that often affect this population, such as the abusive use of alcohol and other drugs or greater exposure to HIV and STIs. The article also highlights the need for governments to promote the continuous education of health professionals, concerning the integral health of LGBTQIA+ people and, specifically, transgender people. Aspects that seem essential to promote better quality of life, avoid social disparities and offer universal and equitable attention in integral health to the Brazilian population. Another analyzed article, with a population cut of trans women and transvestites, was a study that sought to contribute to updating the epidemiology of STIs among transsexual women and transvestites (Bassichetto et al., 2024), confirmed that such sexual health problems present in greater magnitude among these people than in the general population. And, because most do not present symptoms, their treatment continues to be a challenge for public health. In the authors' words, "especially in the youngest, who engage in sex work and who use drugs" (Bassichetto et al., 2024, p. 8). What these analyzed texts contemplate as a common element is the ascertainment that transsexual women and transvestites constitute a vulnerable population and that there are social and economic barriers, anchored in stigmas and prejudices that hinder their access to health services and the labor market, demonstrating that existing legislation is still not sufficient, nor efficient to reverse this situation. This corroborates with findings from research with other members of the LGBTQIA+ population (de Carvalho & Barreto, 2021).

Returning to the reflection that began this chapter, about minority stress, another analyzed article (Souza et al., 2022b) states that the use of alcohol and other drugs emerges in the literature of the area being directly related to minority social stress, but also, to violence, especially physical and sexual, increasing, for example, vulnerabilities in the face of sexual risk exposure, as already discussed in this chapter. In this line of analysis, a cross-sectional and quantitative study with 316 lesbian, gay, bisexual, transvestite, and transsexual individuals, conducted a decade ago in the Brazilian state of Ceará, articulated a reflection around the study's evidence on alcohol, drugs and violence, analyzing the implications for the health of sexual minorities. Thestudy (Parente et al., 2015) shows that the abusive consumption of alcohol and other drugs by sexual minorities is used to deal with the stress produced by occupying a minority position in adverse social contexts resulting from prejudice and stigma related to sexual diversity and gender identities.

11.4 Final Considerations

The aim here was to ascertain whether the texts—which made up the file of the research that originated this chapter—contemplated or not the hypothesis that a hostile and stressful social environment for LGBTQIA+ adolescents and young people—shaped by prejudice and various forms of homophobia—can create conditions of possibility for the abusive use of alcohol and other drugs and the problems resulting from this abuse. And, in this regard, the answer was positive, in most of the studies analyzed. It was also sought to verify if the minority stress appears, in some way, in the bibliographies, which was also demonstrated. About the hypothesis that the harm reduction strategy would appear as a possibility of intervention, this proved to be true, however, without a substantial amount of scientific production in this sense, at least in relation to the LGBTQIA+ population.

Repeated characteristics were identified among the texts. The theme of Men who have Sex with Men (MSM) appeared in more than 50 results from different searches, relating more frequently to the use of alcohol and other drugs and the experience of HIV/Aids, considering inherent the relationship between the two experiences. On the other hand, the term Women who have Sex with Women (WSW) did not appear in any result, which alludes to a context of scientific production still based on the processes of invisibilization of WSW experiences, as already stated in the literature (Alves et al., 2020). In the research with the descriptor "bisexuals," articles were found that only mentioned the group, pointing to a gap in scientific production about bisexuality in Brazil and relating to the difficulties found in the country for the translation and circulation of foreign research (Monaco, 2020). On the other hand, the searches with the descriptors "gender"and "sexuality" resulted in texts mostly related to women (cis), motherhood, heterosexual conjugality, gender disparities between men (cis) and women (cis), and family dynamics. In addition to the pact with cisheteronorma in academic-scientific production and discussions little intersectional, there is the exclusion of the dissident population from the themes discussed there. Another point that should be highlighted is the absence of discussions made by the authors that dealt with the race/color of the population that composed the studies. Racial issues, along with gender, class, territory, ethnicity, education, without establishing hierarchies among such markers, also cross the LGBTQIA+ population and produce different social locations within power relations. What by in turn, will lead to differences in how stigma and prejudice are experienced and yet another factor that can contribute to the use/abuse of alcohol and other drugs. Regarding the LGBTQIA+ population, therefore, elements related to stigma and prejudice appear highly articulated to the vulnerability for the abusive use of alcohol, drugs, and other psychoactive substances.

References

Alves, R. L. V., dos Reis Alves, B. E., & Ferreira, D. T. P. (2020). (R)existência e Invisibilidade Lésbica: Entre conceitos, panoramas e percursos. *Revista Brasileira de Estudos da Homocultura, 2*(8). https://doi.org/10.31560/2595-3206.2019.8.10166

Alves, F. J. O., Fialho, E., Araújo, J. A. P., Naslund, J. A., Barreto, M. L., Patel, V., & Machado, D. B. (2024). The rising trends of self-harm in Brazil: An ecological analysis of notifications, hospitalisations, and mortality between 2011 and 2022. *The Lancet Regional Health – Americas*, 1–11. https://www.arca.fiocruz.br/handle/icict/62724

Bassichetto, K. C., Sperandei, S., McCartney, D. J., Luppi, C. G., Silva, R. J. C., Araújo, S., Magno, L., Bazzo, M. L., Hughes, G., Mayaud, P., Dourado, I., & Veras, M. A. S. M. (2024). Prevalências de clamídia e gonorreia entre mulheres trans e travestis de cinco capitais brasileiras, 2019–2021. *Revista Brasileira de Epidemiologia, 27*, 1–11. https://doi.org/10.1590/1980-549720240006.supl.1

Braga, L. H. R., Menezes, C. S., Martins, I. V., da Silva, J. D. P., & Torres, J. L. (2022). Fatores associados à piora no estilo de vida durante a pandemia de covid-19 na população brasileira de lésbicas, gays, bissexuais, transexuais, travestis e identidades relacionadas: Estudo transversal. *Epidemiologia e Serviços de Saúde, 31*(1), 1–14. https://doi.org/10.1590/s1679-49742022000100005

Bränström, R., Hatzenbuehler, M. L., & Pachankis, J. E. (2016). Sexual orientation disparities in physical health: Age and gender effects in a population-based study. *Social Psychiatry and Psychiatric Epidemiology, 51*(2), 289–301. https://doi.org/10.1007/s00127-015-1116-0

Cabaj, R. P. (2023). *Best practice highlights for working with LGBTQ patients*. American Psychiatric Association. https://www.psychiatry.org/getmedia/1dd0b752-8791-49d0-b8a1-c73d853bd610/Best-Practices-LGBTQ-Patients.pdf

Campos, H. M. N., Mattos, M. P., & Gomes, D. R. (2023). Uso de substâncias psicoativas por universitários da área da saúde antes e durante a pandemia da covid-19: Prevalência e fatores associados. *Revista Baiana de Saúde Pública, 47*(1), 129–148. https://rbsp.sesab.ba.gov.br/index.php/rbsp/article/view/3745

Cardoso, M. R., & Ferro, L. F. (2012). Saúde e população LGBT: Demandas e especificidades em questão. *Psicologia: Ciência E Profissão, 32*(3), 552–563. https://doi.org/10.1590/S1414-98932012000300003

Castoldi, L., Berengan, M. M., Both, N. S., Fortes, S., & Pinheiro, T. V. (2021). Profilaxia pós-exposição ao HIV em populações vulneráveis: Estudo longitudinal retrospectivo em um ambulatório da rede pública do Rio Grande do Sul, 2015–2018. *Epidemiologia E Serviços De Saúde, 30*(2), 1–9. https://doi.org/10.1590/S1679-49742021000200017

Conselho Nacional de Justiça. (2021). *Manual Resolução n° 348/2020*: Procedimentos relativos a pessoas LGBTI acusadas, rés, condenadas ou privadas de liberdade: Orientações a tribunais, magistrados e magistradas voltadas à implementação da Resolução no 348/2020, do Conselho Nacional de Justiça. Conselho Nacional de Justiça. https://www.cnj.jus.br/wp-content/uploads/2021/06/manual_resolucao348_LGBTI.pdf

Cortes, H. M., de Morais, A. V. C., Carnevalli, L. M., & Pinho, P. H. (2022). Saúde mental de mulheres transgêneras: Uma revisão integrativa de literatura/Mental health of transgender women: An integrative literature review. *Journal of Nursing and Health, 12*(3), 1–11. https://periodicos.ufpel.edu.br/index.php/enfermagem/article/view/21706

Coulter, R. W. S., Egan, J. E., Kinsky, S., Friedman, M. R., Eckstrand, K. L., Frankeberger, J., Folb, B. L., Mair, C., Markovic, N., Silvestre, A., Stall, R., & Miller, E. (2019). Mental health, drug, and violence interventions for sexual/gender minorities: A systematic review. *Pediatrics, 144*(3). https://doi.org/10.1542/peds.20183367

Damacena, G. N., Cruz, M. M., Cota, V. L., Souza Júnior, P. R. B., & Szwarcwald, C. L. (2022). Conhecimento e práticas de risco à infecção pelo HIV na população geral, homens jovens e HSH em três municípios brasileiros em 2019. *Cadernos de Saúde Pública, 38*(4), 1–14. https://doi.org/10.1590/0102-311XPT155821

de Carvalho, A. A., & Barreto, R. C. V. (2021). A invisibilidade das pessoas LGBTQIA+ nas bases de dados: Novas possibilidades na Pesquisa Nacional de Saúde 2019? *Ciência & Saúde Coletiva, 26*(9), 4059–4064. https://doi.org/10.1590/1413-81232021269.12002021

de Sousa, A. F. L., Camargo, E. L. S., & Mendes, I. A. C. (2023). Chemsex e suas repercussões na saúde de homens que fazem sexo com homens: Uma perspectiva de saúde global. *Revista Brasileira de Enfermagem, 76*(3). https://doi.org/10.1590/0034-7167-2023-0004

de Souza, D. C., da Silva, M. A., & Beiras, A. (2022). Violência Íntima entre Homens que se Relacionam com Homens – Revisão da Literatura. *Estudos E Pesquisas Em Psicologia, 22*(4), 1709–1728. https://doi.org/10.12957/epp.2022.71775

Evans-Polce, R. J., Veliz, P. T., Boyd, C. J., et al. (2020). Associations between sexual orientation discrimination and substance use disorders: Differences by age in US adults. *Social Psychiatry and Psychiatric Epidemiology, 55*, 101–110. https://doi.org/10.1007/s00127-019-01694-x

Facchini, R., & Barbosa, R. M. (2006). *Saúde das mulheres lésbicas: promoção da eqüidade e da integralidade: Dossiê/[pesquisa, Regina Facchini, Regina Maria Barbosa]*. Rede Nacional Feminista de Saúde, Direitos Sexuais e Direitos Reprodutivos-Rede Feminista de Saúde. https://www.cfess.org.br/arquivos/dossie_da_saude_da_mulher_lesbica.pdf

Falleiros Braga, I., da Silva, J. L., de Souza, G., Santos, Y., dos Santos, M. A., & Iossi Silva, M. A. (2017). Rede e apoio social para adolescentes e jovens homossexuais no enfrentamento à violência. *Psicologia Clínica, 29*(2), 297–318. https://pepsic.bvsalud.org/scielo.php?script=sci_arttext&pid=S0103-56652017000200009

Fontanari, A. M. V., Pase, P. F., Churchill, S., Soll, B. M. B., Schwarz, K., Schneider, M. A., Costa, A. B., & Lobato, M. I. R. (2019). Dealing with gender-related and general stress: Substance use among Brazilian transgender youth. *Addictive Behaviors Reports, 9*, 100166. https://www.sciencedirect.com/science/article/pii/S2352853218301895

Foucault, M. (2020). *História da sexualidade 2: O uso dos prazeres*. 8° ed. Rio de Janeiro: Paz e Terra.

Freitas, L. S. (2020). Minorias sexuais e de gênero, o estigma social e a sociedade de risco. *Saúde & Transformação Social/Health & Social Change, 10*(1/2/3), 001–010. https://incubadora.periodicos.ufsc.br/index.php/saudeetransformacao/article/view/5914

Friedman, R. C. (1999). Homosexuality, psychopathology, and suicidality. *Archives of General Psychiatry, 56*(10). https://doi.org/10.1001/archpsyc.56.10.887

Galvão, T. F., Pansani, T. S. A., & Harrad, D. (2015). Principais itens para relatar Revisões sistemáticas e Meta-análises: A recomendação PRISMA. *Epidemiologia E Serviços De Saúde, 24*(2), 335–342. https://doi.org/10.5123/S1679-49742015000200017

Galvão, M. C. B., & Ricarte, I. L. M. (2019). Revisão sistemática da literatura: Conceituação, produção e publicação. *Logeion: Filosofia da Informação, 6*(1), 57–73. https://doi.org/10.21728/logeion.2019v6n1.p57-73

Gilman, S. E., Cochran, S. D., Mays, V. M., Hughes, M., Ostrow, D., & Kessler, R. C. (2001). Risk of psychiatric disorders among individuals reporting same-sex sexual partners in the national comorbidity survey. *American Journal of Public Health, 91*(6), 933–939. https://doi.org/10.2105/ajph.91.6.933

Goffman, E. (1975). *Estigma: Notas sobre a manipulação da identidade deteriorada*. Márcia Bandeira de Mello Leite Nunes (Trad.). Rio de Janeiro: LTC.

Hatzenbuehler, M. L., Phelan, J. C., & Link, B. G. (2013). Stigma as a fundamental cause of population health inequalities. *American Journal of Public Health, 103*(5), 813–821. https://bit.ly/2DyJYLx

Hendricks, M. L., & Testa, R. J. (2012). A conceptual framework for clinical work with transgender and gender nonconforming clients: An adaptation of the minority stress model. *Professional Psychology: Research and Practice, 43*(5), 460–467. https://psycnet.apa.org/record/2012-21304-001

Hughto, J. M., Reisner, S. L., & Pachankis, J. E. (2015). Transgender stigma and health: A critical review of stigma determinants, mechanisms, and interventions. *Social Science & Medicine, 147*, 222–231. https://doi.org/10.1016/j.socscimed.2015.11.010

Jesus, J. G. (2012). *Orientações sobre identidade de gênero: Conceitos e termos*. EDA/FBN.

King, M., Semlyen, J., Tai, S. S., Killaspy, H., Osborn, D., Popelyuk, D., & Nazareth, I. (2008). A systematic review of mental disorder, suicide, and deliberate self harm in lesbian, gay and bisexual people. *BMC Psychiatry, 8*, 1–17. https://link.springer.com/article/10.1186/1471-244X-8-70

Leal, A. F., Cazeiro, C. C., Mattos, A. C. E., Hentges, B., Teixeira, L. B., Knauth, D. R., Magno, L., Dourado, I., & Veras, M. A. S. M. (2024). Perfil e experiências durante o encarceramento de mulheres trans e travestis (MTT) no Brasil: Um estudo transversal. *Revista Brasileira de Epidemiologia, 27*, 1–9. https://doi.org/10.1590/1980-549720240014.supl.1

Lima, P. K. G. C., Suguyama, P., Guedes, M. R. J., & Oliveira, M. L. F. (2021). Estrutura e antecedentes de famílias de jovens que tentaram suicídio com agentes químicos. *Revista Portuguesa de Enfermagem de Saúde Mental, 26*, 7–20. https://doi.org/10.19131/rpesm.307

Link, B. G., & Phelan, J. C. (2001). Conceptualizing stigma. *Annual Review of Sociology, 27*, 363–385. https://www.jstor.org/stable/2678626

Luiz, O. d. C., & Cohn, A. (2006). Sociedade de risco e risco epidemiológico. *Cadernos de Saúde Pública, 22*(11), 2339–2348. https://www.scielo.br/j/csp/a/86Wndmt9FFbB4SQmCmtMVkm/?lang=pt#

Magno, L., Dourado, I., & Silva, L. A. V. (2018). Estigma e resistência entre travestis e mulheres transexuais em Salvador, Bahia, Brasil. *Cadernos de Saúde Pública, 34*(5) https://www.scielo.br/j/csp/a/3spHF8TDqVCvqwPSMfyZskt/abstract/?lang=pt

Marques, A. L. M., Sorentino, I. S., Rodrigues, J. L., Machin, R., Oliveira, E., & Couto, M. T. (2021). O impacto da Covid-19 em grupos marginalizados: contribuições da interseccionalidade como perspectiva teórico-política. *Interface, 25*, 1–18. https://doi.org/10.1590/Interface.200712

Mendes, J. M. (2015). *Sociologia do risco: Uma breve introdução e algumas lições*. Imprensa da Universidade de Coimbra/Coimbra University Press, Coimbra. https://www.uc.pt/fluc/nicif/riscos/src/SRCII/Sociologia_do_risco.pdf.

Ministério da Justiça e Segurança Pública. (2022). *Dados estatísticos do sistema penitenciário* (Xa ed.). Secretaria Nacional de Políticas Penais. https://www.gov.br/senappen/pt-br/servicos/sisdepen

Ministério da Justiça e Segurança Pública. (2023). *Informação no 95/2022/COAMGE/CGCAP/DIRPP/DEPEN*. Departamento Penitenciário Nacional. Coordenação de Atenção às Mulheres e Grupos Específicos. https://www.gov.br/senappen/pt-br/servicos/sisdepen/relatorios/populacao-carceraria/presos-lgbti/presos-lgbti-2022.pdf

Ministério da Saúde. (2017). *Prevenção Combinada do HIV:* Bases conceituais para profissionais, trabalhadores(as) e gestores(as) de saúde. Secretaria de Vigilância em Saúde. Departamento de Vigilância Prevenção e Controle das Infecções Sexualmente Transmissíveis do HIV/Aids e das Hepatites Virais. https://www.gov.br/aids/pt-br/central-de-conteudo/publicacoes/2017/prevencao_combinada_-_bases_conceituais_web.pdf.

Monaco, H. M. (2020). "A gente existe!": ativismo e narrativas bissexuais em um coletivo monodissidente. *Dissertação de mestrado*, Curso de Antropologia Social, Centro de Filosofia e Ciências Humanas, Universidade Federal de Santa Catarina, Florianópolis. 150 f. https://repositorio.ufsc.br/bitstream/handle/123456789/216098/PASO0512-D.pdf?sequence=-1&isAllowed=y.

Mota, J. C., Sperandei, S., De Boni, R. B., Dourado, I., Veras, M. A. S. M., & Bastos, F. I. (2024). Uso de múltiplas substâncias e fatores associados em mulheres trans e travestis: resultados do estudo TransOdara, Brasil. *Revista Brasileira de Epidemiologia, 27*, 1–9. https://doi.org/10.1590/1980-549720240011.supl.1

Pachankis, J. E., & Safren, S. A. (2019). Adapting evidence-based practice for sexual and gender minorities: The current state and future promise of scientific and affirmative treatment approaches. In J. E. Pachankis & S. A. Safren (Eds.), *Handbook of evidence-based mental health Practice with Sexual and Gender Minorities*. Oxford University Press. https://doi.org/10.1093/med-psych/9780190669300.003.0001

Parente, J. S., Belém, J. M., dos Santos Figueiredo, F. W., da Silva Paiva, L., de Lima Garcia, C., Albuquerque, G. A., Macial, E. S., & Adami, F. (2015). Álcool, drogas e violência: Implicações para a saúde de minorias sexuais. *Reprodução & Climatério, 30*(3), 108–114. https://www.sciencedirect.com/science/article/pii/S1413208715000606

Paveltchuk, F. O., & Borsa, J. C. (2020). A teoria do estresse de minoria em lésbicas, gays e bissexuais. *Revista da SPAGESP, 21*(2), 41–54. http://pepsic.bvsalud.org/scielo.php?script=sci_arttext&pid=S1677-29702020000200004&lng=pt&tlng=pt

Plöderl, M., & Tremblay, P. (2015). Mental health of sexual minorities: A systematic review. *International Review of Psychiatry, 27*(5), 83949. https://doi.org/10.3109/09540261.2015.10

Reback, C. J., & Fletcher, J. B. (2014). HIV prevalence, substance use, and sexual risk behaviors among transgender women recruited through outreach. *AIDS and Behavior, 18*(7), 1359–1367. https://doi.org/10.1007/s10461-013-0657-z

Reisner, S. L., Poteat, T., Keatley, J., Cabral, M., Mothopeng, T., Dunham, E., Holland, C. E., Max, R., & Baral, S. D. (2016). Global health burden and needs of transgender populations: A review. *Lancet, 388*(10042), 412–436. https://doi.org/10.1016/S0140-6736(16)00684-X

Ribas, S. M., & Silva, A. B. (2023). Revisão integrativa: Estudos sobre redução de danos voltada para população de mulheres trans e travestis. *Saúde em Debate, 47*, 1–9. https://www.scielo.br/j/sdeb/a/48JyppskK5LpTxP6fNkMhfz/?format=html&lang=pt#

Sandfort, T. G. M., De Graaf, R., Bijl, R. V., & Schnabel, P. (2001). Same-sex sexual behavior and psychiatric disorders findings from the Netherlands Mental Health Survey and Incidence Study (NEMESIS). *Archives of General Psychiatry, 58*(1), 85–91. https://doi.org/10.1001/archpsyc.58.1.85

Sousa, Á. F. L., Queiroz, A. A. F. L. N., Lima, S. V. M. A., Almeida, P. D., Oliveira, L. B., Chone, J. S., Araújo, T. M. E., Brignol, S. M. S., Sousa, A. R., Mendes, I. A. C., Dias, S., & Fronteira, I. (2020). Prática de chemsex entre homens que fazem sexo com homens (HSH) durante período de isolamento social por COVID-19: Pesquisa online multicêntrica. *Cadernos de Saúde Pública, 36*(12), 1–12. https://doi.org/10.1590/0102-311X00202420

Souza, A. M. A., Moreira, M. M. G., Souza, G. R., & Rocha, N. S. (2022a). Novas perspectivas nas psicoterapias em gays e lésbicas. *Revista brasileira de psicoterapia, 24*(3), 59–72. https://lume.ufrgs.br/handle/10183/259242

Souza, I. C., Tavares, T. M. C. L., Beserra, G. D. L., Araújo Júnior, A. J. L., Sousa, W. M. A., Ribeiro, S. G., Soares, P. R. A. L., & Pinheiro, A. K. B. (2022b). Consumo de drogas e suporte social percebido por minoria sexual. *Revista Gaúcha de Enfermagem, 43*, 1–10. https://doi.org/10.1590/1983-1447.2022.20210151

Valdiserri, R. O., Holtgrave, D. R., Poteat, T. C., & Beyrer, C. (2018). Unraveling health disparities among sexual and gender minorities: A commentary on the persistent impact of stigma. *Journal of Homosexuality, 66*(5), 571–589. https://doi.org/10.1080/00918369.2017.1422944

Vargas, S. M., Wennerstrom, A., Alfaro, N., Belin, T., Griffith, K., Haywood, C., Jones, F., Lunn, M. R., Meyers, D., Miranda, J., Obedin-Maliver, J., Pollock, M., Sherbourne, C. D., Springgate, B. F., Sugarman, O. K., Rey, E., Williams, C., Williams, P., & Chung, B. (2019). Resilience Against Depression Disparities (RADD): A protocol for a randomised comparative effectiveness trial for depression among predominantly low-income, racial/ethnic, sexual and gender minorities. *BMJ Open, 9*(10). https://doi.org/10.1136/bmjopen-2019-031099

Chapter 12
When Drug Addiction Coexists with HIV Infection: The Interaction of Two Powerful Stigmas

Rafael Ballester-Arnal, Maria Dolores Gil-Llario, Cristina Giménez-García, and Estefanía Ruiz-Palomino

12.1 Introduction—Drug Addiction and HIV Infection: The Beginnings of a Toxic Relationship

At the beginning of the 80 s, a new disease made its appearance, HIV infection. Few could suspect that, at that point in the twentieth century, in a time when great epidemics were no longer remembered, a new pathology would be born that would become in just a few years a great pandemic that strained health systems and public health across the world. While in 1981, only 41 cases with symptoms of a clinical presentation that would later be attributed to Human Immunodeficiency Virus had been detected, only a few years later the figure of more than 40 million affected was reached, causing more than five million new infections and three million deaths per year (Ballester, 1999). As expected, a health catastrophe of such magnitude awakened old ghosts and ancient demons, the ancestral tendency of human beings to look for culprits or scapegoats for the disasters that occur in our lives, with the peculiarity that, on this occasion, the blame was placed on the heads of the affected themselves. The more conservative sectors of the United States found it convenient that the first cases were among men who had had sex with other men to rekindle the flame of homophobia. The term "gay plague" gained strength and the idea that a just and in this case "sanitary" God had sent a plague like the one he already sent to the cities of Sodom and Gomorrah, to heal society and punish people who had immoral

R. Ballester-Arnal (✉) · C. Giménez-García · E. Ruiz-Palomino
Department of Basic, Clinical Psychology and Psychobiology, Universitat Jaume I de Castelló, Castelló, Spain
e-mail: rballest@uji.es; gimenezc@uji.es; eruiz@uji.es

M. D. Gil-Llario
Department of Developmental and Educational Psychology, Universitat de València, Valencia, Spain
e-mail: Dolores.Gil@uv.es

T. Mota Ronzani (ed.), *Social Stigma and Drug Use*,
https://doi.org/10.1007/978-3-031-94813-8_12

behaviors began to spread among some conservative sectors of society (Ballester, 1999).

The stigma, in the most original sense of the Greek term, as a mark or stain, found a population to torment again. If for the ancient Greeks this term referred to the tattoos that slaves or criminals received on their bodies to indicate their status or the crime they had committed, a practice likely adopted from the Persians, now suffering from HIV infection or AIDS was the sign that a person had performed shameful behaviors. Thus, the stigma of suffering from HIV, pointed to those already marked from time immemorial for having sexual relations with those of the same sex, although since the beginning of the first millennium, Christianity occupied itself with labeling immoral any sexual conduct outside of reproductive sex within marriage. Shortly, cases of HIV began to be detected in heroin addicts and Haitians, a Caribbean area to which some Americans went to enjoy sex tourism, and thus the expression "Syndrome of the three H's" was coined: homosexuals, heroin addicts, and Haitians. They all had something in common: people seen as morally corrupt or poor immigrants. It took the arrival of HIV to hemophiliacs and especially to the fifth H, that of heterosexuals, for society to understand that this problem could affect any of us. But the stigma is still among us and continues to pursue people living with HIV, adding an additional burden to the stigma that homosexuals or drug addicts already carried.

The transmission routes of HIV are well known, mainly via contact with infected semen, fluids, or blood. The population that used intravenous drugs became an especially socially dangerous group. Not only could they transmit the infection by sharing infected syringes with other people, but they could do so through their sexual relations like any other person. Furthermore, their status as drug users led to a presumption of a general lack of impulse control, not only in drug use but also in condom use practicing risky sexual behaviors, not only in sexual relations with their partners (stable or sporadic) but also in exercising sex work, to which they could resort to pay for drugs (Ballester-Arnal et al., 2013). On the other hand, sex and drugs have long been closely linked, a relationship that has grown stronger over time and is manifested in phenomena such as chemsex, the use of drugs with the aim of prolonging sexual relations or intensifying sexual pleasure. The synergy between the risk of contracting HIV through risky sexual practices or intravenous drug injection was and continues to be present in the drug-dependent population. And to the extent that the consumption of disinhibiting drugs by any means is associated with risky sex, the drug-dependent population becomes a particularly vulnerable target for HIV and also the stigma that accompanies it.

Next, we will analyze the effect that stigma has on the mental and physical health of this population, and the preventive and therapeutic intervention measures, both that we can adopt to confront a "stain" that should never have been associated with this group but rather with the society that pointed fingers at them.

12.2 Impact of Stigma on the Mental Health of Drug-Dependent People with HIV

The scientific advances of antiretroviral therapy and the implementation of integrated models for the combined treatment of HIV and addiction have made HIV a chronic disease, significantly reduced the morbidity and mortality rate, reduced risky behaviors, and improved the quality of life of drug-dependent people living with this disease. These milestones could be promising for the eradication of socially stigmatizing attitudes. However, the social construction related to HIV continues to maintain prejudices, stereotypes, and moralizing beliefs that, as has been said, were born with the epidemic in the 1980s (Batlle, 2021). The so-called third phase of AIDS, the epidemic of social responses to HIV infection, is one of the major obstacles to health equity for people living with this disease (Ballester-Arnal et al., 2016). A greater challenge for public health is the intersectional stigma related to the binomial between HIV and drug use. 40% of people with HIV who inject drugs report having experienced stigma (UNAIDS, 2024). The symbolic dimensions of drug dependence entail a marginalized, criminalized, and conflictive social representation of drug users (Bayat et al., 2020). A study conducted with medical students at Guangzhou University in China concluded that being a drug user is the most stigmatized condition and that, therefore, it is relevant to pay attention to the magnitude of the effect of the interaction of various stigmas (Chan et al., 2007).

Stigma negatively affects psychological well-being, especially in older people (Rzeszutek et al., 2021). A meta-analysis conducted by Logie and Gadalla (2009) determined an association between stigma towards HIV and the self-perception of poor mental health of those with HIV. Stigma is a predictor of being diagnosed with a mental health disorder among people living with HIV (Di Gennaro et al., 2024). The scientific literature shows that depression, anxiety, chronic stress, and suicidal ideation are the most frequent and common problems related to stigma towards HIV, and that social support acts as a buffer factor for the impact of stigma on mental health (Armoon et al., 2022; Rueda et al., 2016). On the other hand, sleep problems seem to mediate the relationship between the experience of stigma and mental health problems, exacerbating the symptoms (Dong et al., 2024). Other psychological problems such as post-traumatic stress disorder, hopelessness, loneliness, or low self-esteem have also been associated with the experience of stigma (Mahajan et al., 2008). The physical and psychological consequences worsen and become chronic when the stigma associated with HIV infection is compounded by prejudices related to other stigmatized identities, such as drug use, which is the focus of this chapter (Dong et al., 2024)., For instance, in a Russian study by Hook et al. (2023), 37% of people with HIV who use drugs reported having experienced intersectional stigma, and it was observed that this fact exacerbates the risk of suffering from anxiety and depression problems compared to other forms of individual stigma.

Stigma is a complex phenomenon studied from multiple approaches. Specifically, the impact of stigma towards HIV on mental health has been attempted to be explained mainly from two theoretical models. In the 1990s, Meyer's (2003) Sexual

Minority Stress Theory was developed. This conceptual model provides a unidirectional explanation, understanding that experiences of stigma affect mental health due to the lasting and cumulative effect of stress experienced by people belonging to groups considered minorities, such as people living with HIV or people who use drugs. More recently, Earnshaw and Chaudoir's Theoretical Framework of HIV Stigma provides a dynamic and reciprocal view of the relationship between different inter and intrapersonal mechanisms of stigma and mental health problems. This model highlights the importance of the individual experience of stigma to adequately explain the psychological consequences derived from its experience.

The mental health of these people, therefore is not only influenced by the prejudices and stereotypes towards HIV that still remain inherent in varied contexts (family, health, work, etc.), but also by the belief that a person with HIV has about the possibility of being stigmatized and rejected in some situations (anticipated stigma) and the acceptance and self-attribution of these negative ideas (internalized stigma). In this sense, having lived situations of discrimination or rejection due to HIV in different significant contexts (perceived stigma) negatively affects the psychological well-being of people with HIV (Chan et al., 2021). In addition, anticipated and internalized stigma can also cause a negative affective state with feelings such as shame, guilt, fear, or worry that, maintained over time, poses a chronic stressor and generates serious coping difficulties and psychological problems (Yuan et al., 2023). Two longitudinal studies, one conducted by Turan et al. (2019) with a sample of women with HIV from the United States and another conducted by Yuan et al. (2024) with a sample of people with HIV from China, showed that internalized stigma towards HIV was a predictor of depressive symptoms. Similarly, there is a body of research that posits that the effect on mental health is due to the dynamic interrelation between different stigma mechanisms. For example, Turan et al. (2017) suggest that perceived stigma would lead to the internalization of stigma and this to the anticipation of stigma experiences.

The consequences of the psychological implications of experiencing stigma are severe for the health and quality of life of people with HIV. The most studied is the lack of optimal adherence to antiretroviral treatment (ART) due to its influence on disease progression (Turan et al., 2019). As observed in Masa et al. (2022), the psychological effects of HIV stigma reduced motivation levels for ART adherence, decreased self-efficacy beliefs, and worsened behavioral skills. The study by Shrestha et al. (2019) in a sample of people with HIV on methadone treatment supported this finding. The motivation for adherence to ART showed a significant mediating effect between stigma and adherence to ART. In addition to the above, stigma can generate adverse health outcomes such as less commitment to the use of health services and greater participation in risk behaviors (Rueda et al., 2016). The constant fear of rejection and the internalization of the feeling of guilt experienced by people with HIV who are drug-dependent influences social isolation and help-seeking. In a study conducted with users of a harm reduction program in New York City, it was reported that almost 60% of participants felt a critical and hurtful attitude due to their condition in the health context and that anxiety at the possibility of being discriminated against led to an avoidance of seeking health assistance

(Muncan et al., 2020). The avoidance of seeking psychological help can also be influenced by the fear of being judged or negatively evaluated by professionals, thus producing an especially severe effect on mental health.

In an attempt to simplify the complexity and diversity of the nature of stigma towards HIV, much of the research evaluates HIV stigma as a single construct or analyzes one type of stigma related to HIV. Despite the evidence that exists about the negative effect of HIV stigma on mental health, the dynamics of functioning that are established between the different stigma mechanisms and the results on mental health remain to be clarified (Masa et al., 2022). Also, it is worth highlighting the complexity of the psychological processes involved in the experience of stigma that develop in a temporally different way and the possible interaction of other variables, such as the experience of intersectional stigmas, when they turn out to be summative experiences as in the case of the drug-dependent person with HIV (Stangl et al., 2023).

12.3 Keys to the Prevention of Stigma and Discrimination in Drug-Dependent People with HIV Infections

The stigma and discrimination towards drug-dependent people with HIV is a multicausal experience that occurs, simultaneously and interactively, at different levels of the system. Consequently, for preventive efforts to be effective, they must be based on a multilevel approach that allows action in each of the dimensions in which it is generated and perpetuated (RIOD, 2019).

To do this, it is necessary to know what strategies and actions have proven to be effective in transforming those variables that predispose to discriminatory behaviors, such as perceived norms and lack of empathy, as well as other interpersonal level variables that reinforce these behaviors in such relevant environments as the family or workplace. At the same time, it is essential to identify which intervention components lead to transforming the stigma that the affected people themselves suffer, without forgetting those structural aspects that legitimize socioeconomic policies that exclude people with HIV, particularly when it interrelates with substance use.

At the interpersonal level, many preventive efforts have focused on improving knowledge and changing attitudes related to transmission routes to reduce the fear associated with the infection process, using psychoeducational approaches, skill development, and psychological support (Brown et al., 2003). Other interventions emphasize improving knowledge, while building compassion, acceptance, and solidarity toward stigmatized people. The evidence supports the utility of interventions based on interpersonal contact (Stutterheim et al., 2023), empathy induction (Batson et al., 2002), and perspective taking (Todd et al., 2012).

In this framework, the use of first-person testimonies has been shown to improve sensitivity and empathy toward people with HIV (Kerr et al., 2020). In addition, small-group participatory methodologies, which require proactivity from participants such as role-playing, debates, reflection exercises, ethical dilemmas, and other experiential activities, have proven to be effective in improving perspective-taking, understanding, and empathy (Ballester-Arnal, et al., 2015, Mak et al., 2015; RIOD, 2019).

As for the self-stigma of the affected people themselves, the literature has found that both psychoeducational and psychotherapeutic interventions are the predominant approaches to reduce internalized stigma, combining information about the problem experienced with the development of communication skills and social support (Ma et al., 2019; Sibley et al., 2024). In addition, proposals designed from the cognitive and acceptance and commitment to values, experiential avoidance, orientation towards change and commitment to meaningful actions for individuals, also improve personal acceptance (Pérez-Pedrogo et al., 2022). Evidence indicates that protective variables for emotional well-being help strengthen people infected with HIV and drug users (Lodi et al., 2022). Furthermore, elements such as starting from a rights-based approach and enhancing the proactive identification of social support optimize empowerment (Molero et al., 2011).

Within this framework, some authors like Zhang et al. (2014), have identified key groups on which to increase efforts. Specifically, they advocate the importance of developing educational interventions and stigma reduction aimed at informal support networks. In this vein, the study by Nabunya et al. (2024), showed the effectiveness of an intervention to reduce the stigma of families that, through 10 fortnightly sessions at their health center, addressed content such as social norms, responsibility in relationships, respectful communication, stress, and social support.

Other interventions have focused on training those who work in organizations and services with substance users and people with HIV (RIOD, 2019). These initiatives have gained more relevance as they have included an intersectional approach, considering aspects such as gender identity and sexual orientation. Specifically, some interventions have focused on the school environment, through training integrated into curricular subjects (Martin et al., 2022) while others have focused on the health and social context, training key agents who have replicated a culture of acceptance and tolerance towards stigmatized people (Li et al., 2014). In this vein, some proposals have included case-based learning and simulations and the participatory design of action plans, including follow-ups, developed in the centers themselves (Watt et al., 2024).

In community settings, the incorporation of spaces for participatory learning and social transformation have been found effective, in which social leaders and people with HIV trained in skills for social justice design a program of community activities designed by, promoting the development of collective strategies to manage the stigma related to HIV and other social inequalities, exacerbated in some contexts such as substance use (Li et al., 2018; Reif et al., 2021). Moreover, given the importance of religious tradition for some communities, other interventions have focused on preventing stigma and discrimination from religious institutions (Cook, 2021; Derose et al., 2016). For instance, after a training program, religious leaders incorporated into their sermons, information about primary and secondary prevention, stigma and its relationship with fear, the impact of HIV on families and communities, and empathy; as well as the relationship between religion and compassion and empathy towards those affected.

At a higher level, some efforts have focused on the role of the media. While research has shown a moderate impact, it stands as a necessary (though not sufficient) strategy to add to other levels of intervention and prevent the stigma associated with drug-dependent people as well as linked to HIV infection (Sola-Morales & Quiroz, 2019). In fact, some of the findings indicate that the effect of the media is sustained in the medium term and could even increase over time.

As in other levels of care, the incorporation of lived experiences by stigmatized people also proves effective in media campaigns (Abroms & Maibach, 2008). Specifically, a study focused on the Latino community showed the challenges of long-term HIV survival of people from the community itself, through digital photography (Witkowski et al., 2021). The testimonies showed empowered and proactive people, focusing on the rights-based approach. Likewise, exposure to accurate information about the phenomenon of drug addiction and HIV in the media is related to less stigma (Sola-Morales & Quiroz, 2019). On the contrary, the visibility of maladjusted models of people with HIV and drug addicts in movies, series, or the news could increase negative emotions (Aghaei et al., 2023; RIOD, 2019).

At a more macro level, the findings propose a reform of policies that discriminate against people living with the infection, taking into account the intersectionality would be necessary for effective reform, from the diversity of origin, to affective-sexual diversity, to transmission routes that, as mentioned in the first section, especially, are penalized as they relate to substance use and/or sexual behaviors. To change this structural stigma, it is proposed to base interventions on environmental theories that can serve to guide the transformation of aspects as diverse as social norms and legislation (Hatzenbuehler & Link, 2014).

Beyond the area and type of intervention, the scientific literature points to some basic aspects for effective stigma prevention and intervention. Efforts should be made to adapt the intervention to the sociocultural context in which it takes place. Such adaptive models have shown their usefulness in reducing stigma, making visible the bystander perspective, and the need to address multiple types of stigma and different levels of intervention, from personal to community (Wingood & DiClemente, 2008).

In general terms, these proposals include a systematic methodology that includes an organized series of stages (Stutterheim et al., 2023). First, evaluation and diagnosis are advised to understand the expressed, perceived, and comparative needs to analyze the problems from a multicausal approach. Second, the delimitation of the expected results and objectives of the intervention both general and specific; that is, defining what should change, for whom, to what extent and in what timeframe. Thirdly, the methodological design of the intervention at different levels is proposed, based on the evidence that guides behavior change. From this approach, moreover, experiences that have proven to be effective also point to some theory or theoretical model that facilitates the identification of key variables and premises such as the Stigma Reduction Theory (Derose et al., 2016; Parker & Aggleton, 2003), or the Social Justice Training approach (Li et al., 2018). Some successful strategies have also taken the Stigma Structuring Theory as a reference, which highlights the role of stigmatized people as change agents who, in the first person, may have the ability to transform prejudices and discrimination (Misir, 2015).

In this way, the configuration of methodologies or contents is not determined by the intuition of those who implement the strategies, but rather the grounded experience facilitated by contrasted theories (Stutterheim et al., 2023). As such, some of the experiences point to the need to incorporate participatory learning adapted to each sociocultural context that, in addition to the transmission of information, allows for the improvement of communication skills and the management of empathy and acceptance both in affected people and in society in general (Nabunya et al., 2024).

To design these preventive programs, it is recommended to create a participatory planning group. In this group, it is essential to incorporate the perspective of stigmatized people, either through the design of content and messages or with their direct involvement in the dissemination of information (RIOD, 2019). In addition to their direct participation, strategies focused on those close to the affected have also favored changes in the environment and helped to detect situations of discrimination (French et al., 2015; Prinsloo et al. 2016). In this type of intervention, it is necessary to foster networks among community organizations and other stakeholders to develop and carry out the strategies to generate trust in neglected communities (Earnshaw et al., 2013, b). For example, in the intervention of Mevissen et al. (2018), the planning group included teachers, a social worker, a public health professional, stigma experts and applied psychology researchers. In others like Cook's (2021), religious centers aligned with community hospitals to address stigma. Toward this goal, audiovisual media and information and communication technologies have also shown to have a relevant role, by allowing to expand influence, reaching different regions and socio-culturally different populations.

After this design phase, a pilot of the intervention should be validated, which allows researchers to test if the materials and dissemination media are adequate. Likewise, in this phase, the evaluation tools that enable the assessment of the effectiveness of the proposed intervention could also be tested.

Finally, the execution, evaluation and follow-up ensure the fulfillment of objectives and expected results, as well as the elaboration of the evaluation and lessons learned. Throughout the design of the intervention, it is essential to have an intersectional approach that makes visible the multiple stigmas that surround drug-dependent people and people with HIV due to their origin, their economic status, their religious beliefs or their sexual orientation (Li et al., 2018; RIOD, 2019).

In this effort, as in other strategies, it is fundamental to contextualize the messages and formats to the sociocultural codes of the environment, aligning communication campaigns and interpersonal actions with the priorities in the prevention of stigma suffered by drug-dependent people and people with HIV at a local, national and international level (Aghaei et al., 2023; Sola-Morales & Quiroz, 2019). Even more so, the evidence shows to what extent the efforts to reduce this stigma should go beyond individual behavior, as the barriers that exist at an institutional and structural level can be more decisive in the long-term effectiveness of an intervention

(Siegel et al., 2015). In this task, all people who could develop actions that contribute to change, regardless of their role, should be involved.

12.4 Final Considerations

As can be seen throughout this chapter, drug-dependent people with HIV infection face a cumulative stigma that includes stigmas associated with any drug dependence, AIDS, sexually transmitted infections in general, homosexuality in some cases and even sometimes sex work or situations of conflict with justice through committing crimes, a situation that sometimes results from the need to get money to consume drugs. These interacting stigmas are too many and generate too much rejection to be processed, digested and neutralized by any human being. On the contrary, in many cases, this stigma is internalized, making the worst enemy oneself, sending self-destructive messages that generate helplessness, low self-esteem, low self-efficacy for change and emotional problems that can even lead to suicide. In the face of such a complex problem, prevention strategies and clinical intervention must necessarily be broad, deep, continuous, multi-componential and coming from multiple sources that have been highlighted throughout this chapter.

Acknowledgements We would like to thank Jacqueline Feldman for her help in revising the English translation of this chapter.

References

Abroms, L. C., & Maibach, E. W. (2008). The effectiveness of mass communication to change public behavior. *Annual Review of Public Health, 29*(1), 219–234. https://doi.org/10.1146/annurev.publhealth.29.020907.090824

Aghaei, A., Sakhaei, A., Khalilimeybodi, A., Qiao, S., & Li, X. (2023). Impact of mass media on HIV/AIDS stigma reduction: A systematic review and meta-analysis. *AIDS and Behavior, 27*(10), 3414–3429. https://doi.org/10.1007/s10461-023-04057-5

Armoon, B., Fleury, M. J., Bayat, A. H., Fakhri, Y., Higgs, P., Moghaddam, L. F., & Gonabadi-Nezhad, L. (2022). HIV related stigma associated with social support, alcohol use disorders, depression, anxiety, and suicidal ideation among people living with HIV: A systematic review and meta-analysis. *International Journal of Mental Health Systems, 16*(1), 17. https://doi.org/10.1186/s13033-022-00527-w

Ballester, R. (1999). *SIDA. Prevención y tratamiento psicológico en la infección por VIH y SIDA*. Universidad Nacional de Educación a Distancia (UNED).

Ballester-Arnal, R., Gil-Llario, M. D., Giménez-García, C., & Kalichman, S. C. (2015). What works well in HIV prevention among Spanish young people? An analysis of differential effectiveness among six intervention techniques. *AIDS and Behavior, 19*(7), 1157–1169. https://doi.org/10.1007/s10461-014-0863-3

Ballester-Arnal, R., Gómez-Martínez, S., Fumaz, C. R., González-García, M., Remor, E., & Fuster, M. J. (2016). A Spanish study on psychological predictors of quality of life in people with HIV. *AIDS and Behavior, 20*(2), 281–291. https://doi.org/10.1007/s10461-015-1208-6

Ballester-Arnal, R., Salmerón-Sánchez, P., Gil-Llario, M. D., & Giménez-Garcia, C. (2013). The influence of drug consumption on condom use and other aspects related to HIV infection among male sex workers in Spain. *AIDS and Behavior, 17*(2), 536–542. https://doi.org/10.1007/s10461-012-0171-8

Batlle, F. M. (2021). Profundizando en las causas y consecuencias del estigma asociado al VIH. *Revista Multidisciplinar del Sida, 24*(9), 3–4.

Batson, C. D., Chang, J., Orr, R., & Rowland, J. (2002). Empathy, attitudes and action: Can feeling for a member of a stigmatized group motivate one to help the group. *Personality and Social Psychology Bulletin, 28*(12), 1656–1666. https://doi.org/10.1177/014616702237647

Bayat, A. H., Mohammadi, R., Moradi-Joo, M., Bayani, A., Ahounbar, E., Higgs, P., Hemmat, M., Haghgoo, A., & Armoon, B. (2020). HIV and drug related stigma and risk-taking behaviors among people who inject drugs: A systematic review and meta-analysis. *Journal of Addictive Diseases, 38*(1), 71–83. https://doi.org/10.1080/10550887.2020.1718264

Brown, L., Macintyre, K., & Trujillo, L. (2003). Interventions to reduce HIV/AIDS stigma: What have we learned? *AIDS Education and Prevention, 15*(1), 49–69. https://doi.org/10.1521/aeap.15.1.49.23844

Chan, R. C., Mak, W. W., Ma, G. Y., & Cheung, M. (2021). Interpersonal and intrapersonal manifestations of HIV stigma and their impacts on psychological distress and life satisfaction among people living with HIV: Toward a dual-process model. *Quality of Life Research, 30*(1), 145–156. https://doi.org/10.1007/s11136-020-02618-y

Chan, K. Y., Yang, Y., Zhang, K. L., & Reidpath, D. D. (2007). Disentangling the stigma of HIV/AIDS from the stigmas of drugs use, commercial sex and commercial blood donation–a factorial survey of medical students in China. *BMC Public Health, 7*, 280. https://doi.org/10.1186/1471-2458-7-280

Cook, L. (2021). HIV stigma reduction and health literacy education program with a cross-generational population in an African American faith-based church. *Journal of Public Health, 29*, 1089–1106. https://doi.org/10.1007/s10389-020-01203-4. Workshop-facilitators-guide.pdf.

Derose, K. P., Griffin, B. A., Kanouse, D. E., Bogart, L. M., Williams, M. V., Haas, A. C., Flórez, K. R., Collins, D. O., Hawes-Dawson, J., Mata, M. A., Oden, C. W., & Stucky, B. D. (2016). Effects of a pilot church-based intervention to reduce HIV stigma and promote HIV testing among African Americans and Latinos. *AIDS and Behavior, 20*(8), 1692–1705. https://doi.org/10.1007/s10461-015-1280-y

Di Gennaro, F., Papagni, R., Segala, F. V., Pellegrino, C., Panico, G. G., Frallonardo, L., Diella, L., Belati, A., Santoro, C. R., Brindicci, G., Balena, F., Bavaro, D. F., Montalbò, D., Guido, G., Calluso, L., Di Tullio, M., Sgambati, M., Fiordelisi, D., De Gennaro, N., & Saracino, A. (2024). Stigma and mental health among people living with HIV across the COVID-19 pandemic: A cross-sectional study. *BMC Infectious Diseases, 24*(1), 423. https://doi.org/10.1186/s12879-024-09315-y

Dong, L., Bogart, L. M., Mutchler, M. G., Klein, D. J., Ghosh-Dastidar, M., Lawrence, S. J., Goggin, K., & Wagner, G. J. (2024). Sleep disturbance mediates the associations between HIV stigma and mental and physical health among black adults with HIV. *Journal of Racial and Ethnic Health Disparities*. https://doi.org/10.1007/s40615-024-02083-0

Earnshaw, V. A., Bogart, L. M., Dovidio, J. F., & Williams, D. R. (2013). Stigma and racial/ethnic HIV disparities: Moving toward resilience. *The American Psychologist, 68*(4), 225–236. https://doi.org/10.1037/a0032705

Earnshaw, V. A., Smith, L. R., Chaudoir, S. R., Amico, K. R., & Copenhaver, M. M. (2013). HIV stigma mechanisms and well-being among PLWH: A test of the HIV stigma framework. *AIDS & Behavior, 17*(5), 1785–1795. https://doi.org/10.1007/s10461-013-0437-9

French, H., Greeff, M., Watson, M. J., & Doak, C. M. (2015). A comprehensive HIV stigma-reduction and wellness-enhancement community intervention: A case study. *Journal of the Association of Nurses in AIDS Care, 26*(1), 81–96. https://doi.org/10.1016/j.jana.2014.03.007

Hatzenbuehler, M. L., & Link, B. G. (2014). Introduction to the special issue on structural stigma and health. *Social Science & Medicine, 103*, 1–6. https://doi.org/10.1016/j.socscimed.2013.12.017

Hook, K., Sereda, Y., Rossi, S., Koberna, S., Vetrova, M. V., Lodi, S., & Lunze, K. (2023). HIV, substance use, and intersectional stigma: Associations with mental health among persons living with HIV who inject drugs in Russia. *AIDS & Behavior, 27*(2), 431–442. https://doi.org/10.1007/s10461-022-03778-3

Kerr, J., Harris, L., Glass, E., Golden, T., & Crawford, T. (2020). "I shall live and not die": Using monologues based on the experiences of older African Americans living with HIV to address HIV-related stigma among African Americans in Louisville, Kentucky. *Family & Community Health: The Journal of Health Promotion & Maintenance, 43*(4), 257–263. https://doi.org/10.1097/FCH.0000000000000268

Li, A. T., Fung, K. P., Maticka-Tyndale, E., & Wong, J. P. (2018). Effects Of HIV stigma reduction interventions in diasporic communities: Insights from the CHAMP study. *AIDS Care, 30*(6), 739–745. https://doi.org/10.1080/09540121.2017.1391982

Li, L., Liang, L. J., Wu, Z., Lin, C., & Guan, J. (2014). Assessing outcomes of a stigma-reduction intervention with venue-based analysis. *Social Psychiatry and Psychiatric Epidemiology, 49*(6), 991–999. https://doi.org/10.1007/s00127-013-0808-6

Lodi, S., Rossi, S. L., Bendiks, S., Gnatienko, N., Lloyd-Travaglini, C., Vetrova, M., Toussova, O., Bushara, N., Blokhina, E., Krupitsky, E., Ekstrand, M. L., Lioznov, D., Samet, J. H., & Lunze, K. (2022). Correlates of intersectional hiv and substance use stigma affecting people with hiv and substance use in st. Petersburg, Russia. *AIDS and Behavior*. https://doi.org/10.1007/s10461-022-03781-8

Logie, C., & Gadalla, T. M. (2009). Meta-analysis of health and demographic correlates of stigma towards people living with HIV. *AIDS Care, 21*(6), 742–753. https://doi.org/10.1080/09540120802511877

Ma, P. H. X., Chan, Z. C. Y., & Loke, A. Y. (2019). Self-stigma reduction interventions for people living with HIV/AIDS and their families: A systematic review. *AIDS and Behavior, 23*(3), 707–741. https://doi.org/10.1007/s10461-018-2304-1

Mahajan, A. P., Sayles, J. N., Patel, V. A., Remien, R. H., & Ortiz, D. J. (2008). Stigma in the HIV/AIDS epidemic: A review of the literature and recommendations for the way forward. *AIDS, 22*(Suppl 2), S67–S79. https://doi.org/10.1097/01.aids.0000327438.13291.62

Mak, W. W., Cheng, S. S., Law, R. W., Cheng, W. W., & Chan, F. (2015). Reducing HIV-related stigma among health-care professionals: A game based experiential approach. *AIDS Care, 27*(7), 855–859. https://doi.org/10.1080/09540121.2015.1007113

Martin, R., Ashimosi, C., Nyandiko, W., Chory, A., Aluoch, J., Scanlon, M., & Vreeman, R. (2022). A systematic review of interventions to reduce HIV-related stigma among primary and secondary school teachers. *AIDS Care, 34*(1), 1–6. https://doi.org/10.1080/09540121.2021.1960264

Masa, R., Zimba, M., Tamta, M., Zimba, G., & Zulu, G. (2022). The association of perceived, internalized, and enacted HIV stigma with medication adherence, barriers to adherence, and mental health among young people living with HIV in Zambia. *Stigma Health, 7*(4), 443–453. https://doi.org/10.1037/sah0000404

Mevissen, F. E. F., Kok, G., Watzeels, A., van Duin, G., & Bos, A. E. R. (2018). Systematic development of a Dutch school-based sexual prejudice reduction program: An intervention mapping approach. *Sexuality Research & Social Policy, 15*(4), 433–451. https://doi.org/10.1007/s13178-017-0301-1

Meyer, I. H. (2003). Prejudice, social stress, and mental health in lesbian, gay, and bisexual populations: Conceptual issues and research evidence. *Psychological Bulletin, 129*(5), 674–697. https://doi.org/10.1037/0033-2909.129.5.674

Misir, P. (2015). Structuration theory: A conceptual framework for HIV/AIDS stigma. *Journal of the International Association of Providers of AIDS Care, 14*(4), 328–334. https://doi.org/10.1177/2325957412463072

Molero, F., Fuster, M. J., Jetten, J., & Moriano, J. A. (2011). Living with HIV/AIDS: A psychosocial perspective on coping with prejudice and discrimination. *Journal of Applied Social Psychology, 41*(3), 609–626. https://doi.org/10.1111/j.1559-1816.2011.00729.x

Muncan, B., Walters, S. M., Ezell, J., & Ompad, D. C. (2020). "They look at us like junkies": Influences of drug use stigma on the healthcare engagement of people who inject drugs in New York City. *Harm Reduction Journal, 17*, 53. https://doi.org/10.1186/s12954-020-00399-8

Nabunya, P., Migadde, H., Namuwonge, F., Mugisha, J., Kirabo, W., Ssentumbwe, V., Claire, N., Raymond, A., Bahar, O. S., Mwebembezi, A., McKay, M. M., & Ssewamala, F. M. (2024). Feasibility and acceptability of group-based stigma reduction interventions for adolescents living with HIV and their caregivers: The Suubi4Stigma randomized clinical trial (2020–2022). *AIDS and Behavior, 28*(5), 1630–1641. https://doi.org/10.1007/s10461-024-04284-4

Parker, R., & Aggleton, P. (2003). HIV and AIDS-related stigma and discrimination: A conceptual framework and implications for action. *Social Science & Medicine, 57*, 13–24. https://doi.org/10.1016/S0277-9536(02)00304-0

Pérez-Pedrogo, C., Planas-García, B. Y., Rivera-Suazo, S., Ortega-Guzmán, J. M., & Albizu-García, C. E. (2022). Preliminary feasibility and acceptability of a cultural adaptation of Acceptance and Commitment Therapy for Latinxs with HIV and drug use disorders in Puerto Rico. *Revista Puertorriqueña de Psicología, 33*(2), 232–243. https://doi.org/10.55611/reps.3302.03

Prinsloo, C. D., Greeff, M., Kruger, A., & Ellis, S. (2016). Psychosocial well-being of people living with HIV and the community before and after a HIV stigma-reduction community "hub" network intervention. *African Journal of AIDS Research, 15*(3), 261–271. https://doi.org/10.2989/16085906.2016.1200640

Reif, S., Cooper, H., Wilson, E., Brown, G., Beckwith, N., & Ward, D. (2021). HIV stigma reduction through peer-led advocacy training. *AIDS Education and Prevention, 33*(4), 303–311. https://doi.org/10.1521/aeap.2021.33.4.303

RIOD/Red Iberoamericana de Organizaciones no Gubernamentales que trabajan en drogas y adicciones. (2019). *Estigma, consumo de drogas y adicciones Conceptos, implicaciones y recomendaciones*. Disponible en https://riod.org/wp-content/uploads/2019/06/ESTIGMA-CONSUMO-DE-DROGAS-Y-ADICCIONES.pdf

Rueda, S., Mitra, S., Chen, S., Gogolishvili, D., Globerman, J., Chambers, L., Wilson, M., Logie, C. H., Shi, Q., Morassaei, S., & Rourke, S. B. (2016). Examining the associations between HIV-related stigma and health outcomes in people living with HIV/AIDS: a series of meta-analyses. *BMJ Open, 6*(7), e011453. https://doi.org/10.1136/bmjopen-2016-011453

Rzeszutek, M., Gruszczyńska, E., Pięta, M., & Malinowska, P. (2021). HIV/AIDS stigma and psychological well-being after 40 years of HIV/AIDS: A systematic review and meta-analysis. *European Journal of Psychotraumatology, 12*(1), 1990527. https://doi.org/10.1080/20008198.2021.1990527

Shrestha, R., Altice, F. L., & Copenhaver, M. M. (2019). HIV-related stigma, motivation to adhere to antiretroviral therapy, and medication adherence among HIV-positive methadone-maintained patients. *Journal of Acquired Immune Deficiency Syndromes, 80*(2), 166–173. https://doi.org/10.1097/QAI.0000000000001891

Sibley, A. L., Colston, D. C., & Go, V. F. (2024). Interventions to reduce self-stigma in people who use drugs: A systematic review. *Journal of Substance Use and Addiction Treatment, 159*, 209284. https://doi.org/10.1016/j.josat.2023.209284

Siegel, J., Yassi, A., Rau, A., Buxton, J. A., Wouters, E., Engelbrecht, M. C., Uebel, K. E., & Nophale, L. E. (2015). Workplace interventions to reduce HIV and TB stigma among health care workers: Where do we go from here? *Global Public Health: An International Journal for Research, Policy and Practice, 10*(8), 995–1007. https://doi.org/10.1080/17441692.2015.1021365

Sola-Morales, S., & Quiroz, C. (2019). Campañas de comunicación para la prevención del consumo de drogas en Chile (2004–2014) entre el prohibicionismo y la estigmatización. *Comunicación y Sociedad, 32*(2), 157–173.

Stangl, A. L., Atkins, K., Leddy, A. M., Sievwright, K. M., Sevelius, J. M., Lippman, S. A., Veras, M. A., Zamudio-Haas, S., Smith, M. K., Pachankis, J. E., Logie, C. H., Rao, D., Weiser, S., & Nyblade, L. (2023). What do we know about interventions to reduce intersectional stigma and discrimination in the context of HIV? A systematic review. *Stigma and Health, 8*(3), 393–340. https://doi.org/10.1037/sah0000414

Stutterheim, S. E., van der Kooij, Y. L., Crutzen, R., Ruiter, R. A. C., Bos, A. E. R., & Kok, G. (2023). Intervention mapping as a guide to developing, implementing, and evaluating stigma reduction interventions. *Stigma and Health*. Advance online publication. https://doi.org/10.1037/sah0000445

Todd, A. R., Galinsky, A. D., & Bodenhausen, G. V. (2012). Perspective taking undermines stereotype maintenance processes: Evidence from social memory, behavior explanation, and information solicitation. *Social Cognition, 30*(1), 94–108. https://doi.org/10.1521/soco.2012.30.1.94

Turan, B., Budhwani, H., Fazeli, P. L., Browning, W. R., Raper, J. L., Mugavero, M. J., & Turan, J. M. (2017). How does stigma affect people living with HIV? The mediating roles of internalized and anticipated HIV stigma in the effects of perceived community stigma on health and psychosocial outcomes. *AIDS and Behavior, 21*(1), 283–291. https://doi.org/10.1007/s10461-016-1451-5

Turan, B., Rice, W. S., Crockett, K. B., Johnson, M., Neilands, T. B., Ross, S. N., Kempf, M. C., Konkle-Parker, D., Wingood, G., Tien, P. C., Cohen, M., Wilson, T. E., Logie, C. H., Sosanya, O., Plankey, M., Golub, E., Adimora, A. A., Parish, C., Weiser, S. D., & Turan, J. M. (2019). Longitudinal association between internalized HIV stigma and antiretroviral therapy adherence for women living with HIV: The mediating role of depression. *AIDS, 33*(3), 571–576. https://doi.org/10.1097/QAD.0000000000002071

UNAIDS (2024). UNAIDS DATA 2024. Joint United Nations Programme on HIV/AIDS. Geneva. https://www.unaids.org/sites/default/files/media_asset/2024-unaids-global-aids-update-summary_es.pdf

Watt, M. H., Marchand, V., Barabara, M. L., Minja, L. M., Stephens, M. J., Hanson, O. R., Mlay, P. S., Olomi, G. A., Kiwia, J. F., Mmbaga, B. T., & Cohen, S. R. (2024). Outcomes of the MAMA training: A simulation and experiential learning intervention for labor and delivery providers to improve respectful maternity care for women living with HIV in Tanzania. *AIDS and Behavior, 28*(6), 1898–1911. https://doi.org/10.1007/s10461-024-04283-5

Wingood, G. M., & DiClemente, R. J. (2008). The ADAPT-ITT model: A novel method of adapting evidence-based HIV interventions. *Journal of Acquired Immune Deficiency Syndrome, 47*(Suppl. 1), S40–S45. https://doi.org/10.1097/QAI.0b013e3181605df1

Witkowski, K., Valerio, R., Samad, A., Matiz-Reyes, A., & Padilla, M. (2021). Aging and thriving with HIV: A photovoice project with long-term HIV survivors in Miami, Florida. *Arts & Health, 13*(3), 329–346. https://doi.org/10.1080/17533015.2020.1821386

Yuan, G. F., Tam, C. C., Yang, X., Qiao, S., Li, X., Shen, Z., & Zhou, Y. (2023). Associations between internalized and anticipated HIV stigma and depression symptoms among people living with HIV in China: A four-wave longitudinal model. *AIDS and Behavior, 27*(12), 4052–4061. https://doi.org/10.1007/s10461-023-04119-8

Yuan, G. F., Zhang, R., Qiao, S., Li, X., Zhou, Y., & Shen, Z. (2024). Longitudinal analysis of the relationship between internalized HIV Stigma, Perceived Social Support, Resilience, and depressive symptoms among people living with HIV in China: A Four-Wave Model. *AIDS and Behavior, 28*(2), 645–656. https://doi.org/10.1007/s10461-023-04251-5

Zhang, Y. X., Golin, C. E., Bu, J., Emrick, C. B., Nan, Z., & Li, M. Q. (2014). Coping strategies for HIV-related stigma in Liuzhou, China. *AIDS and Behavior, 18*(Suppl 2(02)), S212–S220. https://doi.org/10.1007/s10461-013-0662-2

Chapter 13
Intrafamily Violence, Substance Use, and Gender

Marianne Ramos Feijó, Eroy Aparecida da Silva, and Richard Alecsander Reichert

13.1 Introduction

Violence is a complex phenomenon that encompasses multiple dimensions, ranging from macrosocial and structural determinants to intrafamily dynamics. The word *violence* derives from the Latin *violentia*, meaning the act of violating, which includes physical, sexual, moral, and verbal constraints, as well as psychological coercion or force. It is manifested in contexts of unequal power relations, often taking the form of social domination and expropriation, whether political, economic, state, group, or familial. Additionally, violence presents various theoretical perspectives (Amparo et al., 2012; Arendt, 1970/2022; Mbembe, 2020; Minayo & Assis, 2017; Reichert et al., 2024; Zaluar, 1992).

Chauí (1998) asserts that violence is an act of brutality, cruelty, and psychic or physical abuse against a person, characterized by social, intersubjective, and intrafamily relations, defined by fear, terror, and oppression. According to the World Health Organization (WHO), self-directed violence refers to violent acts committed against oneself, including suicide attempts, suicide, and self-inflicted harm. Collective violence is perpetrated by political groups, terrorist organizations, and militias. Interpersonal violence can occur in domestic or community settings and is typically committed by intimate partners or family members (Dahlberg & Krug, 2002).

M. R. Feijó
Department of Psychology, Universidade Estadual Paulista, Bauru, SP, Brazil
e-mail: marianne.r.feijo@unesp.br

E. A. da Silva · R. A. Reichert (✉)
Department of Psychobiology, Universidade Federal de São Paulo, São Paulo, SP, Brazil
e-mail: reichert@unifesp.br

T. Mota Ronzani (ed.), *Social Stigma and Drug Use*,
https://doi.org/10.1007/978-3-031-94813-8_13

This chapter will emphasize interpersonal violence occurring within the context of intimate relationships, also known as domestic violence, as well as interpersonal violence experienced by individuals in street situations. In some cases, this violence occurs between individuals living in the same spaces, making it, therefore, potentially intimate. Intrafamily and interpersonal violence, harmful substance use, and other factors of social vulnerability will be addressed as processes and phenomena that weaken bonds between individuals. Gender constructions, which often lack sufficient equity, hinder the transformation of these relationships into sources of resilience and change (Amato et al., 2015; Malheiro, 2020).

Gender inequalities violate individuals and limit the construction of relationships that promote physical and mental health, which, in turn, depend on opportunities for expression and development being preserved and promoted. In families and in society at large, gender inequality remains the primary context in which violence occurs, and, as such, it has structural aspects. On the streets, conditions are more exposed and unprotected, which exacerbates the living conditions, particularly for women (Hochgraf & Brasiliano, 2023; Malheiro, 2020; Silva & Noto, 2022).

Miura et al. (2018) discussed the use of the terms *Domestic Violence* and *Intrafamily Violence* after conducting a systematic review of academic articles in the field of psychology. According to the authors, the use of the term *Domestic Violence* was unanimous in the articles reviewed when referring to gender-based violence and violence against women. However, when the violence referred to children and adolescents, they observed greater diversity in the terms used. Regarding violence against the elderly, they noted the prevalence of the term *Intrafamily Violence*. The authors emphasized the importance of not reducing the meaning of these terms in ways that limit understanding to the microsocial scope. They also pointed out that the term *domestic*, as addressed in the *Maria da Penha Law*[1] (Brasil, 2006), can refer to violence occurring in living spaces, regardless of whether there is a family bond, as seen in the case of employees and individuals identified as aggregates, who do not necessarily have a parental role and may live sporadically (Brasil, 2002).

[1] In the Brazilian context, the *Maria da Penha Law* (Lei Maria da Penha) is a comprehensive legal framework designed to combat and prevent domestic and family violence against women. Enacted in 2006, it aligns with both national and international Human Rights standards, including the Brazilian Constitution and various treaties such as the Convention on the Elimination of All Forms of Discrimination Against Women and the Inter-American Convention on the Prevention, Punishment, and Eradication of Violence Against Women. The law establishes mechanisms for the protection of women, including the creation of specialized Domestic and Family Violence Courts and measures for providing assistance to women in situations of violence. It ensures that women, regardless of class, race, ethnicity, sexual orientation, or any other factor, can live free from violence, enjoy their fundamental Human Rights, and access justice, health, education, and other essential services. The law emphasizes the importance of creating a supportive environment, with the shared responsibility of the family, society, and the state to ensure women's rights are upheld in both domestic and public spheres (Brasil, 2006).

In this chapter, the terms *intrafamily* and *interpersonal violence* will be used to emphasize that the discussion addresses violence between individuals who interact regularly, either in families or among people in street situations. Intrafamily or interpersonal violence can be characterized as actions or omissions that harm well-being, physical and psychological integrity, freedom, and the right to full development: physical, psychological, sexual, economic, or patrimonial abuse (Brasil, 2002). It is often associated with the use of psychoactive substances and intertwined with social inequalities such as gender (Soares et al., 2021).

Intrafamily violence is a complex and multicausal phenomenon that weakens families and worsens when other vulnerability factors are present. Material poverty, lack of access to rights such as housing, food, health, education, work, coexistence, and leisure can be seen as experiences of violence. When these experiences are associated with violent acts among family members or individuals who interact regularly, they greatly harm people, their development, health, and relationships (Feijó et al., 2017; Soares et al., 2021).

It is worth noting that isolating the effects of a substance as the sole cause of a violent act is not appropriate, as studies indicate that the process of violence, especially when it occurs among family members or intimate individuals, presents a history, the intertwining of various factors, and the relationship itself as aspects that must be considered to understand it. Even when a single violent act is committed by a person who does not know the other, but is carried out under the influence of a psychoactive substance, it is essential to consider that the substance aggravates and triggers aggressiveness and impulsivity, which have certain individual aspects, but also social and cultural dimensions. Racism, sexism, fatphobia, homophobia, transphobia, classism, and other prejudices can be expressed without filter under the influence of substances, by individuals who control or mask their violent and discriminatory actions when sober. The effect of substances, such as alcohol, can exacerbate violence under certain environmental and social conditions, and is therefore not a unique causal factor (Tondowski et al., 2014).

In this framework, social work with families assumes a dual function, as highlighted by Teixeira (2017) and Teixeira and Carloto (2020). It involves both integration into the service network to address vulnerabilities and the implementation of socio-educational actions that foster autonomy, agency, and social participation from an emancipatory standpoint. This mediation is essential in translating public policies into concrete actions within communities, ensuring citizen engagement and participation. It is crucial to distance oneself from theoretical and methodological approaches that perpetuate stereotypes and dominant values regarding family dynamics, framing social issues within a broader context of inequalities and exclusions. In opposition to such reductionist perspectives, the historical-dialectical approach provides a deeper understanding of reality, considering its historical and ontological dimensions. This perspective interprets social needs as expressions of unmet human demands, shaped by the unequal structure of capitalist society, where the concepts of rights and citizenship become central to guiding professional interventions.

13.2 Harmful Use and Dependence on Psychoactive Substances

Scholars, care professionals, and prevention specialists differentiate the terms associated with substance use, avoiding labels, prejudices, discriminatory acts, stigmas, and generalizations, as these distort practices and research related to the topic due to their judgmental nature. Despite this, according to Galduróz (2011) and Schimith et al. (2019), the terms "drug addiction" and "chemical dependence" are still used, and are not always distinguished from substance use. Galduróz (2011) identified the following research parameters: lifetime use, use in the year, use in the month, use in the last 30 days, frequent use (6 or more times in the last 30 days), heavy use (use 20 or more times in the last 30 days), abusive use (when apparent physical, mental, and social problems due to substance use are triggered), and dependence (when the individual can no longer fulfill their daily obligations due to substance use, experiencing adverse effects, and spending almost all of their time either under the influence of the substance, dealing with its effects, or trying to obtain more) (American Psychiatric Association [APA], 2022; World Health Organization [WHO], 2018).[2]

In this chapter, the term "dependence" is adopted, following Galduróz (2011), while the term "harmful use" is used, as it also appears in the scientific literature, to refer to substance use that harms others. Rather than using the term "drugs," the phrase "psychoactive substances"is prioritized, as it is less stigmatizing and encompasses both illicit substances and legal ones, such as alcohol, which affect the central nervous system (Chagas et al., 2021; Reichert et al., 2025). It is emphasized that

[2] Regarding official diagnostic manuals used by a large number of mental health professionals, the fifth revised edition of the DSM (DSM-5-TR), published in 2022, maintained the elimination of the categories of *"abuse"* and *"dependence"* on substances, which were present until the fourth edition of the DSM. The revision integrated recent scientific advancements, such as progress in genetics and neuroimaging, with the aim of improving the diagnosis and understanding of substance use disorders. In DSM-5-TR, the term *"dependence"* continues to be used by some professionals to refer to more severe presentations of substance use (APA, 2022). Regarding the ICD, the WHO revised diagnostic criteria across its versions, with ICD-10 and ICD-11 adopting classifications such as *"harmful use"* and *"dependence."* For the diagnosis of dependence, three or more specific criteria must be present over 12 months, including compulsive desire, difficulties in control, withdrawal symptoms, evidence of tolerance, and persistence in use despite harmful consequences (WHO, 2018). In the context of a biopsychosocial approach aligned with bioethical perspectives and the Harm Reduction approach, terminologies such as *"substance dependence," "drug dependence," "substance use disorder,"* and *"substance-related disorders"* have been gradually adopted to promote a broader and less stigmatized understanding of issues related to substance use. More recently, references to "people who use substances" or "people with substance-related needs" have emerged. These linguistic changes reflect a more comprehensive approach, considering not only biological aspects but also the psychological, social, and cultural factors involved in substance use (Chagas et al., 2021; Nathan et al., 2016; Reichert et al., 2025). This perspective is also aligned with the principles of Psychiatric Reform and the Anti-Asylum Movement, which emphasize human subjects rather than diagnostic categories per se, placing *"mental illness"* in parentheses to address and perceive the individual in their experience of suffering (Amarante, 2017; Reichert et al., 2024).

the situations of use, harmful use, and substance dependence require distinct professional and political responses. Dependence, in particular, necessitates specialized and multi-professional support, as well as specific preventive and protective measures, including harm reduction strategies. Furthermore, it is important to recognize that there is a broad spectrum between use and dependence (Silva et al., 2015). In both harmful use and dependence, the association with violence may occur, leading to significant biopsychosocial consequences (Dahlberg & Krug, 2002; Galduróz, 2011).

Studies on family violence associated with the use of psychoactive substances point to a series of vulnerability factors, which, in a cross-cutting and recursive way, contribute to the maintenance of both the use of violence and the harmful use of psychoactive substances, by people whose relationships and self-views can become increasingly weakened. The aggravation of violence and the progressive increase in the use of psychoactive substances, which are often discriminated behaviors, can generate stigma, which in turn, affects even more the people in question and their relationships (Feijó et al., 2017; Mardani et al., 2023; Monari et al., 2024; Silva & Noto, 2022; Substance Abuse and Mental Health Services Administration, 2020).

Living conditions, relationships, and health influence substance use, while, conversely, the harmful use of psychoactive substances has a reciprocal impact on the health and life of individuals who engage in such use (Ronzani, 2018; Silva et al., 2015). The type of use and the specific substance involved should also be considered. Alcohol, as a legal substance, is widely consumed in society, and the progression of alcohol dependence can be gradual and less perceptible within social groups that normalize its use, despite the potential adverse effects on relationships and the associated risks, such as accidents. Other substances include depressants, such as benzodiazepines, solvents, or inhalants; hallucinogens, such as marijuana, LSD, and ecstasy; and stimulants, such as amphetamines, cocaine, and nicotine. The effects, characteristics, and potential harms of these substances are diverse (Masur, 2004; Masur & Carlini, 2004). In families with children, the use of violence and psychoactive substances by adults significantly affects child development (Silva et al., 2015).

13.3 Integrative Perspective on Health and Bioecological Development

Systemic and new paradigmatic authors offer an integrative perspective on health, encompassing physical, psychological, and social dimensions, which influence each other in a recursive manner (Capra & Luisi, 2014; Morin, 2011). These authors address the concept of "unique health," representing a complex and multifaceted approach (Centers for Disease Control and Prevention [CDC], 2024; Langdon & Wiik, 2010; Morin, 2011), which includes the recursive relationship between humans, as well as the interactions between humans, other animals, and the environment. This perspective aligns with the bioecological view of development (Bronfenbrenner, 1996).

In the fields of Social Psychology, Health Anthropology, and other Health Sciences, the concept of vulnerability can be understood as an "analytical alternative," as described by Oviedo and Czeresnia (2015, p. 238). This perspective is framed as a possibility for understanding human behavior, social practices, and the processes of health and illness, including substance use and dependence, from a relational, complex, and dynamic approach (Reichert et al., 2019; Reichert, 2024). In this regard, it proposes a rupture with the biologicist, universalist, and individualist view of the biomedical model (Alves & Rabelo, 1998; Engel, 1977, 1980; Langdon & Wiik, 2010; Oviedo & Czeresnia, 2015; Sodelli, 2016).

Risk is generally defined as the probability or likelihood that an individual will contract a disease, experience violence, or suffer other forms of harm (Ferreira et al., 2021). Unfavorable social, economic, and political conditions are recognized as factors contributing to social vulnerability, which, in turn, weaken individuals and relationships. According to Ayres et al. (2003), individual vulnerability (including beliefs, knowledge, and behaviors) intersects with relational vulnerability factors (such as family and broader social contexts) and programmatic vulnerabilities, which refer to the needs for public policies, government actions, and social protection networks (Amato et al., 2015; Ayres et al., 2003; Reichert et al., 2019; Silva et al., 2015).

Violence is a factor of vulnerability for harmful use and for dependence on psychoactive substances, which in turn, is a factor of vulnerability for violence. Soares et al. (2021), in an integrative review conducted between 2013 and 2019 on the relationship between psychoactive substance consumption and domestic violence, indicated that psychoactive substances are one of the main factors in the occurrence of domestic violence, insofar as violent acts can be facilitated, influenced, motivated, or triggered by the use of psychoactive substances. They also showed that the use of psychoactive substances can be a consequence of violence, reinforcing that the latter is not a unicausal phenomenon.[3]

Early recreational or sporadic use of psychoactive substances can progress and evolve into dependence, which, in turn, rarely occurs in isolation from broader family and social difficulties. These situations are associated with the expression of psychological distress, which is aggravated by and interconnected with broader social issues, such as consumer culture, as well as ideals of pleasure and beauty (Feijó & Macedo, 2022). However, Walsh (2012) and Reichert et al. (2021a, 2021b) highlight the importance of identifying environmental variables (protective resources) that promote coping and adaptation repertoires, which emerge from

[3] Complementarily, in *Sociologie de la drogue*, Bergeron (2012) argues that the use or dependence on psychoactive substances does not constitute a determining or explanatory factor for violent behaviors or situations in a causal relationship. This is because (1) it is not a necessary condition, given that violence can occur independently of substance use, and (2) it is not a sufficient condition, since the use of psychoactive substances alone does not inherently trigger violent acts.

individuals' interactions with their environment and contribute to dealing with life's challenges—a concept Walsh (2012) refers to as "resilient forces."

Resilience is understood as the process through which individuals, families, or groups continue to develop in the face of adversity, shaped by the social and environmental conditions in which they are embedded, as well as the protective resources available to them (Reichert et al., 2021a, 2021b; Souza, 2011; Walsh, 2012). Resilience and vulnerability are, therefore, interwoven with life contexts and should not be perceived as immutable individual traits, in order to avoid reinforcing prejudices (Amato et al., 2015; Ayres et al., 2003). Factors such as access to secure and meaningful employment for adults, quality education for children and youth, opportunities for continuous learning, healthcare, adequate housing, food security, and well-planned leisure spaces are recognized as protective factors. Furthermore, family bonds and social support networks can serve as protective mechanisms, contributing to resilience processes that may persist across generations (Dalbosco et al., 2019). In contrast, certain relational dynamics and behaviors, such as the use of psychoactive substances and the adoption of violence as strategies to manage conflict and distress, can exacerbate vulnerability (da Silva, 2021; Minayo & Assis, 2017; Silva et al. 2015).

13.4 Substance Use, Violence, Inequalities, and Gender

Tondowski et al. (2014) described intergenerational patterns of family violence associated with harmful alcohol use, evidenced through genograms. In alignment with multigenerational family theories (Bowen, 1978; Cerveny, 2011), the authors demonstrated the intergenerational transmission of family violence associated with harmful alcohol use. This phenomenon involves the recurrence of behaviors, relational dynamics, and family patterns across generations, encompassing ways of managing conflicts, frustrations, deprivations, and difficulties, including relational and marital challenges (Tondowski et al., 2014).

To analyze intergenerational patterns of family violence associated with harmful alcohol use, Tondowski et al. (2014) conducted a study with 42 family members who had a history of such violence across generations. Using genograms constructed through interviews with a semi-structured script, the researchers identified distinct patterns of intergenerational repetition of family violence associated with harmful alcohol use, with more frequent recurrences observed in direct kinship lines (e.g., father-son relationships) and through marriage. The study also highlighted similarities in alcohol consumption patterns, types of violence, family responses, and specific stages of the family life cycle in which family violence associated with alcohol use intensified.

The findings of Tondowski et al. (2014) reinforce the notion of repeated patterns of violence and substance use across generations as a vulnerability factor, as highlighted by Feijó et al. (2017). These aspects contribute to the perpetuation of alcohol use and intimate partner violence, which is often reciprocal between spouses.

However, women tend to be more severely affected due to structural inequalities, including gender disparities (Carvalho et al., 2012; Hochgraf & Brasiliano, 2023; Feijó et al., 2017).

Although violence is a global public health issue, certain populations are disproportionately affected, as social differences are transformed into structural inequalities, exacerbating both suffering and violence itself. The COVID-19 pandemic, which recently impacted populations worldwide, intensified processes of violence and psychological distress, particularly among groups historically marginalized from access to rights and quality of life[4] (Centro de Estudos e Pesquisas em Emergências e Desastres em Saúde [CEPEDES], 2020; Hien et al., 2022; Khanlou et al., 2022).

Women and transgender people are identified as populations in need of continuous prevention and care, sustained by effective public policies and the social deconstruction of stereotypes, prejudices, and power relations that marginalize and leave them unprotected (Carvalho et al., 2012; Conselho Federal de Psicologia [CFP], 2019, 2024a; Oliveira, 2009). Children and the elderly, who are often affected by various forms of domestic violence, are also highlighted in the chapter as groups that should be prioritized in research and interventions. Even when they are not women, these individuals can be subjugated and weakened by power relations that are rooted in expectations of production, income, heteronormativity, and submission within their relationships—dynamics that persist in misogynistic, consumerist, ageist, and structurally violent contexts (Chang et al., 2021; Fang et al., 2022; Niu et al., 2024; Pillemer et al., 2016). Racism, particularly the intersection of conditions targeted by prejudice in society, should also be the focus of attention and serve as a guiding principle for preventive actions and care (Carvalho et al., 2012; CFP, 2017, 2022; Cunningham & Saleh, 2024; Ferrugem, 2019).

[4] In the Brazilian context, the COVID-19 pandemic highlighted significant disparities in access to healthcare services, which severely affected the homeless population (Reichert et al., 2021b; Reichert, 2024). A 2022 survey identified 236,400 individuals experiencing homelessness, representing one in every thousand people in the country. The Southeast region accounted for 62% of this population, with São Paulo having the highest number, housing 95,195 individuals (40% of the total). Key factors associated with homelessness included family problems (44%), unemployment (39%), alcohol and other psychoactive substance use (29%), and loss of housing (23%) (Ministério dos Direitos Humanos e Cidadania [MDHC], 2023). During the pandemic, the homeless population faced increased risks due to the high prevalence of respiratory issues, raising concerns among experts regarding the impact on physical and emotional health, particularly for individuals with anxiety and depression. Additionally, exposure to violence, substance use, and the deprivation of fundamental rights exacerbated this situation, emphasizing the need for public authorities to implement targeted care actions for this vulnerable group (Reichert et al., 2021b; Santiago, 2020). In São Paulo, the *Tem Sentimento* Collective, which supports women and LGBTQIAPN+ people experiencing homelessness and using alcohol, crack, and other substances, provided assistance during the COVID-19 pandemic and continues to engage with this population in the area. Additional information about the Collective can be found in Reichert (2024) and Silva and Campos-Boulitreau (2024). These references offer a comprehensive view of the psychosocial vulnerabilities, social inequalities, and structural violences to which women and LGBTQIAPN+ people are subjected, including gender-based violence and rights violations resulting from prohibitionist policies and the repression of substance use.

In Brazil, a country marked by deep inequalities, social, economic, and political conditions contribute to the exponential increase in violence, including crimes such as rape. At the same time, individuals are exposed to media appeals that equate social status and satisfaction with consumption, while many lack adequate social support, access to leisure opportunities, and essential services and rights necessary for survival (Campello et al., 2018; Ferreira et al., 2021; Magalhães et al., 2007). These dynamics reflect power relations that exacerbate the nature of violent acts and disproportionately impact groups already affected by exclusion and discrimination. Within these contexts, individuals may also internalize violence and perceive the consumption of psychoactive substances as a means of alleviating suffering (Soares et al., 2021; Zaluar, 2004).

Structural and macrosocial aspects further sustain violence, such as the neglect of elderly individuals and children, the exposure of young people to the allure of employment in drug trafficking—particularly those who see no future prospects in education or formal employment—and the precarious working conditions often imposed on Black and Brown individuals, who, when employed, frequently receive lower wages than others (Feijó & Macedo, 2022; Fernandes et al., 2022; Zaluar, 2004).

In a cross-sectional study conducted between 2016 and 2020 in São Paulo, Fernandes et al. (2022) investigated violence against homosexual, bisexual, and transgender individuals. The study analyzed 4828 notifications of suspected or confirmed cases of interpersonal violence, revealing that 51% of reported incidents involved Black and Brown individuals. Furthermore, 64.5% of the violent acts were committed by men, often linked to sexism, homophobia, transphobia, and generational conflicts. The study also identified a correlation between violence and alcohol consumption in many cases, as well as a higher incidence of violence among individuals with fewer years of education.

Although many reports document physical violence, it is important to consider the invisibility of other forms of violence, such as psychological abuse, as well as the underreporting of violence in private or closed environments, such as residences. Sexual violence, in particular, often remains concealed, while other forms of violence may take time to be reported—or may never be—due to psychological and financial factors (Izumi, 2015; Minayo & Assis, 2017; Rutherford et al., 2007; Soares et al., 2021; WHO, 2002).

A recent cross-sectional study (Mota et al., 2024), conducted between 2019 and 2021, examined transvestites and trans women over 18 years of age residing in Brazilian cities, specifically São Paulo, Porto Alegre, Salvador, Manaus, and Campo Grande. The study found that 49.3% of participants reported multiple psychoactive substance use in the past 12 months, with alcohol (65.5%), tobacco (52.9%), and marijuana (40.1%) being the most commonly used substances. The findings indicate that those engaged in multiple substance use were more exposed to situations of violence, unemployment, and unstable employment, in addition to being more frequently involved in transactional sex, possibly due to limited economic opportunities. The authors suggest that this pattern of substance use may serve as a strategy to cope with suffering and social marginalization, despite being associated with various health risks and harms. The study underscores the importance of ensuring comprehensive care for this population, guided by the principles of the Brazilian Unified Health System (SUS) —universality, equality, and integrality—given that transvestites and trans women often face stigma and abandonment, including exclusion from their own family circles.

Regarding domestic violence against children, Domingues (2024) highlights that, despite advancements in child protection laws, the data remain alarming. In 2022, police reports indicated a 16% increase in cases of rape and sexual exploitation of children and adolescents. Among the victims, 90% were female, 61% were under 14 years old, and 56% were Black. In 68% of cases, sexual violence occurred at home, and in 86% of cases, the perpetrators were family members or individuals known to the child or adolescent. A study conducted by the Institute of Applied Economic Research (IPEA, 2021), a Brazilian government-led research organization, found that 29% of sexual violence victims were children under 11 years old, and 45% of perpetrators were family members. Additionally, data from the Ministry of Women, Family, and Human Rights' Dial Denunciation service reported 197,401 violent incidents against children up to nine years old in the first half of 2022. The primary types of violence recorded were physical violence, psychological abuse, and neglect.

Reichenheim et al. (2011) conducted an extensive study on violence and highlighted research on intimate partner violence across sixteen major Brazilian cities. The study revealed that 78.3% of the cases involved psychological violence, 21.5% involved minor physical abuse, and 12.9% involved severe physical abuse. Izumi (2015) provided a detailed sociodemographic profile of women in situations of violence and at risk of death, who were attended at a Women's Reference Center (CRM) and referred to a shelter house between 2011 and 2014. According to the author, power relations are reproduced within the domestic space, reflecting the hierarchical and asymmetric gender roles that have been socially and historically constructed. Men are legitimized to exercise force and power, while women are relegated to positions of subjugation and subordination. An analysis of 967 records of women attended by the CRM Casa Brasilândia from 2011 to 2014 showed that among the 72 women who were sheltered, there was a predominance of those aged between 20 and 29 years, with relatively few years of schooling. Most of the sheltered women (45.8%) had incomplete primary education, meaning less than eight years of schooling. Additionally, 55.6% were Black, and 41.7% did not have formal employment. 63.9% of these women had no income, and 83.3% had between one and four children.

Exclusion, along with the experience of prejudice, discrimination, and stigma, is a factor that increases the potential for exposure to harm (Monteiro & Villela, 2013). For example, people living on the streets may suffer violence from those they interact with daily. This occurs within the microsystem of relationships, as seen in cases of intrafamily violence (Silva & Noto, 2022). In addition to the homeless population, individuals with disabilities, LGBTQIAPN+ people, brown and Black people, Indigenous peoples, immigrants, women, the elderly, and sheltered children may experience violence (CFP, 2017, 2019, 2022, 2024a, 2024b, 2024c, 2024d; Oliveira,

2022; Pagot, 2012). This is especially true when they are deprived of spaces and opportunities for self-expression, legitimacy, work, income, or other means of development. These groups may live in relationships that are violent and devoid of dignity. Such relationships impact their family dynamics and are influenced by them. The internalization of violence and stigma follows individuals in their different living environments. Collectives, however, can act as islands of exception, offering greater protagonism and resilience building (Minayo & Assis, 2017; Silva, 2024). Nevertheless, public policies are essential to ensure access to rights and greater equity. They should be coupled with effective public security that respects and guarantees the dignity of individuals. The diversity of their characteristics, behaviors, and relationships must be valued in interactions between different groups.

13.5 Public Policies and Different Actions of Care with Families

Care for families experiencing suffering, difficulties, and seeking professional help has evolved since the inception of family therapy to the present day. Systemic-cybernetic family therapy, characterized by the greater participation of professionals in interventions aimed at changing family relationships, remained predominant until 1980. At that time, new scientific paradigms, theories, and epistemological foundations began to support practices referred to as new-paradigmatic systemic, constructionist, narrative, collaborative, appreciative, or restorative. These contemporary practices share complex thinking as their foundation, focusing on dialogue and the joint construction of new meanings according to the needs and values of the people involved, as well as their surroundings (Anderson, 2016; Grandesso, 2019). They seek to avoid colonization, blaming, and promote the recognition of different ways of living, loving, and being a family (Feijó & Macedo, 2022). These practices are based on complex systemic thinking, which holds that relationships, processes, and contexts require a careful examination for a multilevel understanding that includes recursive circularity.

An example of such an understanding is Bronfenbrenner's bioecological model (1996) for understanding human development and health, called the PPCT model (Person, Process, Context, and Time). Individual, procedural, micro, meso, exo, and macrosocial aspects intersect at certain times and places and should be considered when a person or family narrates experiences of violence, their needs, and care demands. The professional seeks to identify aspects of vulnerability and resilience intertwined at different instances and levels to collaboratively work with the family in constructing new living possibilities, means of protection, and the interruption of violent processes.

Care for families where violence is present requires, in addition to non-discriminatory dialogue, the avoidance of amplifying stigma in the attempt to build human security (Minayo & Assis, 2017; Monteiro & Villela, 2013; Oliveira, 2020;

Rocha, 2017). This approach aims to guarantee the survival of both individual and relational bonds within the family system, ensuring well-being with dignity in social coexistence. Friede (2021) emphasizes that the existence of a territory with quality of life is related to the expansion of equity and access to rights, such as coexistence and leisure in more peaceful, diverse, and sustainable cities. Public security, integrated and associated with other violence reduction strategies, is ineffective without adequate social, economic, educational, and political conditions that allow families to experience quality of life. The expansion of development perspectives, the preservation of family relationships, access to work, and relationships that allow for greater equity and access to rights are paramount.

Individuals and families present singularities and commonalities, in addition to aspects of resilience and exposure to vulnerability factors. Resilience, according to Souza (2011) and Walsh (2012), is a set of strengths of a person or a group that allow them to face adversities and continue developing despite them. Among the family strengths is the way people take care of each other and how they divide and lead functions and tasks. The family configuration should not be questioned, as there are many types of families,[5] and what matters are their bonds and the sense of belonging of each of its components. The promotion of strengths and the legitimization of the various ways of being a family, of conducting life and facing difficulties, should be the focus of professional action, which collaborates with the construction of new possibilities and new meanings, with support to reduce vulnerability factors that affect people, their relationships, and behaviors (Amparo et al., 2012; Minayo & Assis, 2017; Teixeira, 2017; Teixeira & Carloto, 2020).

It is understood that individual, microsocial (family), macrosocial, and programmatic aspects intersect and result in certain vulnerability factors, which affect individuals and, therefore, families. This aligns with the idea that individuals and

[5] Carloto (2020) e Ceará-Silva et al. (2020) operate under the premise that history is not free from ideological construction and analyze the influence of this ideology on the concept of family, discussing the constitution and definition of the "model family" throughout history. The authors address the importance of a counter-ideological force in public policies related to families, with the aim of promoting social policies linked to counter-hegemonic projects and enabling the construction of new paths. In dialogue with authors such as Bauman (1999), Agamben (2010), Mbembe (2020), and Butler (2017), the authors discuss the paradigms of contemporary society and the way in which policies were constituted, considering that certain lives—those of individuals, social groups, and populations—may be disqualified, invisibilized, or eliminated. Moreover, the critique addresses how affective bonds that sustain families and communities can be undone in favor of economic development within capitalist logic. In this context, it becomes essential to make historical connections, that is, to promote the exercise of thought regarding what is understood as family, avoiding simplifications that do not encompass human plurality and its countless possibilities of arrangements. Thus, it is necessary to engage in a complex process to criticize the hegemonic family model, centered on heterosexual, nuclear, and gendered marriage. In a reality where homocentered, single-parent, Black, and poor families are disregarded, it is essential to qualify their lives so that they are recognized as deserving of protection, paying attention to the diversity of ways of existing and perceiving their real needs, which means recognizing these groups as human beings and subjects of rights (Carloto, 2020; Ceará-Silva et al., 2020).

families should not be blamed but understood in context, taking into account structural issues—therefore, cultural, economic, and political (Silva et al., 2015).

Research on substance dependence, supported by notions of vulnerability and resilience at individual, social, and programmatic levels (Feijó et al., 2017, 2024; Soares et al., 2021), demonstrated that in situations of recurrent violence and psychoactive substance dependence, vulnerability factors stand out compared to resilience factors, which require various care strategies to be enhanced.

Dependence on psychoactive substances, when the reason for seeking health services, should also be understood in a complex and bioecological way, which includes family and macrosocial history. Individual, microsocial, and macrosocial aspects should be understood, considering the process of repeating patterns (behavioral, relational, vital conditions), histories of violence, and family and marital difficulties. Lack of income and work tend to amplify marital and family difficulties, aggravate conflicts, psychological suffering, and the use of violence associated with the progression of psychoactive substance use (Feijó et al., 2017).

The family clinic, an important space for care and interruption of patterns of violence and harmful substance use, should be made more widely and democratically available to the population, which also lacks public policies aimed at equity and various means of reducing social vulnerability. Despite violence being presented as a global phenomenon that affects different groups, those who already suffer from a lack of decent living conditions and who have historically been more frequently victims of discrimination should be prioritized in such policies.

It is also worth noting that, from the point of view of Bioethics, a distinction must be made between existential vulnerability and programmatic vulnerability or violation[6] (Cruz & Taquette, 2020; Junges et al., 2018; de Morais & Monteiro, 2017; Rodrigues & Schramm, 2022). The latter is a condition of social, psychological, and

[6] The scientific bioethics literature distinguishes the concepts of existential vulnerability and programmatic vulnerability or violation (which, in Brazilian bioethics literature, is translated as *"vul neração"*, a new analytical category). *Existential vulnerability* refers to an intrinsic condition of the human experience, while *programmatic vulnerability* or *violation* pertains to exposure that exacerbates this fragility, with implications such as rights violations, intensification of inequalities, and worsening conditions for affected individuals (Cruz & Taquette, 2020; Gomes et al., 2022; Junges et al., 2018; de Morais & Monteiro, 2017; Rodrigues & Schramm, 2022). In the context of substance use, these concepts are particularly relevant, especially when considering programmatic vulnerability, which amplifies the risks and potential harms of substance use, exacerbated by ineffective and iatrogenic policies. The case of women and LGBTQIAPN+ people experiencing homelessness and substance use in the Luz region of São Paulo, pejoratively known as *"Crackland"* (a public space where substances such as alcohol and crack cocaine are openly consumed), exemplifies this dynamic. When analyzing the trajectories of this population, it is observed that many cis, trans, and transvestite women have been marginalized by their families and communities, with the streets becoming the space for survival and socialization, exposing them to risks such as discrimination, physical and psychological violence, sexual abuse, among others (Reichert, 2024). In this context, these people face exclusion in educational, professional, and political spheres, hindering access to social and healthcare services. Prohibitionist policies, often aimed at social and racial hierarchization, intensify repressive measures and deepen inequalities, resulting in violations of the fundamental rights of this population and exacerbating the scarcity of resources, both material and immaterial, such as emotional support, access to information, and support networks (Reichert

physical health misery, that is, complete abandonment. Families in a state of programmatic vulnerability or violation often stay away from inclusive public policies and, therefore, tend to live situations of constant violence and abuse on the streets, which end up reproducing them in their own bonds, thus forming a "spiral of violence". Building public policies for families with their participation in the process is more than necessary in Brazil. This construction goes beyond welfare benefits—also necessary—but the construction of guarantees of legitimate rights to a dignified life.

In the context of international drug[7] policies, significant disparities persist, necessitating an intersectional approach to understanding how gender, race, and class shape the experiences of specific social groups. The intersection of gender and racial biases has a particularly pronounced impact on racialized women, as well as on their children, families, and communities (Csete et al., 2016; Ferrugem, 2019; Perussolo et al., 2019). Given this scenario, the development of gender-sensitive policies is essential to mitigating the adverse effects of drug laws and policies on women and their families. Among the possible strategies, particular emphasis should be placed on reducing prison sentences for women convicted of non-violent offenses. This consideration is especially relevant since women are disproportionately incarcerated for drug-related offenses compared to men. Additionally, expanding access to social and healthcare support services—including substance use treatment tailored to gender-specific needs—is crucial to promoting more equitable and effective drug policies (Csete et al., 2016).

Another possible analysis of the international family-level impacts resulting from prohibition and repression policies on psychoactive substances highlights the adverse consequences of these measures, particularly regarding coercive practices targeting people who cultivate crops used in substance production, such as coca leaf, opium poppy, and cannabis. The forced displacement of rural families in vulnerable situations, often without secure land tenure, exacerbates poverty and food insecurity and, in some cases, leads them to migrate to more marginal regions to sustain cultivation. Furthermore, the geographical isolation resulting from these

---

et al., 2023). These processes generate ethical-political suffering, characterized by the denial of basic rights and the perpetuation of a cycle of exclusion and violence (Sawaia, 2014).

[7] At this point in the text, the use of the term "drug" refers to the arbitrary classification of psychoactive substances in international policies, which divides them into legal and illegal categories, with moral, medicinal, and legal implications (Bergeron, 2012). However, there are numerous controversies in the health field regarding its definition, as pointed out by Fiore (2006). Etymologically, "drug" originates from the Dutch word *"droog,"* meaning "dry products," a term associated with cultural exchanges during the Crusades and the Age of Exploration. Throughout history, cultural and political factors, such as cosmological, aesthetic, and hygienist views, have influenced the use and conceptions of substances, leading to the eradication of local psychoactive plants by colonizers and the consolidation of a coloniality of knowledge. This process was marked by the opposition of Christianity to other religions, the pursuit of a monoculture of Christian thought, and economic and geopolitical interests. Currently, the knowledge about "drugs" is largely influenced by the biomedical perspective and criminalization, with social and structural impacts that primarily affect vulnerable individuals, families, and communities (Costa, 2021).

dynamics compromises cultivators' access to state-led public health and education campaigns while also distancing them from basic healthcare services (Csete et al., 2016).

Regarding young people, Zaluar (2004) argues that prohibitionist policies have fostered the consolidation of a "*warrior ethos*," sustained by a repressive logic linked to the "war on drugs." Among the factors contributing to violence, the author points to the disintegration of community organizations and socializing agencies, as well as exclusion from educational, professional, and political spheres. The continuous diffusion of capitalist values through the media also fosters a scenario in which ethical principles are subordinated to immediate gratifications. Furthermore, the historical subordination of social policies to the capital accumulation process undermines social development in Brazil, particularly in areas such as education, work, and health. The absence of socio-familial support and future prospects can lead young people to reproduce violent patterns and engage in illicit activities, in which, according to Bourgois (2003), extreme violence becomes functional and rewarded, a dynamic that Becker (2008) defines as "motivation for a deviant act." As an alternative, Zaluar (2004) proposes intersectoral projects that integrate public participation, the implementation of decentralized ombudsman networks, the expansion of educational opportunities, and the provision of professional and sports training programs, focusing on promoting values of peaceful relationships and collective cooperation. These initiatives strengthen family and community bonds, stimulate the active participation of children, young people, and adults, and contribute to the development of citizenship and democratic coexistence.

13.6 Final Considerations

Violence arises when there is a lack of words, dignified expression, and rights. It emerges when dialogue is insufficient to guarantee the development of each person in the family and society, as well as the free expression of ideas. Harmful use and dependence on substances also manifest in more severe forms, associated with violence, when living conditions are unsatisfactory and freedom is restricted.

The cultivation of democracy and dialogue in conflict resolution, as well as the confrontation of issues that generate suffering and misunderstandings, is necessary. The appreciation of people with different identities—gender, ethnicity, generation, and ways of presenting and relating—should also be fostered. This goes beyond promoting spaces of separate coexistence, which segregate groups in families, schools, workplaces, and other public spaces such as the city itself. Exclusion is a form of violence that internalizes and underlies many other forms of violence, both suffered and perpetrated. Therefore, peaceful coexistence and the legitimization of differences should be valued and encouraged through the construction of inclusive public policies. These policies should broadly involve support for solidarity-based economies, art and culture, access to health, education, and the guarantee of rights (Silva & Campos-Bolitreau, 2024).

In unequal societies with a lack of opportunities for study, employment, and qualified income, young people and other groups are often poorly understood in their needs, including how they love and build families. The demands between partners and between parents and children, who live in a consumerist, individualistic, and meritocratic society, present rigid challenges that cannot be resolved through dignified coexistence for those who do not conform to media and heteronormative standards.

As briefly discussed in this chapter, there are many factors of vulnerability or violations that perpetuate violence associated with harmful use of psychoactive substances. However, the lack of decent work, income, and the guarantee of basic rights should be highlighted. The overlap of roles, especially for women, is also a factor of individual, couple, and family weakening, hindering the balance between family, work, leisure, and rest, which is essential for health. Parallel, but not dissociated from such difficulty, the appeal to consumption and financial dependence are aspects that oppress people and limit autonomy, which is also necessary for development, expression, and the transformation of patterns that maintain violence and harmful substance use.

The experiences of discrimination and internalized stigma by populations victimized by prejudice and lack of decent conditions—such as food, housing, health, and education—need to remain at the center of discussions in the construction, expansion, review, and monitoring of public policies.

References

Agamben, G. (2010). *Homo Sacer: O poder soberano e a vida nua*. Editora UFMG.

Alves, P. C. B., & Rabelo, M. C. (Eds.). (1998). *Antropologia da saúde: Traçando identidade e explorando fronteiras*. Editora FIOCRUZ. https://doi.org/10.7476/9788575414040

Amarante, P. (2017). *Teoria e crítica em saúde mental: textos selecionados*. Zagodoni.

Amato, T. C., Ronzani, T. M., & Noto, A. R. (2015). Resiliência: Contribuições das evidências científicas para a construção do conceito. In E. A. Silva, Y. G. Moura, & D. Zugman (Eds.), *Vulnerabilidades, resiliência e redes – Uso, abuso e dependências de drogas* (pp. 171–180). Red.

American Psychiatric Association (APA). (2022). *Diagnostic and statistical manual of mental disorders* (5th ed., text rev.). American Psychiatric Association.

Amparo, D. M., Almeida, S. F. C., Brasil, K. T. R., Conceição, M. I. G., & Marty, F. (2012). *Adolescência e violência: Intervenções e estudos clínicos, psicossociais e educacionais*. Editora UnB.

Anderson, H. (2016). Algumas considerações sobre o convite ao diálogo. *Nova Perspectiva Sistêmica, 25*(56), 49–54.

Arendt, H. (2022). *Sobre a violência*. Civilização Brasileira. (Originally published in 1970).

Ayres, J. R. C. M., Franca Junior, I., Calazans, G. J., & Saletti Filho, H. C. (2003). O conceito de vulnerabilidade e as práticas de saúde: Novas perspectivas e desafios. In D. Czeresnia & C. M. Freitas (Eds.), *Promoção da saúde: Conceitos, reflexões, tendências* (pp. 117–138). FIOCRUZ.

Bauman, Z. (1999). Globalização: As consequências humanas. .

Becker, H. (2008). *Outsiders: Estudos de sociologia do desvio*. Zahar. (Trabalho original publicado em 1963).

Bergeron, H. (2012). *Sociologia da droga*. Ideias & Letras.
Bourgois, P. (2003). *In search of respect: Selling crack in El Barrio*. Cambridge University Press.
Bowen, M. (1978). *Family therapy in clinical practice*. Jason Aronson.
Brasil. (2002). *Violência intrafamiliar: Orientações para a prática em serviço*. Secretaria de Políticas de Saúde, Ministério da Saúde. Recuperado de http://bvsms.saude.gov.br/bvs/publicacoes/cd05_19.pdf
Brasil. (2006). *Lei n. 11.340, de 7 de agosto de 2006. Dispõe sobre a Lei Maria da Penha*. Recuperado de http://www.planalto.gov.br/ccivil_03/_ato2004-2006/2006/lei/l11340.htm
Bronfenbrenner, U. (1996). *A ecologia do desenvolvimento humano: Experimentos naturais e planejados*. Artes Médicas.
Butler, J. (2017). *Quadros de Guerra: Quando a vida é possível de luto?* Civilização Brasileira.
Campello, T., Gentili, P., Rodrigues, M., & Hoewell, G. R. (2018). Faces da desigualdade no Brasil: Um olhar sobre os que ficam para trás. *Saúde em Debate, 42*, 54–66. https://doi.org/10.1590/0103-11042018S305
Capra, F., & Luisi, P. L. (2014). *A visão sistêmica da vida: Uma concepção unificada e suas implicações filosóficas, políticas, sociais e econômicas*. Cultrix.
Carloto, C. M. (2020). Cuidados, produção e reprodução social: Uma abordagem a partir da economia feminista. In S. M. Teixeira & C. M. Carloto (Eds.), *Família, cuidado e políticas sociais* (pp. 49–63). Papel Social.
Carvalho, A. P. C., Salaini, C. J., Allebrandt, D., Meinerz, N. E., & Weisheimer, N. (2012). *Desigualdades de gênero, raça e etnia*. Intersaberes.
Ceara-Silva, G. L., Freitas, R. C. S., & Barros, N. V. (2020). Nós bem efeitos em fios puídos: Famílias enredadas em tempos de exceção. In S. M. Teixeira & C. M. Carloto (Eds.), *Família, cuidado e políticas sociais* (pp. 27–47). Papel Social.
Centers for Disease Control and Prevention (CDC). (2024). *About CDC's One Health Office*. Recuperado de https://www.cdc.gov/one-health/php/about/?CDC_AAref_Val=https://www.cdc.gov/onehealth/who-we-are/index.html
Centro de Estudos e Pesquisas em Emergências e Desastres em Saúde (CEPEDES). (2020). *Saúde mental e atenção psicossocial na pandemia COVID-19: Violência doméstica e familiar na COVID-19*. Fundação Oswaldo Cruz. Recuperado de https://www.fiocruzbrasilia.fiocruz.br/wp-content/uploads/2020/04/Sa%C3%BAde-Mental-e-Aten%C3%A7%C3%A3o-Psicossocial-na-Pandemia-Covid-19-viol%C3%AAncia-dom%C3%A9stica-e-familiar-na-Covid-19.pdf
Cerveny, C. (2011). *A família como modelo: Desconstruindo patologias* (2a ed.). Livro Pleno.
Chagas, C., de Paula, T. C. S., & Galduróz, J. C. F. (2021). A linguagem e o estigma: Os termos utilizados na área de álcool e outras drogas. *Epidemiologia e Serviços de Saúde, 30*(1). https://doi.org/10.1590/S1679-49742021000100024
Chang, E. S., Monin, J. K., Zelterman, D., & Levy, B. R. (2021). Impact of structural ageism on greater violence against older persons: A cross-national study of 56 countries. *BMJ Open, 11*(5), e042580. https://doi.org/10.1136/bmjopen-2020-042580
Chauí, M. (1998). Ensaio ética e violência. *Revista Teoria e Debate, 11*(39).
Conselho Federal de Psicologia (CFP). (2017). *Relações raciais: Referências técnicas para atuação de psicólogas/os*. CFP.
Conselho Federal de Psicologia (CFP). (2019). *Tentativas de aniquilamento de subjetividades LGBTIs*. CFP.
Conselho Federal de Psicologia (CFP). (2022). *Psicologia brasileira na luta antirracista*. CFP e Comissão de Direitos Humanos do Conselho Federal de Psicologia.
Conselho Federal de Psicologia (CFP). (2024a). *Mulheres, psicologia e enfrentamento às violências*. CFP.
Conselho Federal de Psicologia (CFP). (2024b). *Nota técnica sobre atuação de psicólogas (os) junto aos povos indígenas*. CFP.
Conselho Federal de Psicologia (CFP). (2024c). *XII Seminário de Psicologia e Políticas Públicas: interface entre psicologia e populações em situação de refúgio, migração e apatridia*. CFP.

Conselho Federal de Psicologia (CFP). (2024d). *Referências técnicas para atuação de psicólogas(os) no atendimento às mulheres em situação de violência*. CFP.

Costa, J. A. C. (2021). A colonialidade do saber sobre as drogas. In B. G. S. Favaretto & P. G. Marson (Eds.), *Drogas: O que sabemos sobre?* (pp. 15–35). Appris.

Cruz, J. D. R., & Taquette, S. R. (2020). Viver na rua: Vulnerações e a bioética da proteção. *Revista Bioética, 28*(4), 427–436. https://doi.org/10.1590/1983-80422020284427

Csete, J., Kamarulzaman, A., Kazatchkine, M., Altice, F., Balicki, M., Buxton, J., Cepeda, J., Comfort, M., Goosby, E., Goulão, J., Hart, C., Kerr, T., Lajous, A. M., Lewis, S., Martin, N., Mejía, D., Camacho, A., Mathieson, D., Obot, I., Ogunrombi, A., et al. (2016). Public health and international drug policy. *Lancet (London, England), 387*(10026), 1427–1480. https://doi.org/10.1016/S0140-6736(16)00619-X

Cunningham, J. K., & Saleh, A. A. (2024). Structural stigma, racism, and sexism studies on substance use and mental health: A review of measures and designs. *Alcohol Research: Current Reviews, 44*(1), 08. https://doi.org/10.35946/arcr.v44.1.08

da Silva, E. A. (2021). Conceptual and practical horizons of systemic family psychotherapy and substance use. In A. L. M. Andrade, D. De Micheli, E. A. da Silva, F. M. Lopes, B. d. O. Pinheiro, & R. A. Reichert (Eds.), *Psychology of substance abuse* (pp. 289–299). Springer. https://doi.org/10.1007/978-3-030-62106-3_20

Dahlberg, L. L., & Krug, E. G. (2002). Violência: Um problema global de saúde pública. In E. G. Krug, L. L. Dahlberg, J. A. Mercy, A. B. Zwi, & R. Lozano (Eds.), *Relatório mundial sobre violência e saúde* (pp. 1–22). OMS.

Dalbosco, C., Veiga, J., & Sudbrack, M. F. O. (Eds.). (2019). Prevenção ao uso de álcool e outras drogas em contexto escolar e outros espaços: Fortalecendo as redes sociais e de cuidados. Technopolitik.

de Morais, T. C. A., & Monteiro, P. S. (2017). Conceitos de vulnerabilidade humana e integridade individual para a bioética. *Revista Bioética, 25*(2), 311–319. https://doi.org/10.1590/1983-80422017252191

de Oliveira, M. R. (2009). *No limiar da memória: Estudo antropológico sobre mulheres e violências na metrópole contemporânea* (Tese de Doutorado), Universidade Federal de Santa Catarina). Retireved from https://repositorio.ufsc.br/xmlui/handle/123456789/89718.

Domingues, T. L. C. (2024). *Saúde pública na atenção individual e familiar de criança vítima de violência doméstica* (Tese de Doutorado), Universidade Estadual Paulista "Júlio de Mesquita Filho."

Engel, G. L. (1977). The need for a new medical model: a challenge for biomedicine. *Science (New York, NY), 196*(4286), 129–136. https://doi.org/10.1126/science.847460

Engel, G. L. (1980). The clinical application of the biopsychosocial model. *The American Journal of Psychiatry, 137*(5), 535–544. https://doi.org/10.1176/ajp.137.5.535

Fang, Z., Cerna-Turoff, I., Zhang, C., Lu, M., Lachman, J. M., & Barlow, J. (2022). Global estimates of violence against children with disabilities: An updated systematic review and meta-analysis. *The Lancet. Child & Adolescent Health, 6*(5), 313–323. https://doi.org/10.1016/S2352-4642(22)00033-5

Feijó, M. R., & Macedo, R. M. S. (2022). Adolescentes na contemporaneidade: Resiliência, vulnerabilidade e necessidades. In R. M. S. Macedo & I. Kublikowski (Eds.), *Família e comunidade: Interfaces da psicologia clínica* (pp. 45–56). CRV.

Feijó, M. R., Noto, A. R., Silva, E. A., Locatelli, D. P., Camargo, M. L., & Gebara, C. F. P. (2017). Álcool e violência das relações conjugais: Um estudo qualitativo com casais. *Psicologia em Estudo, 21*(4), 581–592. https://doi.org/10.4025/psicolestud.v21i4.31556

Fernandes, H., Bertini, P. V. R., Hino, P., Taminato, M., Silva, L. C. P., Adriani, P. A., & Ranzani, C. M. (2022). Interpersonal violence against homosexual, bisexual and transgender people. *Acta Paul Enferm, 35*, eAPE01486. https://doi.org/10.37689/acta-ape/2022AO014866

Ferreira, B. S., Melo, A. F., Guarino, P. C., & Jordão, M. P. D. (2021). Crimes violentos letais e intencionais (CVLI): Fatores e motivações que os influenciam em consonância com as políticas

de segurança pública. *Revista Brasileira de Segurança Pública, 15*(2), 12–27. https://doi.org/10.31060/rbsp.2021.v15.n2.1174
Ferrugem, D. (2019). *Guerra às drogas e a manutenção da hierarquia racial*. Letramento.
Fiore, M. (2006). *"Drogas": Controvérsias médicas e debate público*. Mercado de Letras.
Friede, R. (2021). A segurança humana no contexto de uma cidade educadora. *Revista Brasileira de Segurança Pública, 15*(2), 28–43. https://doi.org/10.31060/rbsp.2021.v15.n2.1202
Galduróz, J. C. F. (2011). Epidemiologia do uso de substâncias psicotrópicas no Brasil: Dados recentes. In *Secretaria Nacional de Políticas sobre Drogas, Prevenção ao uso indevido de drogas: Capacitação para Conselheiros e Lideranças Comunitárias* (pp. 55–72). SENAD. Recuperado de https://www.uniad.org.br/wp-content/uploads/2011/12/livro_completoiv_oficial-copia.pdf#page=55
Gomes, D., Molina, L. R., & Finkler, M. (2022). Vulneração social e problemas ético-políticos transversais à saúde bucal na Atenção Primária à Saúde. *Saúde Debate, 46*(133), 392–404. https://doi.org/10.1590/0103-1104202213310
Grandesso, M. (2019). *Contrucionismo social e práticas colaborativo-dialógicas: Contextos de ações transformadoras*. CRV.
Hien, D. N., Bauer, A. G., Franklin, L., Lalwani, T., & Pean, K. (2022). Conceptualizing the COVID-19, opioid use, and racism syndemic and its associations with traumatic stress. Psychiatric services (Washington, D.C.), 73(3), 353–356. doi:https://doi.org/10.1176/appi.ps.202100070.
Hochgraf, P. B., & Brasiliano, S. (Eds.). (2023). *Álcool e drogas: Uma questão feminina*. Red Publicações.
Instituto de Pesquisa Econômica Aplicada (IPEA). (2021). *Atlas da violência 2021*. Recuperado de https://www.ipea.gov.br/atlasviolencia/publicacoes/212/atlas-da-violencia-2021
Izumi, M. N. C. (2015). O perfil das mulheres em risco de morte atendidas no Centro de Referência da Mulher Casa Brasilândia. In T. S. A. M. Brabo (Ed.), *Educação, mulheres, gênero e violência* (pp. 133–152). Oficina Universitária/Cultura Acadêmica. https://doi.org/10.36311/2015.978-85-7983-713-5.p133-152
Junges, J. R., Barbiani, R., & Zoboli, E. L. C. P. (2018). Vulneração programática como categoria explicativa dos problemas éticos na atenção primária à saúde. *Trabalho, Educação e Saúde, 16*(3), 935–953. https://doi.org/10.1590/1981-7746-sol00149
Khanlou, N., Vazquez, L. M., Pashang, S., Connolly, J. A., Ahmad, F., & Ssawe, A. (2022). 2020 Syndemic: Convergence of COVID-19, gender-based violence, and racism pandemics. *Journal of Racial and Ethnic Health Disparities, 9*(6), 2077–2089. https://doi.org/10.1007/s40615-021-01146-w
Langdon, E., & Wiik, F. (2010). Anthropology, health and illness: An introduction to the concept of culture applied to the health sciences. *Revista Latino-Americana de Enfermagem, 18*(3), 459–466. https://doi.org/10.1590/S0104-11692010000300023
Magalhães, R., Burlandy, L., & Senna, M. C. M. (2007). Desigualdades sociais, saúde e bem-estar: Oportunidades e problemas no horizonte de políticas públicas transversais. *Ciência & Saúde Coletiva, 12*(6), 1415–1421. https://doi.org/10.1590/S1413-81232007000600002
Malheiro, L. (2020). *Tornar-se mulher usuária de crack: Cultura e política sobre drogas*. Telha.
Mardani, M., Alipour, F., Rafiey, H., Fallahi-Khoshknab, M., & Arshi, M. (2023). Challenges in addiction-affected families: A systematic review of qualitative studies. *BMC Psychiatry, 23*(1), 439. https://doi.org/10.1186/s12888-023-04927-1
Masur, J. (2004). *O que é toxicomania*. Brasiliense.
Masur, J., & Carlini, E. (2004). *Drogas: subsídios para uma discussão*. Brasiliense.
Mbembe, A. (2020). *Políticas da inimizade*. N-1.
Minayo, M. C. S., & Assis, S. G. (Eds.). (2017). *Novas e velhas faces da violência no século XXI: visão da literatura brasileira do campo da saúde*. FIOCRUZ.
Ministério dos Direitos Humanos e da Cidadania (MDHC). (2023). *População em Situação de Rua no Brasil: Relatório Nacional 2023*. Recuperado de https://www.gov.br/mdh/pt-br/navegue-

portemas/populacao-em-situacao-de-rua/publicacoes/relat_pop_rua_digital.pdf. Acesso em 04 de janeiro de 2024.

Miura, P. O., Silva, A. C. d. S., Pedrosa, M. M. M. P., Costa, M. L., & Nobre Filho, J. N. (2018). Violência doméstica ou violência intrafamiliar: Análise dos termos. *Psicologia & Sociedade, 30*, e179670. https://doi.org/10.1590/1807-0310/2018v30179670

Monari, E. N., Booth, R., Forchuk, C., & Csiernik, R. (2024). Experience of family members of relatives with substance use disorders: An integrative literature review. *Creative Nursing, 30*(3), 232–244. https://doi.org/10.1177/10784535241252169

Monteiro, S., & Villela, W. (Eds.). (2013). *Estigma e saúde*. FIOCRUZ.

Morin, E. (2011). *Introdução ao Pensamento Complexo*. Sulina.

Mota, J. C., Sperandei, S., De Boni, R. B., Dourado, I., Veras, M. A. S. M., & Bastos, F. I. (2024). Uso de múltiplas substâncias e fatores associados em mulheres trans e travestis: Resultados do estudo TransOdara, Brasil. *Revista Brasileira de Epidemiologia, 27*, e240011.supl.1. https://doi.org/10.1590/1980-549720240011.supl.1

Nathan, P. E., Conrad, M., & Skinstad, A. H. (2016). History of the concept of addiction. *Annual Review of Clinical Psychology, 12*, 29–51. https://doi.org/10.1146/annurev-clinpsy-021815-093546

Niu, L., Li, Y., Bai, R., Pagán, J. A., Zhang, D., & Diaz, A. (2024). Global prevalence of violence against children and adolescents during COVID-19: A meta-analysis. *Child Abuse & Neglect, 154*, 106873. https://doi.org/10.1016/j.chiabu.2024.106873

Oliveira, E. (2020). *O universo da segurança humana*. Juruá.

Oliveira, R. G. (2022). *Vidas em exclusão e a reinvenção do cuidado*. FIOCRUZ.

Oviedo, R., & Czeresnia, D. (2015). O conceito de vulnerabilidade e seu caráter biossocial. *Interface – Comunicação, Saúde, Educação, 19*(53), 237–250. https://doi.org/10.1590/1807-57622014.0436

Pagot, A. M. (2012). *O louco, a rua, a comunidade: As relações da cidade com a loucura em situação de rua*. FIOCRUZ.

Perussolo, A., Oliveira, M. R., Guerini, E., Reichert, K. G., & Reichert, R. A. (2019). A política criminal de drogas e o encarceramento de mulheres: Impactos do proibicionismo e do sistema prisional. In A. Zaluar, E. Guerini, M. R. de Oliveira, & R. A. Reichert (Eds.), *Drogas, ciências e políticas públicas: Discussões interdisciplinares e práticas de saúde* (pp. 189–209). Recanto das Letras.

Pillemer, K., Burnes, D., Riffin, C., & Lachs, M. S. (2016). Elder abuse: Global situation, risk factors, and prevention strategies. *The Gerontologist, 56*(Suppl 2), S194–S205. https://doi.org/10.1093/geront/gnw004

Reichenheim, M. E., de Souza, E. R., Moraes, C. L., Jorge, M. H. P. M., da Silva, C. M. F. P., & Minayo, M. C. d. S. (2011). Violence and injuries in Brazil: The effect, progress made, and challenges ahead. *The Lancet, 377*(9781), 1962–1975. https://doi.org/10.1016/S0140-6736(11)60053-6

Reichert, R. A. (2024). *Amidst the flow: Biographical narratives, social trajectories, and urban itineraries of crack cocaine users in São Paulo*. Ethics Press.

Reichert, R. A., Marques, M. W. C., Comis, M. A. C., Silva, E. A., Sudbrack, M. F. O., & De Micheli, D. (Eds.). (2024). *Substance use, public policy and harm reduction: Social and health studies and interventions*. Ethics Press.

Reichert, R. A., Oliveira-Ramos, A., Andrade, A. L. M., & De Micheli, D. (2021a). Resiliência: Aspectos comportamentais e componentes neurais. In M. Rodrigues & D. S. Pereira (Eds.), *Psicologia Positiva: Dos conceitos à aplicação* (pp. 169–187). Sinopsys.

Reichert, R. A., Ramos de Oliveira, M., De Micheli, D., & Aparecida da Silva, E. (2023). Trajetórias sociais e vulnerabilidades associadas ao uso de crack e outras drogas: Um estudo na cidade de São Paulo, Brasil. *Revista Cultura y Droga, 28*(36), 206–235. https://doi.org/10.17151/culdr.2023.28.36.9

Reichert, R. A., Silva, E. A., Andrade, A. L. M., & De Micheli, D. (2019). Conceitos de dependência e vulnerabilidade ao uso de drogas. In C. Dalbosco, J. Veiga, & M. F. O. Sudbrack (Eds.),

Prevenção ao uso de álcool e outras drogas no contexto escolar e outros espaços: Fortalecendo as redes sociais e de cuidados (pp. 35–58). Technopolitik.

Reichert, R. A., Silva, E. A., De Micheli, D., Noto, A. R., Skinstad, A. H., & Galduróz, J. C. (2025). Substance use disorders: History, theoretical models and diagnostic criteria (ICD-11 and DSM-5-TR). In R. A. Reichert, A. L. M. Andrade, & D. De Micheli (Eds.), Neuropsychology and substance use disorders. Springer. https://doi.org/10.1007/978-3-031-82614-6

Reichert, R. A., Silva, E. A., Ronzani, T. M., & Amarante, P. (2021b). Barreiras de acesso e o papel da psicologia na adesão de usuários de drogas na atenção básica à saúde. In F. M. Lopes et al. (Eds.), *Psicoterapias e abuso de drogas: Uma análise a partir de diferentes perspectivas teórico-metodológicas* (pp. 441–472). CRV. https://doi.org/10.24824/978652511044.8.441-472

Rocha, R. M. d. A. (2017). O histórico da segurança humana e o (des)encontro das agendas de desenvolvimento e segurança. *Carta Internacional, 12*(3), 104–129. https://doi.org/10.21530/ci.v12n3.2017.676

Rodrigues, C. A. B., & Schramm, F. R. (2022). Bioética de proteção: Fundamentos e perspectiva. *Revista Bioética, 30*(2), 355–365. https://doi.org/10.1590/1983-80422022302531PT

Ronzani, T. M. (Ed.). (2018). *Drugs and social context: Social perspectives on the use of alcohol and other drugs*. Springer. https://doi.org/10.1007/978-3-319-72446-1

Rutherford, A., Zwi, A. B., Grove, N. J., & Butchart, A. (2007). Violence: A glossary. *Journal of Epidemiology and Community Health, 61*(8), 676–680. https://doi.org/10.1136/jech.2005.043711

Santiago, H. (2020). *Novo coronavírus é "barril de pólvora" para população de rua em São Paulo*. Portal UOL. Recuperado de https://tab.uol.com.br/noticias/redacao/2020/03/26/coronavirus-e-barril-de-polvora-para-populacao-de-rua-em-sao-paulo.htm.

Sawaia, B. (Ed.). (2014). *As artimanhas da exclusão: Análise psicossocial e ética da exclusão*. Vozes.

Schimith, P. B., Murta, G. A. V., & de Queiroz, S. S. (2019). A abordagem dos termos dependência química, toxicomania e drogadição no campo da Psicologia brasileira. *Psicologia USP, 30*, e180085. https://doi.org/10.1590/0103-6564e180085

Silva, A. M. (2024). *Inclusão racial e mercado de trabalho: Perspectivas de atuação por intermédio de práticas coletivas* (Tese de Doutorado). Universidade Estadual Paulista "Júlio de Mesquita Filho."

Silva, E. A., & Campos-Bolitreau, A. R. (Eds.). (2024). *Artistação com a comunidade: A arte no processo de cuidado com pessoas em sofrimento psíquico*. Devires.

Silva, E. A., Moura, Y. G., & Zugman, D. (Eds.). (2015). *Vulnerabilidades, Resiliência e Redes – Uso, Abuso e Dependências de Drogas*. Red.

Silva, E. A., & Noto, A. R. (2022). *Famílias e uso de drogas: Paradigmas da pós-modernidade*. Red.

Soares, G. N., Fernandes, M. M., Ko da Cunha, A. M. F., & Souza e Souza, L. P. (2021). Ocorrência de violência intrafamiliar relacionada ao consumo de álcool e outras drogas no Brasil. *Revista Brasileira de Segurança Pública, 15*(2), 44–73. https://doi.org/10.31060/rbsp.2021.v15.n2.1212

Sodelli, M. (2016). *Uso de drogas e prevenção: Da desconstrução da postura proibicionista às ações redutoras de vulnerabilidade*. Via Verita.

Souza, M. (2011). Resiliência e desastres naturais. *Ciência e Cultura, 63*(3), 4–5. https://doi.org/10.21800/S0009-67252011000300002

Substance Abuse and Mental Health Services Administration. (2020). *Substance use disorder treatment and family therapy: Updated 2020* (Treatment Improvement Protocol (TIP) Series, No. 39). Chapter 2—Influence of substance misuse on families. Substance Abuse and Mental Health Services Administration. https://www.ncbi.nlm.nih.gov/books/NBK571087/

Teixeira, S. M. (2017). *Trabalho social com família: Fundamentos históricos, teórico-metodológicos e técnico-operativos*. EDUFPI.

Teixeira, S. M., & Carloto, C. M. (2020). *Família, cuidado e políticas sociais*. Papel Social.

Tondowski, C. S., Feijó, M. R., Silva, E. A., Gebara, C. F. d. P., Sanchez, Z. M., & Noto, A. R. (2014). Intergenerational patterns of family violence related to alcohol abuse: A genogram-based study. *Psicologia: Reflexão e Crítica, 27*(4), 806–814. https://doi.org/10.1590/1678-7153.201427421

Walsh, F. (2012). *Normal family processes*. Guilford Press.
World Health Organization (WHO). (2002). *World report on violence and health*. World Health Organization.
World Health Organization (WHO). (2018). *International Classification of Diseases for Mortality and Morbidity Statistics* (11th Revision). World Health Organization. Recuperado de https://icd.who.int/browse11/l-m/en
Zaluar, A. (1992). *Violência e educação*. Cortez.
Zaluar, A. (2004). *Integração perversa: Pobreza e tráfico de drogas*. Editora FGV.

Chapter 14
Accessibility Barriers to Treatment from a Gender Perspective

Antonio Vidal Infer, Juan Carlos Valderrama-Zurián, and Andrea Sixto-Costoya

14.1 Introduction

Ana is a person like you or me. Some time ago, she realized that she had difficulty restraining herself when drinking. Once she started, she couldn't stop and, increasingly, she took any opportunity to continue consuming. She lied to everyone: her partner, her family, her friends, at work… Everything would have remained the same if it weren't for the day her partner discovered a lie and, from then on, her lies were uncovered one by one and her reality collapsed like a house of cards. Forced by circumstances, she had no choice but to start treatment to stop her alcoholism. But Ana was aware of her alcohol dependence long before. If she had started at that time, the damage would have been much less. And, why didn't she start treatment then?

Ana is a fictional character. However, what is happening to her is very real and common in people who suffer from addictions. Access to treatment implies a necessary change in lifestyle that has led people with addictions to immerse themselves

A. V. Infer (✉) · J. C. Valderrama-Zurián
Grupo UISYS, Departamento de Historia de la Ciencia y Documentación, Facultad de Medicina y Odontología, Universitat de València, Valencia, Spain
e-mail: antonio.vidal-infer@uv.es; juan.valderrama@uv.es

A. Sixto-Costoya
Grupo UISYS, Departamento de Trabajo Social y Servicios Sociales, Facultad de Ciencias Sociales, Universitat de València, Valencia, Spain
e-mail: andrea.sixto@uv.es

T. Mota Ronzani (ed.), *Social Stigma and Drug Use*,
https://doi.org/10.1007/978-3-031-94813-8_14

in a problem over which they have little control and that is pushing them to the limit in every sense. This lifestyle change also has a series of consequences, such as the abandonment of routines, certain social contacts (probably most of them) and, above all, feeling the judgment of others on their backs, which can be even harder in the case of women. This judgment is based on societal moral models, which makes them face intersectional discrimination that pushes them to hide their problem or not seek treatment for fear of being rejected or misunderstood. In the case of women, it is related to their role as caregivers and the fundamental pillar of the family, resulting in greater difficulty in accessing treatment services than in the case of men and, when they do, they usually have to face additional barriers (Torrens-Melich et al., 2021), as will be seen in this chapter. To all this, is added the lack of self-confidence, due to a very reduced sense of self-efficacy and almost non-existent self-esteem. Too many challenges at the same time.

Just like in Ana's case, the barriers are not always visible; they are not physical walls or obvious restrictions, but more subtle obstacles that appear in their minds, or from the society that surrounds them. We could assume that Ana is not a heterosexual woman or that, for example, she is transgender; these people would not only experience oppression or rejection for being women consumers, but this would be compounded by the fact of not being heteronormative (Loo et al., 2021; Romero-Mendoza et al., 2018). In addition, we could imagine that Ana is a migrant and has language difficulties or feels a cultural barrier in her host country, or that her socioeconomic level is low. That is, multiple situations that can occur at the same time and that multiply the difficulty of each step toward treatment, which could be halted by feelings of shame and guilt, emotions that isolate those seeking help, caused by the weight of social stigmas, silent judgment, and misinformation.

Close people and their social environment are also conditioned by the same invisible barriers. In addition, they do not fully understand the nature of an addiction and this lack of knowledge places individuals with substance use disorder in a position of vulnerability and isolation that reinforces the fear of people like Ana of failure and guilt, not knowing how to address a situation that is perceived more as a personal failure than as a health problem, making her feel increasingly alone in her battle. And, for this reason, at the time she was not able to find a way to ask for help…

In addition, the barriers are also found in the system itself. In health centers, the particularities of people like Ana, who are not only fighting against addictions, but also against many aspects of their life, prejudices, ignorance and, in short, the fear that surrounds them and hinders their access to the path of recovery, are not always seen and can be even greater when people are immigrants, belong to an ethnic minority or have been victims of gender violence. We will start by describing the system, that is, the elements that make up a process of addiction treatment.

14.2 Addiction Treatment

When Ana starts to think about starting a treatment for her addiction, she gets chills. She doesn't know anyone who has gone through it. She imagines it will be very costly and that it will be an experience similar to being confined in a penitentiary. She doesn't know what she's up against and she's scared.

The first thing people like Ana, who want to start a treatment, encounter is a lack of information. They don't know what a treatment program is, how to access it, how long it lasts, whether it will cost them money, or what their day-to-day will be like. The very configuration of treatment programs can in itself be an obstacle to starting one. Addiction treatment is based on a combination of pharmacological strategies, psychological interventions, and rehabilitation actions, which vary depending on the nature of the addiction, the characteristics of the patient, and the available resources (NIDA, 2018). Moreover, as these are chronic disorders, addictions require long-term treatments. Care circuits must therefore be designed to offer a continuous process of care through the different phases of treatment: detoxification, habituation, and recovery/reintegration into society, counting on primary, specialized, and community care services and resources.

The admission criteria for the different treatment programs vary depending on the nature of the program and the profile of the patient (López-Goñi et al., 2017). For example, hospital detoxification is aimed at people with high levels of dependence, or serious medical comorbidities. However, patients with moderate dependence are treated in outpatient care services, with residential programs for people who have repeatedly failed in outpatient treatments or are at high risk of relapse.

Treatment programs can be public or private, that is, either funded by the State or paid for by the users. In any case, even though they may be public, the casuistry in the field of addictions is very diverse and, therefore, there are many particularities due to the profile of the user and their environment that can influence access to a treatment program. Certain groups or populations are exposed to greater difficulties in accessing addiction treatment. Among the most vulnerable groups are people in situations of poverty or exclusion; for example, homeless people (Collard et al., 2014). This group has a lower probability of accessing socio-health resources, which complicates both the identification of the addiction and its treatment. The lack of a stable environment and support also increases the risk of relapse in these groups (Paquette & Pannella Winn, 2016).

Another particularly affected group is the prison population, given that the incidence of psychoactive substance use in prison is usually high, although the availability of treatment is limited and focused on immediate abstinence, not on comprehensive rehabilitation. Therefore, upon leaving prison, many people find difficulties in continuing their treatment, which can lead to an increase in relapses and, as a result, in criminal recidivism (Leukefeld et al., 2009).

Another vulnerable group is adolescents. At this life stage, emotional and cognitive development can be affected by the onset of an addictive disorder (Anderson et al., 2006). In addition, the adolescent is often reluctant to seek treatment, due to a lack of awareness of their problem and fear of stigma.

People with comorbid mental disorders also face specific difficulties, as addictions and mental disorders (depression, anxiety, or schizophrenia among others) interact in complex ways, complicating treatment. Integrated approaches, based on dual pathology, are essential to improve outcomes (Kelly & Daley, 2013), although their availability is also often limited.

Finally, we understand that gender is also relevant when identifying vulnerabilities in the treatment of addictions, due to certain specific and differentiated barriers and obstacles that women or people from the LGBTQIA+ community face throughout the treatment process. Addiction is still perceived in some cases as a vice or a lack of willpower, rather than a treatable medical disease; therefore, people who suffer from an addiction, especially women and LGBTIQA+ people, would be blamed for their situation and deserve to be punished or marginalized (Siddiqui & Rutherford, 2023). Therefore, these groups, when suffering from an addiction, are more likely to hide their problem for fear of judgment or rejection. Often, this social stigmatization is added to having been victims of gender violence or abuse, which creates a very complex situation to face. The lack of specific treatment resources and programs that take into account their particular needs, such as attention to motherhood, the possible loss of custody of their children, or support in cases of violence, further complicates their access to treatment. This phenomenon is known as intersectional stigma and is reflected in the marginalization and discrimination they experience in health services (Paschen-Wolff et al., 2024). This chapter focuses especially on the attention to the gender perspective in access to addiction treatment. To do this, we will follow Ana's thread and the different types of barriers that a person like her could encounter when accessing treatment for her addiction, grouping them into two main blocks: barriers related to the care system and socio-health resources and barriers related to the person and their environment.

14.3 Barriers Related to Socio-Health Resources

The very socio-health resources dedicated to addressing addictions can in themselves, directly or indirectly, constitute a barrier to access to treatment for certain patient profiles, especially women and vulnerable groups. Below, this type of accessibility barriers.

14.3.1 Informative and Administrative

We already know that the first barrier Ana encountered was a lack of information. Once she overcame her fear, Ana wanted to inform herself, but she didn't know how to do it or where to start. Given her emotional state, the fact of seeing difficulties even to find information on how access to treatment works made her give up and desist.

The health system does not always provide people with necessary and understandable information that allows them to access care, including addiction-related information, something that conditions effective access to health services. In addition, although it is not Ana's case, these difficulties should be added to the case where there are difficulties related to language knowledge, or the complicated bureaucratic procedures, increasingly greater, which are not preceded by adequate information or training for administrative and health personnel (Médicos del Mundo, 2022). In cases like these, the main victims of this lack of knowledge are people belonging to especially vulnerable groups, such as migrants, especially those in an irregular situation, and the homeless (without these two situations being exclusive), to which other factors such as gender, age, educational level, or social class are added (Médicos del Mundo, 2022; Nichols & Malenfant, 2022). Additionally, in these (and other) groups there may also be technological barriers that prevent them from accessing online administrative procedures, such as the lack of a device to access the Internet or complete ignorance of electronic processing procedures.

14.3.2 Training and Capacity Building of Professionals

To get better informed, Ana has gone to her health center. Once there, she did not feel confident to talk to the staff who attended her. When she asked, they responded loudly so that everyone could hear what they were saying, and she was very uncomfortable with the situation. Again, she thought it would be best to leave.

The first contact of people suffering from addiction with the care circuit is not always made in a specialized resource; in many cases, this contact is made through primary care resources, although also in other services, such as Cardiology, Respiratory or Neurology, and even in hospital emergencies. In all these resources, it is very likely that the staff working there have little training, even nonexistent, in the management of the patient with an addiction. This can result in difficulty in identifying the disorder effectively, making erroneous diagnoses and inappropriate treatments (Nyaku et al., 2024), or even dismissing the problem, (Adeniran et al., 2023). In the case of women and LGBTQIA+ people, these types of barriers are harder to overcome. Women encounter throughout their lives not only more barriers to health services, but with less understanding and adaptation once they can access them (Organización Mundial de la Salud, 2018). It is also known that much of the information, training and clinical perception is insensitive to sex differences and, above all, gender (Montesó-Curto et al., 2014; Vázquez-Santiago & Garrido Peña, 2016), including aspects related to sexual and gender diversity (Rider et al., 2019; Valenzuela & Cartes, 2019).

Also, prejudices and lack of skills in managing patient with substance use disorder of some health professionals, like the person who attended Ana at the counter and did not hesitate to speak loudly about her addiction, can represent another significant barrier and that their lack of empathy affects the quality of treatment and its success (Loo et al., 2021). This lack of empathy is particularly severe with bisexual people, as they are discriminated against both within and outside of the LGBTQIA+ community, a phenomenon called "binegativity," which increases the propensity to develop addiction problems and avoids accessing treatment (Rothstein et al., 2024). It has also been described the convenience of service providers having adequate training for the management of transgender patients and thus avoid anti-trans stigma (Baguso et al., 2022). On the contrary, when the staff shows empathy and compassion, the likelihood of stigma is reduced and fear of starting treatment is lost (Steinhauser et al., 2024)

14.3.3 Geographical

Ana lives in a small city, where there are only two outpatient health centers. When she obtained information about the treatment, she discovered that the nearest resource is 40 km away.

The degree of proximity to a socio-health resource can be determining in the decision to access a treatment. The areas furthest from urban centers have fewer resources in general and health and addiction-related services in particular (Fredericksen et al., 2024). And it is even more complicated to find providers trained in gender and sexual diversity issues. This forces patients to travel long distances to receive care (Parker et al., 2024) or to depend on virtual services, which are not always accessible. As mentioned earlier, the costs associated with transportation or the use of a own car can be high and affect not only access to treatment but adherence to it (Pouille et al., 2024). Also, reasons like the lack of childcare services, can be definitive in making the decision to start the process. Likewise, when a displacement is necessary, the partner can also become an interference for the woman to go to the center, especially when she is also suffering from addiction and does not want her to have access to treatment: for example, by taking away her car keys or not allowing her to take it to the treatment center (Fusco et al., 2024).

All of this causes that, when people have low economic income and a lack of personal and logistical resources, they face additional barriers such as lack of transportation, the cost of medications and lack of health insurance, which directly affects their ability to access continuous treatment (Adeniran et al., 2023).

Also, the lack of integration between mental health services and addiction treatment programs forces people with dual pathology to seek treatment in different places, which complicates their access to comprehensive care. Agterberg et al. (2020) point out that the lack of coordination between these services creates additional barriers for people who need a treatment that addresses both problems simultaneously.

The reason that geographical location can be a barrier to access is not solely the responsibility of the Public Administration. The shortage of health personnel specialized in addictions is more critical in rural areas; professionals are not always willing to travel to very distant locations. On the other hand, private companies do not usually consider it profitable to establish specialized resources in these types of municipalities. This resulting shortage contrasts with urban areas, where there are multidisciplinary teams that provide comprehensive care for addictions (Parker et al., 2024). All of this perpetuates to some extent the difficulty of access and, at times, the exclusion from the health system of people who live in these areas (James et al., 2024).

14.3.4 Structural

> Ana has made the decision to start a treatment to recover from her alcohol addiction. After consulting the addiction specialist, they inform her that in her case she would have to be admitted to a therapeutic community, but there is a waiting list and it seems that she will still have to wait.

One of the most evident structural barriers is the lack of places in treatment centers, which causes long waiting lists, delays access to treatment and increases the risk of relapse (Schettini et al., 2024). The lack of adequate infrastructure and complementary services, such as temporary housing or job support, hinders the reintegration of people in recovery. Also negatively influences the little flexibility that centers sometimes have, when they do not offer schedules that adapt to the needs of the service users, which decreases therapeutic adherence.

To all this is added that some people who belong to the LGBTIQA+ collective, especially trans people, face discrimination in traditional treatment centers, which are designed from a cisnormative and heteronormative perspective, including segregation by sex in facilities such as bathrooms and dormitories, which causes transgender people not to feel safe or comfortable receiving treatment and fear being discriminated against or not recognized for their gender identity (Matsuzaka, 2018). In addition, as mentioned earlier, the structural barriers are not only related to the lack of resources, but also with the invisibility of their needs within conventional treatment programs. Many trans or non-binary people, for example, may feel that care services do not respect their gender identity, which can generate great discomfort and even previous traumas, such as medical discrimination (Loo et al., 2021).

In the case of patients with comorbidities there is an additional barrier, which is the lack of coordination between mental health services and other specialties, as well as the shortage of specialized personnel and resources, all of which hinder their comprehensive treatment (Knopf, 2024).

14.4 Barriers Related to the Person and Their Environment

14.4.1 Economic

Ana has a doubt. She already knows that she has to enter a treatment program, but she is not sure if it has a cost, if she will have enough money to travel every day, if she will be able to continue working or will have to take leave, etc. In short, she does not know if she can afford it…

As mentioned earlier, people who are in the same situation as Ana barely have information about the cost of treatment. Ignorance about economic conditions can be somewhat deterrent. In fact, the cost of rehabilitation programs, both outpatient and residential, can be prohibitive, especially in private resources or in health systems where services are not fully covered by public health or medical insurance. The problem of expenses goes further: for example, the loss of income from being absent from work (Schettini et al., 2024), or the additional costs of transportation and accommodation to receive treatment that patients living in areas far from urban centers must face (Parker et al., 2024). When women have no income, they face additional financial barriers that prevent them from paying for treatment or temporarily leaving work to undergo rehabilitation programs (Greenfield et al., 2007). Additionally, the difficulty in finding suitable services causes non-conforming gender people to often face prohibitive treatment costs, which forces them to seek less effective alternatives or to not receive treatment at all.

In the case of women and some cases of the LGTBQIA+ collective such as trans people, economic barriers may be even more accentuated due to the structural inequalities that exist in regarding income and employment. These populations often have greater difficulties in finding stable and well-paid jobs, which limits their ability to afford relocation or treatments. Women are often employed in poorly paid and precarious jobs that do not offer them the necessary economic security to take a leave to enter a rehabilitation program, and the fear of losing their job or facing work repercussions for seeking treatment, acts as a significant barrier (Agterberg et al., 2020). In addition, trans and non-binary people, in particular, face high levels of job discrimination, which exacerbates their economic situation.

Finally, the lack of available places and the limited duration of publicly funded treatments (often insufficient for severe cases of addiction) can prolong the waiting time and increase the risk of relapse (Schettini et al., 2024).

14.4.2 Cultural and Ethnic Barriers

Cultural and ethnic barriers play an important role in the accessibility to treatment, especially for women from ethnic minorities or migrant backgrounds. What would happen if Ana were an immigrant, of a different religion or with a skin color different from the majority in the society where she lives? In these cases, she would probably experience, in addition to the stigma that exists toward substance use, the one related to her cultural or ethnic condition. Social norms within communities can impose additional restrictions for them to seek treatment, especially when these norms punish female behavior that deviates from the "expected." For example, some migrant women may find themselves trapped in a situation of financial and emotional dependence on their partners, which prevents them from accessing external support resources.

In addition, the language barrier and the lack of health staff trained to work with culturally diverse populations accentuate the exclusion of these women from the health system (Médicos del Mundo, 2022; Paschen-Wolff et al., 2024). This lack of inclusive and culturally competent programs reinforces distrust in health services, leading many people from the LGBTIQA+ community to avoid or delay treatment, which often results in a worsening of their health problems (Reisner et al., 2015).

14.4.3 Childcare

> Ana has to leave her daughter Marta with some neighbors from her farm. She has no choice, as she has to attend afternoon sessions and has no one else to leave her with. She also can't take her with her. She worries, because her neighbors don't know the reason for leaving Marta with them, and she fears that her daughter might tell them by accident, or that they find out through other means, and she is saddened by not being able to spend time with her.

A significant obstacle, particularly in the case of women who have children, is their care. The responsibility they have toward them makes them feel ashamed of their consumption and fear losing their custody or being perceived as "bad mothers"; all this becomes a significant psychological and structural barrier (Fusco et al., 2024), which is even greater if the socio-health center is linked to the Public Administration (Svensson et al., 2023). Women who face these fears often choose not to seek treatment until the situation becomes critical; the pressure of caring for their children, relatives or dependents, limits their ability to fully participate in rehabilitation programs and postpones access to treatment (McNeely et al., 2018). Obviously, in the case of single mothers, everything is more complicated, as they are the main caregivers in their families. Also, non-conforming gender people face challenges related to caregiving responsibilities, especially when their gender identity is not respected by the family or the community, which adds an additional layer of stress and isolation (Loo et al., 2021)

As mentioned earlier, many women prioritize the well-being of their children over their own, but treatment programs do not usually offer nurseries or support services that allow women to participate in treatment sessions without the worry of who will take care of their children. In short, the dual role of caregiver and patient with treatment needs creates a conflict that many women cannot resolve, especially in contexts where there is no social or family support to distribute these responsibilities (Sajjad et al., 2024).

14.4.4 Psychosocial

Ana is about to start treatment. For now, it will be outpatient, because there are no places in the therapeutic community yet. She has to access the center, but fears that someone might recognize her. In fact, every time she enters the resource, she has the feeling that they are looking at her and she feels judged. It is not a pleasant situation and, every day, she thinks about quitting the treatment to avoid the ordeal.

Since the end of the last century, one of the fundamental aspects of addressing addictions was their progressive medicalization: they gradually stopped being a vice to be considered as a chronic disease. This change in approach significantly improved the application of therapies to address this disorder. Despite this, the traditional gender expectations can reinforce the stigma toward women, who are often perceived as "bad mothers" or "neglectful" if they prioritize their health over family responsibilities (Fusco et al., 2024), which generates shame and guilt, preventing them from seeking help. Even the very designation as "drug addicts" results in an increase in perceived stigma, (Goodyear et al., 2018). This stigma not only comes from society, but also from the patient themselves (self-stigma), and even from healthcare personnel, which reduces confidence in the system and the patient's willingness to participate in treatment (Luoma et al., 2007). In Ana's case, she feels observed and judged, despite not having seen any objective expression of disapproval from anyone at the center.

The family and peers also suffer this shame in relation to the problem, a phenomenon also known as courtesy stigma. In the early stages of an addictive process, there is a denial or lack of awareness about the addiction problem on the part of the social and family network, which becomes a crucial psychological barrier, delaying early intervention, key to successful treatment. Moreover, when family and social support is scarce, the rehabilitation process becomes much more complex, as the lack of healthy personal relationships can have negative consequences on the emotional well-being of the person suffering from addiction: the social isolation associated with addiction increases feelings of loneliness and hopelessness, which causes a greater desire to consume the substance as a form of escape.

A critical aspect in the treatment of women with addictions is the impact of trauma, especially that related to gender violence. There is a bidirectional relationship between drug use and gender violence, and in the case of women, the consumption of substances such as alcohol is fundamental in the persistence of these types of violent behaviors and coping with victimization (Shiva et al., 2021). In fact, women, in particular, are more likely to develop substance use disorders in response to previous traumas, such as gender violence or sexual abuse, which hinders the recovery from their addiction by not adequately addressing these traumas in traditional treatment programs (Romero-Mendoza et al., 2018; Tirado-Muñoz et al., 2018). In addition, it is worth mentioning the power that their partners exert over them, sometimes in the form of abuse, which can prevent their women from accessing treatment resources; it is their partners who control access to medical services and the money to pay for them if necessary. All this creates a double barrier: they not only fight against their addiction, but also against untreated trauma and against their consumption as a coping method. The fear of revictimization within the healthcare system, especially when a trauma-sensitive treatment approach is not offered, prevents them from seeking help.

In short, if Ana did not ask for help before, it was because having an addiction is bad, but it is even worse when it is a woman. This stigma, present both in society and within families, as a result of cognitive biases regarding gender (Vázquez-Santiago & Garrido Peña, 2016), reinforces isolation and guilt, preventing many women from seeking help for fear of being judged, because they are also expected to assume caregiver roles and, therefore, it is even less understood when they become addicts. And this process is more pronounced when it comes to transgender people, where 50% of them feel unmotivated to access treatment programs (Matsuzaka, 2018).

14.5 Final Considerations: Proposals to Improve Accessibility

In recent years, the availability of treatments has markedly improved thanks to the expansion of telemedicine and online care programs, especially due to the pandemic caused by Covid-19, which have facilitated access, among others, to mental health and addiction treatment services, especially in areas geographically distant from these services. This modality of remote treatment has become an effective tool to eliminate physical and economic barriers, improving adherence to treatment. In fact, the use of these approaches can also facilitate access to treatment for women who either suffer geographical barriers or prefer to be attended without being seen when accessing resources in person.

Another issue that can be improved is the lack of training of non-specialized health professionals in addictions. For this, training curricula have been designed that train this professional group in the management of the patient with substance use disorder, allowing for effective screening, brief intervention, and referral to specialized treatment (SAMHSA, 2017). It is therefore necessary to have the largest number of health professionals for the challenge of an integral intervention aimed at the person, ensuring that patients not only receive medical treatment, but also comprehensive social support in order to effectively connect patients with health services (D'Ippolito et al., 2015). Additionally, policies can be developed that include the creation of financial incentives to encourage the specialization of professionals in addiction treatment, as well as the implementation of educational campaigns at the national level that seek to destigmatize addiction treatment, as well as communication campaigns to demystify addiction and highlight recovery stories, thus bringing the problem of addictions closer to the non-specialized health professional collective and the general public. These policies can help reduce the social and health stigma that limits access to treatment for many people, especially gender minorities (Bodkin et al., 2015; Reisner et al., 2015). In this line, the implementation of programs that integrate a gender approach, such as the use of harm reduction models and non-judgmental care, has proven to be effective in increasing adherence to treatment in vulnerable women, such as people in situations of prostitution and sexual exploitation. These multidisciplinary approaches ensure that patients not only receive medical care, but also psychological and social support that considers the complexities of their lives.

The fact of using models considered as asexual, but which are clearly androcentric, has influenced the creation of clinical frameworks loaded with significant gender biases, and that is why much of the information, training, and clinical perception are insensitive to sex differences and, above all, gender (Montesó-Curto et al., 2014; Vázquez-Santiago & Garrido Peña, 2016). Therefore, initiatives that promote empathy and a greater understanding of the specific barriers that women face (Bodkin et al., 2015) and the LGBTQIA+ community (Reback et al., 2018) can help to reduce stigma and foster a supportive and understanding environment. Lastly, the involvement of translators, cultural mediators, and educational resources adapted to cultural diversity, to overcome the barriers that arise in cases where there are differences in culture and language.

Facilitating comprehensive treatment that addresses addictions and mental pathology can help overcome the structural barriers related to the treatment of dual pathology, something that according to scientific literature improves adherence to treatment and reduces relapse rates (Schettini et al., 2024). Likewise, a key aspect is the design and implementation of policies that promote a gender approach in addiction care. It is essential that governments develop regulatory frameworks that include specific programs for women and non-conforming gender individuals, integrating psychological support, reproductive health services, and resources for victims of gender violence (Organización Mundial de la Salud, 2018; Rider et al., 2019). Also, the creation of treatment spaces that include trauma-focused interventions, as well as staff sensitization, is fundamental to break this cycle of violence and substance dependence, as well as the implementation of inclusive and culturally competent programs that include specific support groups for women and non-conforming gender individuals. The importance of designing measures to overcome gender inherent barriers, such as the inclusion of daycare services in treatment centers, financial support for women in situations of economic vulnerability, or providing flexible therapy schedules (Paschen-Wolff et al., 2024). Similarly, it would be beneficial to create spaces that include specific support groups, trained staff, and non-discriminatory policies are key measures to ensure that LGBTQA+ individuals can access the care they need without fear of being judged or mistreated (Reback et al., 2018).

References

Adeniran, E., Quinn, M., Wallace, R., Walden, R. R., Labisi, T., Olaniyan, A., & Brooks, B. (2023). A scoping review of barriers and facilitators to the integration of substance use treatment services into US mainstream health care. *Drug and Alcohol Dependence Reports, 7*, 100152. https://doi.org/10.1016/j.dadr.2023.100152

Agterberg, S., Schubert, N., Overington, L., & Corace, K. (2020). Treatment barriers among individuals with co-occurring substance use and mental health problems: Examining gender differences. *Journal of Substance Abuse Treatment, 112*, 29–35. https://doi.org/10.1016/j.jsat.2020.01.005

Anderson, K. G., Ramo, D. E., & Brown, S. A. (2006). Life stress, coping and comorbid youth: An examination of the stress-vulnerability model for substance relapse. *Journal of Psychoactive Drugs, 38*(3), 255–262. https://doi.org/10.1080/02791072.2006.10399851

Baguso, G. N., Aguilar, K., Sicro, S., Mañacop, M., Quintana, J., & Wilson, E. C. (2022). "Lost trust in the system": System barriers to publicly available mental health and substance use services for transgender women in San Francisco. *BMC Health Services Research, 22*, 930. https://doi.org/10.1186/s12913-022-08315-5

Bodkin, K., Delahunty-Pike, A., & O'Shea, T. (2015). Reducing stigma in healthcare and law enforcement: A novel approach to service provision for street level sex workers. *International Journal for Equity in Health, 14*, 35. https://doi.org/10.1186/s12939-015-0156-0

Collard, C. S., Lewinson, T., & Watkins, K. (2014). Supportive housing: an evidence-based intervention for reducing relapse among low income adults in addiction recovery. *Journal of Evidence-Based Social Work, 11*(5), 468–479. https://doi.org/10.1080/15433714.2013.765813

D'Ippolito, M., Lundgren, L., Amodeo, M., Beltrame, C., Lim, L., & Chassler, D. (2015). Addiction treatment staff perceptions of training as a facilitator or barrier to implementing evidence-based practices: A national qualitative research study. *Substance Abuse, 36*(1), 42–50. https://doi.org/10.1080/08897077.2013.849646

Fredericksen, R. J., Mixson, L. S., Estadt, A. T., Leichtling, G., Bresett, J., Zule, W., Walters, S. M., Friedmann, P. D., Romo, E., Whitney, B. M., Delaney, J. A. C., Crane, H. M., Tsui, J. I., Young, A., Seal, D., & Stopka, T. J. (2024). Barriers to retention in inpatient and residential drug treatment among persons who use opioids and/or injection drugs living in the rural U.S. *Journal of Substance Use and Addiction Treatment, 165*, 209453. https://doi.org/10.1016/j.josat.2024.209453

Fusco, R. A., Kulkarni, S. J., & Pless, J. (2024). "He gets mad that I'm sober": Experiences of substance use coercion among postpartum women in recovery. *Journal of Substance Use and Addiction Treatment, 164*, 209407. https://doi.org/10.1016/j.josat.2024.209407

Goodyear, K., Haass-Koffler, C. L., & Chavanne, D. (2018). Opioid use and stigma: The role of gender, language, and precipitating events. *Drug and Alcohol Dependence, 185*, 339–346. https://doi.org/10.1016/j.drugalcdep.2017.12.037

Greenfield, S. F., Brooks, A. J., Gordon, S. M., Green, C. A., Kropp, F., McHugh, R. K., Lincoln, M., Hien, D., & Miele, G. M. (2007). Substance abuse treatment entry, retention, and outcome in women: a review of the literature. *Drug and Alcohol Dependence, 86*(1), 1–21. https://doi.org/10.1016/j.drugalcdep.2006.05.012

James, P. D., Nash, M., & Comiskey, C. (2024). Barriers and enablers for adolescents accessing substance-use treatment: A systematic review and narrative synthesis. *International Journal of Mental Health Nursing*. (early access). https://doi.org/10.1111/inm.13378

Kelly, T. M., & Daley, D. C. (2013). Integrated treatment of substance use and psychiatric disorders. *Social Work in Public Health, 28*(3–4), 388–406. https://doi.org/10.1080/19371918.2013.774673

Knopf, A. (2024). Why physicians don't want to treat addiction: Emotional and system barriers. *JAMA Network Open, 36*(31), 1–3. https://doi.org/10.1002/adaw.34212

Leukefeld, C., Oser, C. B., Havens, J., Staton Tindall, M., Mooney, J., Duvall, J. B., & Knudsen, H. (2009). Drug abuse treatment beyond prison walls. *Addiction Science & Clinical Practice, 5*(1), 24–30. https://doi.org/10.1151/ascp095124

Loo, S., Almazan, A. N., Vedilago, V., Stott, B., Reisner, S. L., & Keuroghlian, A. S. (2021). Understanding community member and health care professional perspectives on gender-affirming care: A qualitative study. *PLoS One, 16*(8), e0255568. https://doi.org/10.1371/journal.pone.0255568

López-Goñi, J. J., Fernández-Montalvo, J., Arteaga, A., & Esarte, S. (2017). Searching objective criteria for patient assignment in addiction treatment. *Journal of Substance Abuse Treatment, 76*, 28–35. https://doi.org/10.1016/j.jsat.2017.02.014

Luoma, J. B., Twohig, M. P., Waltz, T., Hayes, S. C., Roget, N., Padilla, M., & Fisher, G. (2007). An investigation of stigma in individuals receiving treatment for substance abuse. *Addictive Behaviors, 32*(7), 1331–1346. https://doi.org/10.1016/j.addbeh.2006.09.008

Matsuzaka, S. (2018). Transgressing gender norms in addiction treatment: Transgender rights to access within gender-segregated facilities. *Journal of Ethnicity in Substance Abuse, 17*(4), 420–433. https://doi.org/10.1080/15332640.2016.1264338

McNeely, J., Kumar, P. C., Rieckmann, T., Sedlander, E., Farkas, S., Chollak, C., Kannry, J. L., Vega, A., Waite, E. A., Peccoralo, L. A., Rosenthal, R. N., McCarty, D., & Rotrosen, J. (2018). Barriers and facilitators affecting the implementation of substance use screening in primary care clinics: A qualitative study of patients, providers, and staff. *Addiction Science & Clinical Practice, 13*, 1–15. https://doi.org/10.1186/s13722-018-0110-8

Médicos del Mundo. (2022). *Informe de barreras de acceso al sistema sanitario, mayo 2023*. Médicos del Mundo.

Montesó-Curto, P., Ferré-Grau, C., Lleixà-Fortuño, M., Albacar-Riobóo, N., & Lejeune, M. (2014). Diagnosed, identified, current and complete depression among patients attending primary care in Southern Catalonia: Different aspects of the same concept. *Archives of Psychiatric Nursing, 28*(1), 50–54. https://doi.org/10.1016/j.apnu.2013.10.002

National Institute on Drug Abuse (NIDA). (2018). *Principles of drug addiction treatment: A research-based guide* (3rd ed.). National Institute on Drug Abuse. Disponible en: https://nida.nih.gov

Nichols, N., & Malenfant, J. (2022). Health system access for precariously housed youth: A participatory youth research project. *Society and Mental Health, 12*(2), 137–154. https://doi.org/10.1177/21568693221082206

Nyaku, A. N., Zerbo, E. A., Chen, C., Milano, N., Johnston, B., Chadwick, R., & Crystal, S. (2024). A survey of barriers and facilitators to the adoption of buprenorphine prescribing after implementation of a New Jersey-wide incentivized DATA-2000 waiver training program. *BMC Health Services Research, 24*(1), 10648. https://doi.org/10.1186/s12913-024-10648-2

Organización Mundial de la Salud. (2018). Género y salud. https://www.who.int/es/news-room/fact-sheets/detail/gender

Paquette, K., & Pannella Winn, L. A. (2016). The role of recovery housing: Prioritizing choice in homeless services. *Journal of Dual Diagnosis, 12*(2), 153–162. https://doi.org/10.1080/15504263.2016.1175262

Parker, S., Reichley, N., Biello, K. B., Goldman, J., Buxton, J. A., Hadland, S. E., Sherman, S. G., & Marshall, B. D. L. (2024). Differences by race and ethnicity in drug use patterns, harm reduction practices and barriers to treatment among people who use drugs in Rhode Island. *Research Square*. https://doi.org/10.21203/rs.3.rs-4768821/v1

Paschen-Wolff, M. M., DeSousa, A., Paine, E. A., Hughes, T. L., & Campbell, A. N. C. (2024). Experiences of and recommendations for LGBTQ+-affirming substance use services: An exploratory qualitative descriptive study with LGBTQ+ people who use opioids and other drugs. *Substance Abuse Treatment, Prevention, and Policy, 19*(1), 2. https://doi.org/10.1186/s13011-023-00581-8

Pouille, A., De Ruysscher, C., van Selm, L., van Amsterdam, J., van den Brink, W., Busz, M., Perez Gayo, R., Atzemis, M., & Vanderplasschen, W. (2024). Challenges and support needs among persons with a migration background who use drugs in four European metropolitan cities. *Research Square*. https://doi.org/10.21203/rs.3.rs-4732446/v1

Reback, C. J., Clark, K., Holloway, I. W., & Fletcher, J. B. (2018). Health disparities, risk behaviors and healthcare utilization among transgender women in Los Angeles County: A comparison from 1998–1999 to 2015–2016. *AIDS and Behavior, 22*, 2524–2533. https://doi.org/10.1007/s10461-018-2165-7

Reisner, S. L., Pardo, S. T., Gamarel, K. E., White Hughto, J. M., Pardee, D. J., & Keo-Meier, C. L. (2015). Substance use to cope with stigma in healthcare among U.S. female-to-male trans masculine adults. *LGBT Health, 2*(4), 324–332. https://doi.org/10.1089/lgbt.2015.0001

Rider, G. N., McMorris, B. J., Gower, A. L., Coleman, E., Brown, C., & Eisenberg, M. E. (2019). Perspectives from nurses and physicians on training needs and comfort working with transgender and gender-diverse youth. *Journal of Pediatric Health Care, 33*(4), 379–385. https://doi.org/10.1016/j.pedhc.2018.11.003

Romero-Mendoza, M., Lozano-Verduzco, I., Saldivar, G., & Manriquez Montiel, Q. (2018). "Something that could get rid of the cold inside" Women's motives for using addictive substances from a gender perspective. *Journal of Substance Use, 23*(5), 466–470. https://doi.org/10.1080/14659891.2017.1397209

Rothstein, M. C., Schulz, C. T., Todaro, S. M., Stamates, A. L., Ehlke, S. J., & Kelley, M. L. (2024). An examination of protective factors for bisexual stigma and alcohol use among heavy drinking young bisexual women. *Journal of Bisexuality, 24*(1), 56–73. https://doi.org/10.1080/15299716.2023.2296892

Sajjad, A., Shah, S., Abbas, G., Aslam, A., Randhawa, F., Khurram, H., & Assiri, A. (2024). Treatment gap and barriers to access mental healthcare among women with postpartum depression symptoms in Pakistan. *PeerJ, 12*, e17711. https://doi.org/10.7717/peerj.17711

Schettini, G., Lindner, P., Ekström, V., & Johansson, M. (2024). A mixed method study exploring similarities and differences in general and social services-specific barriers to treatment-seeking among individuals with a problematic use of alcohol, cannabis, or gambling. *BMC Health Services Research, 24*(970). https://doi.org/10.1186/s12913-024-11304-5

Shiva, L., Shukla, L., & Chandra, P. S. (2021). Alcohol use and gender-based violence. *Current Addiction Reports, 8*, 71–80. https://doi.org/10.1007/s40429-021-00354-y

Siddiqui, H., & Rutherford, M. D. (2023). Belief that addiction is a discrete category is a stronger correlate with stigma than the belief that addiction is biologically based. *Substance Abuse Treatment, Prevention, and Policy, 18*(1), c1–11. https://doi.org/10.1186/s13011-022-00512-z

Steinhauser, S., Haroz, R., Jones, I., Skelton, W., Fuller, B. M., Roberts, M. B., & Trzeciak, S. (2024). Emergency department staff compassion is associated with lower fear of enacted stigma among patients with opioid use disorder. *Academic Emergency Medicine, 31*(12), 1204–1211. https://doi.org/10.1111/acem.14970

Substance Abuse and Mental Health Service Administration (SAMHSA). (2017). Screening, brief intervention, and referral to treatment (SBIRT). Disponible en: https://www.samhsa.gov/sbirt

Svensson, M., Jönson, H., & Johansson, S. (2023). Stigma-related barriers to participation in support groups for children: Social workers' experiences and destigmatizing strategies. *Child & Family Social Work, 29*, 24–34. https://doi.org/10.1111/cfs.13048

Tirado-Muñoz, J., Gilchrist, G., Fischer, G., Taylor, A., Moskalewicz, J., & Torrens, M. (2018). Psychiatric comorbidity and intimate partner violence among women who inject drugs in Europe: A cross-sectional study. *Archives of Women's Mental Health, 21*(3), 259–269. https://doi.org/10.1007/s00737-017-0800-3

Torrens-Melich, M., Orengo, T., Rodríguez de Fonseca, F., Almodóvar, I., Baquero, A., & Benito, A. (2021). Gender perspective in dual diagnosis. *Brain Sciences, 11*(8), 1101. https://doi.org/10.3390/brainsci11081101

Valenzuela, A., & Cartes, R. (2019). Perspectiva de género en la educación médica: Incorporación, intervenciones y desafíos por superar. *Revista Chilena de Obstetricia y Ginecologia, 84*(1), 82–88. https://doi.org/10.4067/S0717-75262019000100082

Vázquez-Santiago, S., & Garrido Peña, F. (2016). El enfoque de género en las necesidades de atención sociosanitaria. *Enfermeria Clinica, 26*(1), 76–80. https://doi.org/10.1016/j.enfcli.2015.09.003

Chapter 15
The Role of the Caregiver in the Addiction Treatment Process

Antonio Vidal Infer, Juan Carlos Valderrama-Zurián, and Andrea Sixto-Costoya

15.1 Introduction

The care, accompaniment, and support of a person suffering from any type of disease is a hard and exhausting process. From the recognition of the problem, to the diagnosis and subsequent actions, all stages are more bearable if they have the presence of a support figure. This reality is easy to understand because any person, regardless of geographical location, age, gender, social class, or ethnicity, has experienced the illness of a loved one and has felt the need to accompany them.

However, not all diseases are conceptualized in the same way, nor are they understood in the same way. In other words, there are "first" and "second" class diseases, depending on the knowledge about them, their prevalence, causes and consequences, and the level of empathy and understanding. Although this undoubtedly affects the person suffering from the disease, it also affects the people who care for and accompany them. The stigma, prejudices, and lack of understanding about some diseases impact the caregiver in a particularly painful way, activating feelings of guilt and shame, resulting in a delay in action and a lack of tools on how to proceed. This is the case with mental illnesses, sexually transmitted diseases, infectious diseases such as the human immunodeficiency virus (HIV) or the human papillomavirus (HPV), and, of course, addictive disorders.

A. V. Infer (✉) · J. C. Valderrama-Zurián
Grupo UISYS, Departamento de Historia de la Ciencia y Documentación, Facultad de Medicina y Odontología, Universitat de València, Valencia, Spain
e-mail: antonio.vidal-infer@uv.es; juan.valderrama@uv.es

A. Sixto-Costoya
Grupo UISYS, Departamento de Trabajo Social y Servicios Sociales, Facultad de Ciencias Sociales, Universitat de València, Valencia, Spain
e-mail: andrea.sixto@uv.es

T. Mota Ronzani (ed.), *Social Stigma and Drug Use*,
https://doi.org/10.1007/978-3-031-94813-8_15

For this reason, it is essential to address the problem that arises with the caregivers of others with addiction problems, as this is a particularly vulnerable group dealing with the complexity of a disease that carries stigma and a lack of understanding.

15.2 What Do We Mean by Caregiver in the Context of Addictions?

The onset of an addiction marks a before and after in the life of the person who suffers from it. It does not happen overnight, but it is a process in which the person with an addictive disorder suffers the consequences of it in each of the areas of their life, and it tends to be seen as a first-person disease. Nothing could be further from the truth. The entire close environment of the person with an addictive disorder is greatly affected when the disorder sets in. It is duly recognized in the scientific literature the important role that family support plays in the recovery of those suffering from an addiction (Lozano et al., 2023), although the consequences that this disease has on the people who take care of them have not been studied to the same extent. In the text of this chapter, reference is made to the figure of the caregiver, although this does not mean that the role falls solely on one person, as there may be several collaborating in the role's development.

As for their typology, it could be said that there are two main types of caregivers, formal and informal, with the latter being the most common (Catalán & Garrote, 2012):

1. Formal caregiver: A person professionally trained to offer care to people with specific needs, such as those related to addiction, usually linked to health institutions or rehabilitation centers, where they receive financial compensation for their work.
2. Informal caregiver: This role, generally assumed by close family members, faces the responsibility of offering emotional support, ensuring therapeutic compliance, and generally facilitating the patient's daily life. These burdens have a significant impact on their own life and well-being, as they also have to balance the care of the person with an addictive disorder with their own personal and work responsibilities, which is why they must reorganize their family life and learn to handle difficult situations related to the addiction.

The constant support of the caregiver can make a difference in terms of the success or failure of recovery, because they not only help in treatment, but they reduce the likelihood of relapse by acting as a permanent support network. However, this role can generate negative effects, such as physical and emotional exhaustion, due to the constant burden of caring for someone with a chronic disease like addiction. This can translate into physical and mental health problems, such as increased stress, anxiety, and depression. All of this will be discussed in depth later.

For this reason, the caregiver must receive both training and professional support to prevent burnout and ensure their well-being. This social and professional support is essential to prevent consequences on the mental and physical health of the caregiver.

15.3 Why Is It Important to Discuss the Role of Support in Addictions?

In scientific literature, it is easy to find evidence that discusses the advantages of social and family support in the prevention, treatment, and reintegration of addictive behaviors (Candil, 2016; Edwards & Steinglass, 1995; SAMHSA, 2024). This is not surprising, addictions, like any other health-related issue, are better addressed if the person feels accompanied and supported.

Family support is therefore considered a protective factor against the development of an addictive behavior, so, at a preventive level, it has great value. In this sense, there is the study by Catanzaro and Laurent (2004), which two decades ago stated that the greater the family support in adolescence, the lower the risk of developing a future addiction, understanding family support as the perception that the person with an addictive disorder has about protection and understanding in the family. In this way, the family environment becomes a safe environment in which to grow and develop and family support is assumed as a multidimensional variable that is related to low levels of perceived family conflicts, and high levels of cohesion and expressiveness. These dimensions of the family environment have been associated with greater adaptation in both adolescents and adults (Catanzaro & Laurent, 2004). In addition to the relevance of family support as a protective and preventive factor, another study highlighted the extent to which informal support and community services modulate the course of alcohol addiction, as well as the fundamental role that social relationships acquire (Weisner et al., 2003). Likewise, some experiences show that patients whose relatives were the subject of psychoeducational interventions adapted to the patients' problems, showed better perception of family support throughout the treatment (Martínez-González et al., 2012) and that the family acted as a protective factor in terms of adherence to treatment (Nelson et al., 2024).

However, the consequences for the family and the close social environment of a person suffering from addictive disorders are negative in terms of their quality of life, affecting social and family dynamics (Kalra & Tung, 2024; Maina et al., 2021). In the following lines, a journey is made through the impact of addictions on caregivers, focusing on the description of their situation, the different areas of their life affected and, also, in some ideas and proposals to improve their quality of life.

15.4 Responsibilities and Functions of the Caregiver

Just as addiction is a process in which the patient with an addiction changes, so does the role of the caregiver evolve through this process. Their responsibilities and functions are different depending on the stage of the treatment:

- Before treatment: the caregiver plays a crucial role for the person with an addictive disorder to recognize their problem and be encouraged to seek help, as they often deny the severity of their situation and, therefore, find it difficult to start a treatment on their own initiative; for example, by detecting signs, such as sudden changes in behavior or excessive and out of context consumption of a substance. When addressing the issue, it is important that the caregiver does so from empathy and without judging, creating an environment in which the person feels heard. The family environment is particularly relevant because, according to Miller and Rollnick (2023), it fosters an atmosphere of support, understanding, and emotional stability that can significantly contribute to the individual's commitment to change. In addition, these same authors have shown that motivational interventions led by caregivers can significantly increase treatment readiness.
- During treatment: the constant support of the caregiver is essential, especially accompanying the person to the treatment sessions and being present throughout the process. Patients who have a family support system have better outcomes during rehabilitation (SAMHSA, 2024). This support helps to reduce the feeling of isolation and, in addition, is useful for the caregiver by strengthening emotional tools and stress management. The caregiver must be available for the patient in times when emotions are difficult to handle and temptations to relapse appear.
- After treatment: the work of the caregiver does not end, but is fundamental to prevent relapses and assist in the social reintegration of the patient (Nattala et al., 2010). The risk of relapse is higher during the first weeks after treatment. At this point, the caregiver must supervise a new routine that does not include the use of substances and promoting participation in healthy activities, whether they are work-related, social or recreational, as well as identifying early signs of relapse.

Next, the two main functions of the caregiver are described: emotional support and logistical support.

15.4.1 *Emotional Support*

The quality of emotional support can directly influence the patient's motivation to continue with treatment and their ability to cope with stressful situations. In this sense, the caregiver acts as a source of security, helping to reduce the fear and anxiety that often accompany the treatment of an addiction. Likewise, it also helps the person with an addictive disorder to manage their emotions, especially those that increase the risk of relapse, such as stress, frustration, or despair, among others.

Emotional support is also essential in the stage after treatment, where the risk of relapse is high, as has been mentioned. The person with an addictive disorder needs at this point an environment of stability and understanding. A context of prolonged emotional stability strengthens the patient's skills to handle stressful situations and thus reduces the likelihood of relapse.

Occasionally, episodes of crisis may unexpectedly arise due to the mere appearance of withdrawal symptoms, or the confrontation of intense emotional situations, or when a relapse has occurred. People with addictions tend to experience difficulties in regulating their emotions and controlling impulses, which leaves them vulnerable to relapse when they appear. At this point, the caregiver must provide emotional support and help stabilize the person with an addictive disorder. Crisis management techniques, such as intervention in times of high emotional distress, can help reduce the negative impact of these episodes on the recovery process. In addition, the caregiver must be able to recognize the signs prior to a crisis, such as drastic changes in behavior or mood, and act before the situation worsens.

15.4.2 Logistical Support

The role of the caregiver within the routine procedures in the life of someone suffering from an addiction is fundamental. Regarding surveillance and control, they are key aspects within the functions that a caregiver must perform in accompanying someone with an addiction. Supervision of the patient's habits and behaviors is essential to detect early signs of relapse and for the patient to feel greater responsibility towards their actions. In addition, if the caregiver combines surveillance with emotional support, the effectiveness of the treatment increases.

Surveillance should not focus exclusively on the person with an addictive disorder, but also on their environment: access to substances, friendships, relatives or objects associated with consumption. An environment free of stimuli associated with consumption can decrease the likelihood of relapse and the caregiver must take measures to limit the patient's contact with those elements that can trigger the addiction.

The caregiver must also establish clear boundaries and control strategies that contribute to the patient's autonomy; the long-term goal is for the patient to gain control over their own behavior. Activities such as promoting self-control skills in the patient and participating in healthy activities that promote a new routine free of addictions, can be a fundamental pillar to prevent relapses.

Logistical support also translates into adopting the role of liaison between the person with an addiction and health professionals, facilitating the exchange of information and understanding of the recommendations provided. Effective communication between the caregiver and the medical team can significantly improve adherence to treatment. In addition, the caregiver also explains to health professionals the particularities of the life and environment of the person being cared for, which allows for more effective and personalized care.

It is important that the caregiver participate as much as possible in therapy sessions to provide information that can be valuable to the therapist, as the person with an addictive disorder is likely to hide or omit certain key issues related to their addiction due to shame or denial of the problem.

Finally, the caregiver must also be responsible for managing and coordinating the administrative part of the treatment: for example, the schedule of medical appointments, the control of the administration of medications, ensuring participation in certain additional therapeutic activities, among others.

15.5 Impact of Addictions on Caregivers

Next, we delve into the impact that addiction has on those who care for the person with an addictive disorder. It should be noted that the consequences of addictions on the formal caregiver will not be addressed, as they are professionals with specialized training that allows them, unlike the informal caregiver, to disconnect from work as soon as their working hours end.

15.5.1 Economic Impact

The impact of addiction on the family economy is significant in the balance of income and expenses (Sharma et al., 2019). If the person with an addiction is gainfully employed, they may stop earning and generate a loss of profit that affects the family's livelihood. Of course, it is the family in general and the caregiver in particular who have to assume, not only the role of emotional and physical support, but also must cover the economic needs of the home, which is another addition in the general computation of stress and overload. In addition, it is not only the work of the person with an addictive disorder that is in danger, as the hourly dedication of the caregiver can also have consequences on their work.

In addition to the reduction of income, there may be an increase in medical and rehabilitation expenses, with the consequent financial strain on the family economy. In fact, the costs associated with the treatment of addiction can also be high, not only in private health care centers, but in public health systems that do not cover this type of treatment. The cost of therapies, admissions, medications and other specialized services can sometimes become an insurmountable obstacle for families, forced to resort to loans, sell assets or make significant sacrifices in other aspects of their lives to be able to afford the treatment of the person with an addictive disorder. This prolonged financial pressure can affect the quality of life of all household members, generating a cycle of economic stress that can further aggravate family dynamics.

To all this, we must add the cases where the person with an addiction has access to the current account or credit cards and makes improper and sometimes reckless uses of family money, either to sustain substance consumption, or to cover previously contracted debts. This not only aggravates economic difficulties, but can also generate serious family conflicts, eroding trust and the sense of financial security in the home.

15.5.2 Impact on Family Structure and Relationships

The appearance of an addictive disorder deeply affects the family relationships, transforming the dynamics as the caregiver assumes new responsibilities. These responsibilities increase as the person with addictive behavior loses functionality in their daily life, which often generates an imbalance in power relations and the distribution of tasks within the home (Edwards & Steinglass, 1995). Consequently, this imbalance can produce significant emotional wear among family members, especially in the primary caregiver, and thus contribute to the emergence of problems such as chronic stress, anxiety, and depression among caregivers (Marín-Navarrete et al., 2016).

It should be remembered that addiction does not appear suddenly, but has a trajectory and, therefore, is not the same at every stage of the process. In fact, as addiction progresses, family relationships can deteriorate due to the feeling of abandonment experienced by other household members, who often perceive that the needs of the person with an addiction are prioritized over family needs (Brown et al., 2015). The time the caregiver spends with their own family can be threatened and, as a result, generate intrafamily conflicts that result in a progressive emotional distancing, even leading in some cases to definitive breaks in affective relationships (Orford, 2013). Children, in particular, may experience feelings of abandonment or neglect, as the caregiver is focused on the needs of the person with an addictive disorder. This situation can lead to behavioral problems and poor school performance.

15.5.3 Impact on the Mental Health of the Caregiver

The responsibility of caring for someone with a dependency generates an intense emotional and psychological burden, so the impact of addiction on the mental health of the caregiver is considerable. As seen earlier, the consequences of an addictive disorder on daily life, relationships, and the economy result in high levels of stress and anxiety, due to the unpredictable nature of addiction and the constant attention required by the person with an addictive disorder. All of this leads to an emotional burden that can deteriorate the general well-being of those who care for them. Being a process, in which more time in treatment is required as a predictor of therapeutic success, the stressful situation can last for weeks or months. Continuous exposure to stressful situations, beyond the onset of anxiety disorders, can lead to a prolonged release of the hormone cortisol, whose excessive release is associated with various health problems, including a deficient functioning of the immune system (Sapolsky, 2004). Chronic stress can lead to generalized exhaustion, also known as Burnout Syndrome.

Also, the overload of care can lead to symptoms of depression, due to the feeling of guilt and failure that has been previously discussed. These feelings, along with emotional exhaustion, increase the vulnerability of the caregiver to mood disorders. To all this is added a perception of low social support, that is, caregivers feel that they cannot share their difficulties with others for fear of being judged or misunderstood (Brown et al., 2015).

The courtesy stigma, which affects people close to the person with addictive disorders, is also often suffered by the caregiver (Favina et al., 2024; Maldonado et al., 2023). When the person with an addiction is a family member, this courtesy stigma can spread to the rest of the family nucleus, causing conflict situations, a greater emotional burden, and repercussions on the well-being of the family environment.

Also, the mental health of the caregiver can be compromised when their relationship with the person with an addiction reaches a point of codependency, that is, the commitment to their recovery becomes personal and with blurred boundaries. In these cases, caregivers personally assume the responsibility for the patient's recovery; if the person with an addiction relapses or does not progress as expected, it can generate frustration and feelings of guilt (Lowang & Singh, 2023).

15.6 Care of the Caregiver

One of the key elements regarding the role of the caregiver is, precisely, their care. As described in the previous section, each of the responsibilities and functions performed by the caregiver carries a physical and emotional burden that is difficult to manage, especially when it comes to relatives or close friends of the person with an addictive disorder and who are not care professionals. Therefore, it is necessary to address the health of the caregiver and, next, some strategies will be proposed for this purpose.

15.6.1 Regarding Emotional Coping

Those who care for people with addictions must face an intense and prolonged emotional burden, which produces emotional exhaustion, which can become pathological, with the development of disorders such as anxiety and depression. It is essential that the health system and addiction professionals recognize the needs of the caregiver and offer emotional and therapeutic support to manage stress and exhaustion. The well-being of the caregiver is not only crucial for their own mental health, but it is also key to the success in the treatment of the person with an addictive disorder; an exhausted or sick caregiver cannot respond to the needs of the person with an addictive disorder to recover from their addiction. In fact, previous studies have determined that the caregiver of a person with an addictive disorder suffers more emotional burden than people who care for those who suffer from other mental pathologies, such as dementia (Soellner & Hofheinz, 2024). Moreover, this burden is even greater in situations where there is domestic violence (Hsu, 2024). Psychological interventions aimed at the caregiver are, therefore, essentials. These interventions, such as cognitive-behavioral therapy or support groups, have proven to be effective in helping caregivers manage their emotions and develop strategies to cope with stress (Sampogna et al., 2023). When caregivers feel guilt or overwhelmed by their role, they need to be provided with skills for emotional management, training, and ongoing support to learn to take care of themselves while caring for their loved ones. The emotional well-being of the caregiver will result in greater therapeutic efficacy.

Another source of emotional tension arises when the patient expresses wishes contrary to medical recommendations, something that forces the caregiver to make difficult decisions, considering the patient's physical well-being, mental health, and autonomy. Adequate training on handling conflict situations can be key to minimizing the consequences of all these types of sources of emotional stress (Marín-Navarrete et al., 2016). In this regard, it is interesting to mention initiatives like that of Renati et al. (2022), which present the design of an application that serves to offer tools for emotional management, self-care, or information on how to deal with stress, which seems to be yielding good results.

15.6.2 Regarding Codependency and Personal Boundaries

The relationship between the caregiver and the person suffering from an addictive disorder can reach a point of codependency, where, due to a lack of clear boundaries, the emotional dynamic leads the caregiver to become excessively involved in the life of the person with an addiction. Therefore, it is essential that training and psychological support also focus on recognizing the signs of codependency and establishing healthy boundaries, in order to experience less emotional exhaustion. For example, one of these healthy boundaries should be aimed at not personally assuming responsibility for the patient's recovery.

The acquisition of self-care skills, with activities such as physical exercise, meditation, and access to psychological therapies is a convenient and beneficial process to avoid the consequences of codependency. Likewise, the establishment of own support networks can be a space where they can share their experiences and feelings without fear of being judged. Similarly, therapeutic interventions aimed at caregivers, such as family therapy or support groups for codependents, are essential to help them understand the boundaries between their own well-being and the recovery process of the person with an addictive disorder.

15.6.3 Regarding Chronic Stress (Burnout)

As mentioned in the previous section, burnout or emotional exhaustion is a set of symptoms, common among caregivers of people with addictions, caused by chronic stress due to emotional and physical overload, which can lead to a feeling of helplessness, chronic fatigue, and even end up in a depression (Shishkova & Bocharov, 2022). Caregivers must develop strategies to prevent burnout, such as the development of skills to manage stress and the implementation of clear boundaries. Dedicating time to recreational activities, regular physical exercise, healthy eating, and adequate rest, can be useful activities to maintain mental and physical well-being.

In cases where burnout has already set in the caregiver, psychological therapies, such as cognitive-behavioral therapy or acceptance and commitment therapy, have proven to be effective in helping them develop coping strategies for difficult situations (Levin et al., 2024; Ng et al., 2024). Psychotherapy also offers a safe space where caregivers can express their frustrations and concerns.

15.6.4 Regarding Stigma and Isolation

The social stigma inherent in addictions not only affects the people who suffer from them, but also the people who accompany them in their recovery process who often experience social isolation, shame, or even rejection from friends and family, the so-called courtesy stigma, mentioned earlier. Caregivers who feel stigmatized are more prone to develop symptoms of anxiety and depression. Therefore, they must have access to support networks that offer them a safe space where they can share their experiences and thus break with isolation.

The development of a strong support network, informal (family and friends) or formal (support groups), is essential to decrease the impact of stigma and isolation on caregivers. In fact, support groups for caregivers have proven to be effective in reducing stress and isolation, by allowing them to connect with other people going through similar situations. In addition, community resources, especially NGOs, also play a crucial role in providing education and tools for caregivers to have more coping skills for the burden of taking care of a person with an addictive disorder. Interventions that focus on strengthening the social skills of the family, such as the one proposed by Hatmanti et al. (2023), in which they propose organizing a family nursing method with a support-based educational system focused on families supporting teenagers addicted to smartphones. Or the one proposed by Kalra and Tung (2024), where they emphasize the importance of interventions that emphasize strengthening support systems and various aspects of families with personalized approaches.

Regarding stigma, it is worth noting that women often take on the role of caregivers in a more intense way, which aggravates the burden they bear. The traditional concept of women as being protective, the fundamental pillar of the family, unconditional lover, and with unlimited capacity for self-sacrifice, has been an image generated by the dominant social representations and gender stereotypes. (Negrete Carballo & Edith García Cerón, 2023). In a landscape where it is still difficult to disassociate from the idea of the man as the provider and the woman in charge of the home and domestic care, women, both in their role as mothers and wives, have predominantly carried the responsibility of supporting family members with addictions, often being the last and most unconditional resource. According to Santos and Martin (2009), who focus on the case of relatives with alcoholism, the situation can lead caregivers to isolation and exhaustion, possibly leading them to stop frequenting social environments for fear that the patient will drink and cause humiliating scenes. Therefore, the care and attention to caregivers must necessarily have a gender perspective, which allows a deeper understanding of the roles and the physical, psychological, and social overload that falls on women.

15.7 Final Considerations

Throughout the chapter, an attempt has been made to break down, from different perspectives, the role of informal caregivers of other people with addictive behaviors. This is a role not chosen, imposed by circumstances, and often invisible, which is very difficult to face. Therefore, an attempt has been made to respond to the different challenges that a caregiver must face. These challenges involve, first of all, as precise a conceptual approach as possible, where it is understood what responsibilities the caregiver is assuming without any type of training, ranging from logistical support in day-to-day life, to purely emotional support. On the other hand, there has been an in-depth discussion about another key aspect, which is the impact, more direct or indirect, on the life of the caregiver, in the economic, family, and psychological areas. Taking into account all of the above, if anything stands out from this chapter, it is the section dedicated to the care of the caregiver. The informal caregiver needs tools and specific attention on how to deal with the situation that has arisen, without losing their own health along the way. They must, therefore, have access to emotional coping tools, how to establish personal boundaries, deal with stress, cope with the stigma associated with addictions, and not fall into the isolation that can be caused by having a relative or close person with addictive behaviors, whether out of shame, the aforementioned stigma, or simply not knowing how to deal with complex situations in social environments.

Finally, and by way of conclusion, it is worth noting that the care of a person with an addictive disorder is not only the responsibility of the family or the close social environment that suffers from this problem. Society as a whole and Public

Administrations must assume their part of the responsibility in the care and attention to the needs of caregiver families. The family or the close environment will not ask for help if they do not know they can ask for it because they are unaware of the services available to them. Addictions arise, in part, because there is a social context that encourages or facilitates them; therefore, the responsibility in dealing with them must be collective.

References

Brown, S., Tracy, E. M., Jun, M., Park, H., & Min, M. O. (2015). Personal network recovery enablers and relapse risks for women with substance dependence. *Qualitative Health Research, 25*(3), 371–385. https://doi.org/10.1177/1049732314551055

Candil, A. L. (2016). Acompañar a usuarios intensivos de drogas: el papel de las redes de proximidad en los tratamientos ambulatorios. *Antípoda. Revista de Antropología y Arqueología, 1*(26). https://doi.org/10.7440/antipoda26.2016.08

Catalán, M. P., & Garrote, A. I. (2012). Revisión de los cuidados informales. Descubriendo al cuidador principal. *NURE Inv [edición electrónica], 9*(57), 1–12. Disponible en: http://www.fuden.es/FICHEROS_ADMINISTRADOR/ORIGINAL/NURE57_origi-nal_revis.pd

Catanzaro, S. J., & Laurent, J. (2004). Perceived family support, negative mood regulation expectancies, coping, and adolescent alcohol use: Evidence of mediation and moderation effects. *Addictive Behaviors, 29*(9), 1779–1797. https://doi.org/10.1016/j.addbeh.2004.04.001

Edwards, M. E., & Steinglass, P. (1995). Family therapy treatment outcomes for alcoholism. *Journal of Marital and Family Therapy, 21*(4), 475–509. https://doi.org/10.1111/j.1752-0606.1995.tb00176.x

Favina, A., Munaru, G., Muwanguzi, M., Rubega, A., Lutasingwa, D., Maling, S., & Ashaba, S. (2024). Psychometric evaluation of the affiliate stigma scale for caregivers of people with mental illness in Uganda. *BMC Psychology, 12*, 450. https://doi.org/10.1186/s40359-024-01947-8

Hatmanti, N. M., Sari, R. Y., Septianingrum, Y., Setiyowati, E., & Maimunah, S. (2023). Supportive educative system based on the integration of family centered care and family tasks towards family support in adolescents with smartphone addiction. *Bali Medical Journal, 12*(3), 2896–2900. https://doi.org/10.15562/bmj.v12i3.4351

Hsu, W. Y. (2024). Occurrence and correlates of domestic violence among Asian patients with alcohol use disorder seeking treatment for cessation. *Alcohol (Fayetteville, N.Y.), 120*, 59–64. https://doi.org/10.1016/j.alcohol.2024.01.002

Kalra, H., & Tung, S. (2024). Mediating role of social support and family functioning on quality of life of family caregivers of individuals with alcohol use disorder. *Indian Journal of Psychological Medicine, XX*(X), 1–7. https://doi.org/10.1177/02537176241275566

Levin, M. E., Krafft, J., & Twohig, M. P. (2024). An overview of research on acceptance and commitment therapy. *The Psychiatric clinics of North America, 47*(2), 419–431. https://doi.org/10.1016/j.psc.2024.02.007

Lowang, C., & Singh, K. P. (2023). Co-dependents' awareness on addiction: scope of social work intervention with family members of substance dependent in Arunachal Pradesh. *Towards excellence, 15*(3), 186–199. https://doi.org/10.37867/te150317

Lozano, A., Estrada, Y., Scott, D., Tapia, M. I., Santos, H. P., Jr., Carrico, A. W., Zolobczuk, J., Manker, A., & Prado, G. (2023). Familias con Orgullo: Study protocol for an efficacy study of a family-based intervention for Hispanic sexual minority youth. *PLoS One, 18*(12), e0295683. https://doi.org/10.1371/journal.pone.0295683

Maina, G., Ogenchuk, M., Phaneuf, T., & Kwame, A. (2021). "I can't live like that": the experience of caregiver stress of caring for a relative with substance use disorder. *Substance Abuse Treatment, Prevention, and Policy, 16*(1), 11. https://doi.org/10.1186/s13011-021-00344-3

Maldonado, D., Ronzani, T. M., & Fernandes, L. (2023). Estigma de cortesia e condições de saúde: revisão sistemática de literatura. *Psicologia Em Estudo, 28*. https://doi.org/10.4025/psicolestud.v28i0.52111

Marín-Navarrete, R., Medina-Mora, M. E., & Tena-Suck, A. (2016). Addiction care in Mexico: A challenge for non-specialized health professionals. *Salud Mental, 39*(5), 241–242. https://doi.org/10.17711/SM.0185-3325.2016.027

Martínez-González, J. M., Albein-Urios, N., Munera, P., & Verdejo-García, A. (2012). Psychoeducation as a strategy to improve family support perceived from patient with alcohol dependence and personality disorder. *International Journal of Psychological Research, 5*(1), 18–24. https://doi.org/10.21500/20112084.745

Miller, W. R., & Rollnick, S. (2023). *Motivational interviewing: Helping people change* (4th ed.). Guilford Press.

Nattala, P., Leung, K. S., Nagarajaiah, & Murthy, P. (2010). Family member involvement in relapse prevention improves alcohol dependence outcomes: a prospective study at an addiction treatment facility in India. *Journal of Studies on Alcohol and Drugs, 71*(4), 581–587. https://doi.org/10.15288/jsad.2010.71.581

Negrete Carballo, L. A., & Edith García Cerón, M. d. l. Á. (2023). Intervención sistémica en mujeres familiares de personas con abuso de sustancias adictivas. *Revista Internacional de Investigación en Adicciones, 9*(1), 51–60. https://doi.org/10.28931/riiad.2023.1.06

Nelson, D. D., McDaniel, J. T., McIntosh, S., Godinet, M., & Albright, D. L. (2024). Family support and treatment completion for unhealthy alcohol use in a SBIRT program. *Journal of Social Work Practice in the Addictions, 25*(1), 100–118. https://doi.org/10.1080/1533256X.2024.2351366

Ng, L., Adams, E., Henderson, D., Donaghy, E., & Mercer, S. W. (2024). Interventions for burnout and well-being in homelessness staff: a systematic scoping review. *medRxiv*. https://doi.org/10.1101/2024.08.21.24312389

Orford, J. (2013). *Addiction dilemmas: Family experiences from literature and research and their lessons for practice*. Wiley-Blackwell.

Renati, R., Bonfiglio, N. S., & Rollo, D. (2022). Dealing with loved ones' addiction: Development of an app to cope with caregivers' stress. *International Journal of Environmental Research and Public Health, 19*(23). https://doi.org/10.3390/ijerph192315950

Sampogna, G., Brohan, E., Luciano, M., Chowdhary, N., & Fiorillo, A. (2023). Psychosocial interventions for carers of people with severe mental and substance use disorders: a systematic review and meta-analysis. *European Psychiatry : The Journal of the Association of European Psychiatrists, 66*(1), e98. https://doi.org/10.1192/j.eurpsy.2023.2472

Santos, E. C. V. d., & Martin, D. (2009). Cuidadoras de pacientes alcoolistas no município de Santos, SP, Brasil. *Revista Brasileira de Enfermagem, 62*(2), 194–199. https://doi.org/10.1590/s0034-71672009000200004

Sapolsky, R. M. (2004). *Why zebras don't get ulcers* (3rd ed.). Henry Holt.

Sharma, A., Sharma, A., Gupta, S., & Thapar, S. (2019). Study of family burden in substance dependence: A tertiary care hospital-based study. *Indian Journal of Psychiatry, 61*(2), 131–138. https://doi.org/10.4103/psychiatry.IndianJPsychiatry_123_15

Shishkova, A. M., & Bocharov, V. V. (2022). The burnout concept as a theoretical framework for investigating the caregiving impact of relatives of patients with addictive disorders. *Psychology in Russia: State of the Art, 15*(3), 111–132. https://doi.org/10.11621/pir.2022.0307

Soellner, R., & Hofheinz, C. (2024). Burden and satisfaction with social support in families with a history of problematic substance use or dementia—A comparison. *BMC Psychology, 12*(1), 448. https://doi.org/10.1186/s40359-024-01940-1

Substance Abuse and Mental Health Services Administration [SAMHSA]. (2024). Recovery and recovery support. U.S. Department of Health and Human Services. https://www.samhsa.gov/find-help/recovery

Weisner, C., Delucchi, K., Matzger, H., & Schmidt, L. (2003). The role of community services and informal support on five-year drinking trajectories of alcohol dependent and problem drinkers. *Journal of Studies on Alcohol, 64*(6), 862–873. https://doi.org/10.15288/jsa.2003.64.862

Chapter 16
Stigmatization of Women Who Consume Alcohol in a Rural Indigenous Community in Central Mexico

Marcela Tiburcio Sainz, Jazmín Mora Ríos, and Pilar Bernal Pérez

16.1 Introduction

The word "stigma" comes from the Greek *στίγμα*, Latin stigma, which refers to the tattoos given to slaves and criminals to mark their status or crime. These tattoos were brief inscriptions or initials, mainly on the forehead, and marked the greatest type of social degradation in Greek and later Roman civilization (Setién-García, 2020). One of the principal scholars on the subject was the sociologist Erving Goffman, who defined social stigma as an attribute or mark carried by some individuals, whose "discrediting effect is very extensive; sometimes it is also called a failing, a shortcoming, a handicap" (Goffman, 2022, p. 2). According to Goffman, when these marks are related to psychology, they are called character defects.

Nowadays, a mark on some aspect of identity that is considered negative places a heavy burden on a person; it causes others to disapprove and point them out, which limits and devalues them. That is, the negative value carried by stigma exists in close relation to the norms, beliefs, and attitudes in the context surrounding the person affected.

The aim of this chapter is to explore the experiences of stigma of women in an Indigenous community in central Mexico who use alcohol. It first presents a review of the literature on the subject, followed by an analysis of the narratives of women from the community, where the production and consumption of the traditional

M. Tiburcio Sainz (✉) · P. Bernal Pérez
Department of Social Sciences in Health, Ramón de la Fuente Muñiz National Institute of Psychiatry, Mexico City, Mexico
e-mail: tibsam@inprf.gob.mx; pilar.bp@tec.mx

J. Mora Ríos
Direction of Epidemiological and Psychosocial Research, Ramón de la Fuente Muñiz National Institute of Psychiatry, Mexico City, Mexico
e-mail: morarj@inprf.gob.mx

T. Mota Ronzani (ed.), *Social Stigma and Drug Use*,
https://doi.org/10.1007/978-3-031-94813-8_16

alcoholic beverage pulque is an ancestral practice, with particular beliefs and values that accept and privilege men who drink it, but disapprove of and condemn women who do.

In recent years, the United Nations, through the United Nations Office on Drugs and Crime (UNODC, 2020), has called on member countries to combat the stigmatization of people who use substances. Such stigma is a global problem with numerous effects on the lives of users that interfere with getting appropriate care. In Mexico, a study of the perceptions of people who use substances found that there is greater negative perception of illegal drug users than of those who use alcohol (Bustos et al., 2022). Social tolerance towards alcohol is greater, mainly in rural areas of the country, and is present in people's lives, so that when there are problems related to its use, it takes up to 10 years for them to seek help (Natera et al., 2007).

In an interesting review, Davis and O'Neill (2022) identified some barriers to treatment for alcohol use in rural communities. Prominent among these are the doctor-patient relationship, barriers with health service providers, the remoteness of care services, lack of privacy, internalized stigma, social prejudice, addiction as a moral rather than health issue, and health care workers' stigmatization of patients. Lipsky et al. (2016) understand discrimination as one or more stressful events that can affect people's well-being; their research suggests that discrimination is related to alcohol abuse and mental disorders, and that Hispanic women who use substances suffer greater discrimination.

16.2 The Social Burden of Being a Woman in Minority Ethnic Groups

There are certain factors that characterize ethnic minorities in Mexico, specifically the Indigenous population: (a) social marginalization, (b) the stigmatization of difference, (c) inequality and lack of recognition, (d) scarcity of material resources, and (e) challenges to survival (Bari, 2002; Navarrete, 2008). These factors contribute to precarious living conditions for the community in general, and for those with alcohol use problems in particular. In the case of Indigenous women, discrimination is associated with) symptoms and manifestations of mental health problems such as depression and anxiety in vulnerable populations (Romer, 2003). The disadvantages are even greater due to gender differences in social and cultural roles (Camacho et al., 2022). Generally speaking, in various ethnic groups and societies, being a woman implies a disadvantageous social burden, and it therefore creates a social problem.

There is growing interest in the question of gender inequalities in health care. It is becoming increasingly important to understand the impact of these inequalities on various areas of women's lives, for example in access to health resources, in cultural diversity, in social inequality, and in their interconnections (Llort-Suárez et al., 2013). While there have been advances in legislation, and in the recognition of the need to address health problems from a perspective of gender and human rights, it remains a challenge to implement actions that have a real impact on women's lives. This is particularly true in spaces where traditional gender assumptions are deeply rooted and assign women to private spaces (the home, the family, and reproduction) while men dominate the public sphere as economic providers. In practice, these stereotyped gender roles are unsustainable because families require resources to survive, and women's economic participation is important in supporting their homes. The persistence of these cultural premises in the social imaginary affects women's emotional well-being and translate into violence of all kinds when they are perceived to transgress these roles.

Many of the approaches in the social sciences and in epidemiological studies have been characterized by an androcentric perspective (Esteban, 2006), in concepts that describe women's role in the home, the family, motherhood, sexuality, reproduction, and the domestic and public spheres, attributing them to a certain gender role reserved just for women (Llort-Suárez et al., 2013). This perspective has legitimized inequalities between men and women, and promoted the idea that certain behaviors or situations are allowed for men, but not for women. The result has been an invisibilization of women's legitimate needs outside of the traditionally imposed roles, or that even seem to contradict such roles, such as alcohol use. Sweetnam and Morrissette (2018), for example, explored the factors involved in the recovery of women who consumed alcohol in an aboriginal community in Manitoba, Canada. Among the major barriers women identified to receiving treatment for alcohol use were: (a) stigma and social disapproval, (b) a high unemployment rate, (c) economic barriers, (d) the responsibilities of care for family members, and (e) opposition and lack of support from friends and family. The authors note that women who enter treatment for alcohol use have different needs than men, and that the perception of alcohol abuse among women contrasts with society's perception of femininity, which contribute to women's secrecy about alcohol abuse and their hesitation in seeking help.

Epidemiological data allows us to know precisely the differences in alcohol use between men and women. The Mexican survey of alcohol and tobacco use (Villatoro, et al., 2017) shows that 48.1% of men used alcohol in the previous month, 19.8% excessively; the figures for women were 24.4% and 10.3%, respectively. Men's alcohol use is thus almost double that of women; however, since 2011, there has been an increase in women's use.

In the state of Hidalgo, this same survey reports a prevalence of daily alcohol use in men of 3.2 and 0.9% in women, and the figures for excessive alcohol use are 45.6% for men and 21.9% for women (Villatoro, et al., 2017). Both nationally and in Hidalgo, women's use is almost half that of men. Vega et al. (2015), in a study of the Indigenous population living in and native to Mexico City, found that the prevalence of alcohol use for Indigenous women was 22.9%, as compared with 21% for non-Indigenous women. Indigenous populations suffer from little or no direct access to health services, at the same time that the repercussions of alcohol use affect them more severely because of malnutrition and extreme poverty.

Vázquez et al. (2022), in a study of alcohol and other substance use by Indigenous women aged 18–69 in the state of Tabasco found that 34.5% presented a low risk of use, 46% a moderate risk, and 19.5% a high risk. These data make visible the fact that women use alcohol with different levels of risk. The need thus arises to address and analyze the dichotomy present in the social construction of the roles assigned to men and women in terms of alcohol use and their respective consequences of social discrimination (Llort-Suárez et al., 2013).

16.3 Indigenous Women and Alcohol Use

Closely related to the norms and cultural values around alcohol use is the fact that women who drink excessively experience a greater number and severity of associated problems than men. Gender differences also occur around recovery; in a study of the natural remission of alcohol dependence it was found that women experience less social pressure than men to seek help, since their closest social network ignores or denies the problem of alcohol use and thus receives less support to maintain abstinence (Bischof et al., 2000).

The situation of female drinkers living in rural areas has been even less explored, but some studies suggest that like urban women, they suffer greater stigmatization than men (Weisner & Schmidt, 1992; Wilsnack et al., 2000), and are morally and socially penalized (Llort-Suárez et al., 2013). Rural women may present more severe problems related to use than their urban counterparts, including greater comorbidity, and the barriers to seeking treatment may be greater in rural areas. However, it is possible that the differences with urban women in stigmatization are smaller than expected (Booth & McLaughlin, 2000).

In summary, alcohol use among the rural female population is a little-studied phenomenon, and even less is known about Indigenous women in Mexico. However, anthropologists have made important contributions in this regard, including the work of Berruecos and Velasco (1977) in the Sierra de Puebla; of García-Alcaraz (1972) in Estado de Mexico, of Pozas (1957) among the Chamula, and of Eber (1995) among the Pedranos of Chiapas, as well as of others who have documented a high level of alcohol use among Indigenous adults of both sexes.

16.4 Female Drinkers in the Otomí Indigenous Community of the Mezquital Valley

Some years ago, a study was carried out in an Indigenous community of the municipality of Cardonal, in the state of Hidalgo, located in the region known as the Mezquital Valley (Tiburcio Sainz, 2009). The municipality has been inhabited by Otomí people since the sixteenth century (INFDM, 2002). Today, about 6.2% of the population over 5 years old speaks an Indigenous language, mainly Otomí (INEGI, 2020). Franco (1992) explains that the isolation of Cardonal has left it one of the municipalities where the Otomí language and culture have been best preserved. According to INEGI (2020), the total population of the community is 745 inhabitants, 55% women and 45% men. The economically active population is 39% of the total, and 290 individuals 15 years or older are literate. However, it is also an area with a high level of excessive alcohol use.

The consumption of pulque as a traditional cultural practice has been maintained for many years among the people of the Mezquital Valley. Pulque is considered a food, a traditional drink, and a product that can be traded. It is consumed at family gatherings and village ceremonies, but it is also part of daily consumption. Until recently, some mothers even gave young children aguamiel,[1] as if it were a harmless drink, and even believed that it was nutritious. The consumption of pulque and alcohol in general has been normalized as a widespread practice in the population, almost entirely accepted and approved for men, but not for women.

An ethnographic investigation in this community, carried out by a research team from the National Institute of Psychiatry (Natera et al., 2007), found that in the community of the Mezquital Valley, as in many other Indigenous communities in Mexico, women are given attributions and responsibilities related to the care of others, as well as to modesty, self-denial, obedience toward men, and an implicit duty to remain silent. A woman who drinks alcohol is stigmatized with disapproval, discrimination, segregation, and doubts about her morality. Although some women hide their drinking, precisely because they are pointed out and judged by the rest of the community, their level of use can be high or excessive, so that some of them meet the diagnostic criteria for incipient dependence, such as an inability to abstain, increased tolerance, lack of control, and effects on other areas of life.

The following section presents the experience of two Indigenous women from this community who have consumed a significant amount of alcohol from a very early age, who have been stigmatized, and who have suffered the consequences both of their drinking and of the associated stigma.

16.5 The Stigma Associated with Alcohol Use: Two Women's Experiences

Cristina and Bertha are two friends in their twenties who live in one of the municipalities of the Mezquital Valley. Knowing that a study was being carried out about families and alcohol use in the area, they themselves approached the researchers to ask for help and to be given "pills to stop drinking pulque." They were aware that

[1] Aguamiel is the sap of the maguey plant, from which pulque is made. It is extracted from the heart of the maguey through an artisanal process of scraping the inside of the plant. It contains a large quantity of sugars and proteins. Pulque is the alcoholic beverage that is obtained from the fermentation of aguamiel.

they had a problem with alcohol use, but they did not know what to do about it, and their request for help provided an opportunity to learn their stories. Both had been drinking pulque since they were little girls; like many people in the community they were raised with this tradition that can become a serious problem. Now they are adults with their own children, and their drinking have been getting worse, both in quantity and in frequency.

Although there are differences, the women's stories have elements in common: alcohol use from an early age, influence from family members to drink, social stigma from the community and its consequences, inability to control their current alcohol use, and its effect on their children.

16.5.1 The Case of Bertha

Bertha is an Indigenous woman who grew up in a large family including her parents and several siblings. Bertha mentions an important detail that she associates with her start of alcohol use: having had a distant mother. In Bertha's own words:

> [I started drinking pulque] when I was little. It's that my grandmother... my mom lived with my grandmother and, well, my mom didn't hold me, she hung me in the hammock up on the roof and gave me a bottle of aguamiel, and, well, there I was and they left, they went to work or to herd the animals and they left me hanging there alone. I didn't walk until I was three years old, pure pulque, and well, yes, the truth is, I grew up on pure pulque, almost... yes. My brothers and sisters didn't, just me, I'm the only one who drank pulque, because, well, they didn't like it, and because my mom... What can I say? She loved them more. (Bertha)

Bertha's pulque consumption continued throughout her childhood without necessarily being excessive, as there were social controls that helped to keep it within certain limits. She said she drank less as a teenager; in high school, she was embarrassed that her classmates might find out that she liked to drink it. She says: "You see, talking to someone, it smells a lot like pulque."

Having a partner seemed to be the moment when Bertha's consumption increased considerably. She says she went to live with her husband after finishing junior high school: "I was embarrassed, I'd better not drink pulque until we were together. Now my husband knows very well that I drink pulque."

16.5.2 The Case of Cristina

Cristina was the one who took the initiative to approach the research team. She said she had wanted to talk about her alcohol use for a long time but she was embarrassed and didn't know how to do so. The conversation took place near the kiosk,[2] as she wanted to avoid anyone hearing her.

Cristina says that she began drinking pulque when she was a child: "The truth is, [I have drunk it] since I was little because my mom and dad gave me pulque." Paradoxically, she remembers that her father didn't let her drink much, and he told her not to drink it "because you're not a man." When she got married, her husband also drank excessively—in fact, he died for reasons related to his drinking. While they were married, Cristina and her husband had serious arguments that led to physical violence when both got drunk:

> The truth is, when we both got drunk we fought, and my children sometimes got scared because the truth is, we fought with one another, and, well, they got scared. And then, well, I... I won't deny it, I tell the truth, we fought, then neither of us ate... He slapped me and kicked me and I pulled his hair... Yes, we hit one another like that, and the one who won, he would win and leave, and I would stay there in my house with my children, waiting. The truth is, we fought over pure jealousy, pure jealousy and being drunk, jealousy both of us. And from there, things would calm down for a couple of weeks, a week, and then we would fight again when he came home drunk. (Cristina)

Cristina and Bertha say they are very close friends, but above all they share drinking together and their stigmatization from the community. They drink pulque every day, and beer only occasionally, when someone else invites them. Each of them drinks an average of 2–3 l of pulque daily, and up to 4 or 5 l when they drink together: "if it's the two of us I drink a lot; if I'm alone, less," "alone it almost doesn't happen."

Since they developed this pattern of drinking, neither of the two has tried to reduce it. Nor have they had periods when they stop drinking, even if they are sick or under medical treatment: "Not even a year or two months, instead I'll put the pills aside and drink my pulque. I don't even finish the medicine... not even one or two days" (Cristina). Both drink their first glass of pulque at midday after having eaten, never on an empty stomach. Both women refer to experiencing an inability to stop drinking once they start:

> If I drink just a little sip I want more until I feel that I can't anymore... I mean, until I feel I want more, until I get drunk, or until I feel sleepy or I don't know... but, well, I feel that I can't anymore, because I... I go to sleep, yes, but I get up and I want more. (Bertha)

They usually drink pulque together at one of their homes, and occasionally, when they go to the nearest city, they drink discreetly at the market, as it is forbidden to do so in public. When someone invites them, they drink beer in a shop in their town or one nearby.

---

[2] In Mexico, there are often kiosks in parks, generally open on all sides, which are traditionally used for community events or as a place for socializing.

Both their mothers also drink pulque and are sometimes enablers and drinking companions. According to Cristina "My mom lets me drink, we drink when she comes to my house." "She doesn't drink much anymore, just two or three liters, but she gets drunk quickly, because now she doesn't drink much. When she was here she used to drink a lot but now she doesn't." Bertha, in turn, begins to play the role of enabler of her daughter's drinking and attributes her daughter's drinking to the fact that she drank during pregnancy:

> Sometimes [my daughter] tells me, "Mom, I want a little bit of pulque," she says, I feed her and give her pulque, and, well... she drinks, but just a little, not even a glass, just a little bit, but now that I think about it, she is too young to give it to her, I need to give her something so that she dislikes it. I think that she liked it from a young age because I drank pulque and I imagine... I drank pulque and I was pregnant. (Bertha)

Neither woman has received any help or advice about how to stop drinking; there are no specialized treatment centers in their community or in nearby towns.

In Cristina's case, drinking precipitated physical violence between her and her husband. Bertha attributes to alcohol two significant incidents in her life that are related: she mentioned having "given away" her daughter (who currently lives with her husband's family), as a result of an episode of infidelity on her part that almost ended her marriage.

A woman drinking pulque excessively generates the rejection of the community, expressed not only in criticism, but also in mistreatment, disparagement, and sexual harassment. Both women said that there have been numerous occasions when men have come to knock on their door at night with the intention of sexually abusing them:

> He knocks on the door to see if I'm going to come out so he can grab me I think, I think he wants to rape me, but I don't, I don't get up, I don't get up and I bolt the door. (Cristina)

Women also marginalize them:

> They criticize us a lot, that we are drunks, that we're crazy, or who knows what, people hardly talk to us, ever, because they're mad that we drink, and we drink a lot of pulque, that we're drunks, that we're crazy, who knows what, and sometimes I feel very ashamed to go to a meeting or wherever I go, since people see me, who knows what they're whispering, they look me over from head to toe to see if I'm okay or not okay, I feel very ashamed. (Cristina)

> They criticize us, that we're a couple of drunkards that... they even make up gossip that isn't true, that we're with who knows who... they hardly talk to us, they don't say hello to us, if we say hello to them they don't respond... So I even tell her that we should get out of this town so they can relax. My mom left, she left, she also drank pulque, they said that she was taking people's husbands, and I don't know what kind of gossip there was, what there was, until she left. (Bertha)

These manifestations of the community's displeasure can take on more aggressive characteristics, such as insults, and on one occasion a woman tried to bewitch Cristina, apparently so she would stop drinking:

> I just remember that I drank a little bit of pulque and then I felt something, yes, and then I went to a doctor or I don't know what these people are called who know about something

> you feel or what you drank, or what you did or who hates you or who loves you, then I went, and I was left all alone because of that, I felt like I was going to die, right here in my chest I felt something like I don't know what, and then I threw up... he told me to take some fucking thing that I shouldn't take so sometimes I'm very well and sometimes I'm not very well, but just my head... he told me that I would throw that thing up and I did throw it up, it was dirt from the cemetery.

The negative consequences of these women's drinking also affect the well-being of their families and the community. Children seem to be the main victims, and they too receive signs of rejection and aggression from members of the community:

> They always hit my children, the older kids, they always hit him in the stomach, kick him, they hit him very hard when he no longer... my son comes into the kitchen, crying, he's already crying but what can I do? If I don't have money to say to people, You know what? Why are you hitting my daughter, I'm coming right now, I'm going to tell the judge, I'm going to go to court... No, why should people make fun of me? (Cristina)

16.6 Final Considerations

The brief literature review presented here shows how inequities between men and women affect various areas of a woman's life: social and economic relationships, access to health care, and especially access to care relative to substance use, in this particular case, alcohol, whose use in Mexico is accepted and tolerated in men, but is stigmatized and punished in women. This dichotomy seems to be more clearly defined among some ethnic minorities.

For the women interviewed, the main consequences of alcohol use are observed in the social sphere. Thus, there is disapproval from the community, through moralistic finger-pointing and its punishment of the woman who drinks, the social "stain" on what is culturally considered womanly virtue: kindness, selflessness, and a lack of desire, including a desire for alcohol. The findings of this study highlight the importance of including sociocultural and contextual factors in the development of interventions aimed at women, a conclusion that coincides with those found in previous studies (Espinosa Cortés, 2020).

In Bertha's story, there is a background of neglect and abuse in her childhood, and her parents used alcohol when she was a child, so she learned from a very young age to use alcohol to deal with loneliness when she was left alone at home. It has been found in Hispanic women that post-traumatic stress disorders predict harmful alcohol use (Lipsky et al., 2016), as observed in her narrative. The planning of culturally relevant care programs requires further research on post-traumatic stress and its close relationship with subsequent alcohol use, as well as the specificities of this health problem according to ethnicity. As part of such an effort, it is important to encourage the participation of communities, in order to reduce the stigmatization of those who present this and other mental health problems. Psychoeducation on these topics is one way in which this might be accomplished. It is also necessary to train health providers working in these communities to correctly identify those at risk because of alcohol use, and to destigmatize the practice of excessive drinking by understanding it not as a moral problem, but as a health problem, and by providing them with intervention strategies and resources for referrals to specialized care when required.

References

Bari, C. (2002). La cuestión étnica: Aproximación a los conceptos de grupo étnico, identidad étnica, etnicidad y relaciones interétnicas. *Cuadernos de Antropología Social N° 16*, 149–163, 20.

Berruecos, L., & Velasco, P. (1977). *Patrones de ingestión de alcohol en una comunidad indígena de la Sierra Norte de Puebla*. México.

Bischof, G., Rumpf, H., Hapke, U., Meyer, C., & John, U. (2000). Gender differences in natural recovery from alcohol dependence. *Journal of Studies on Alcohol, 61*, 783–786.

Booth, B. M., & Mclaughlin, Y. S. (2000). Barriers to and need for alcohol services for women in rural populations. *Alcoholism: Clinical and Experimental Research, 24*(8), 1267–1275.

Bustos, M., Mora-Rios, J., Villatoro, J., Fleiz Bautista, C., Molina, A., & Medina-Mora, M. E. (2022). Changes in attitudes toward people with substance use disorder: A drug dependence: A comparative study of the general population in Mexico. *International Journal of Environmental Research and Public Health, 19*, 8538. https://doi.org/10.3390/ijerph19148538

Camacho, J., López, K., Guzmán, F., Alonso, M., & González, P. (2022). Identidad étnica y consumo de alcohol en una población indígena de México. *Ciencia Latina Revista Científica Multidisciplinar, 6*(2). https://doi.org/10.37811/cl_rcm.v6i2.2089

Davis, C., & O'Neill, S. (2022). Treatment of alcohol use problems among rural populations: a review of barriers and considerations for increasing access to quality care. *Current Addiction Report, 9*, 432–444.

Eber, C. (1995). *Women and alcohol in a highland Maya town: Water of hope, water of sorrow*. University of Texas Press. 342 p.

Espinosa Cortés, L. M. (2020). Pobreza, estigma y salud. Experiencias vivenciales en tres comunidades de la Costa Chica de Oaxaca, México. In J. Mora Ríos & G. Nateras (Coords.), *Estigma y discriminación en salud. Escenarios y contextos de investigación internacional* (pp. 93–129). UNAM, Instituto Nacional de Psiquiatría y UNAM-PUIS.

Esteban, M. (2006). El estudio de la Salud y el Género: Las ventajas de un Enfoque Antropológico y feminista. *Revista Salud Colectiva, 2*(1), 9–20.

Franco, P. V. (1992). *Grupo doméstico y reproducción social. Parentesco, economía e ideología de una comunidad Otomí del Valle del Mezquital*. Centro de Investigaciones y Estudios Superiores en Antropología Social. Ediciones de la Casa Chata, México, 258 p.

García-Alcaraz, A. (1972). El maguey y el pulque en Tepetlaoxtoc. *Comunidad, 7*(38), 461–474.

Goffman, E. (2022). *Stigma: Notes on the management of spoiled identity*. Penguin.

Instituto Nacional de Estadística, Geografía e Informática (INEGI). (2020). Lengua Indígena. https://www.inegi.org.mx/temas/lengua/

Instituto Nacional para el Federalismo y el Desarrollo Municipal. (2002). *Enciclopedia de los Municipios de México. Hidalgo*. Gobierno del Estado de Hidalgo.

Lipsky, S., Kernic, M., Qiu, Q., & Hasin, D. (2016). Posttraumatic stress disorder and alcohol misuse among women: effects of ethnic minority stressors. *Social Psychiatry Psychiatr Epidemiol, 51*, 407–419.

Llort-Suárez, A., Ferrand-Esquerré, S., Borrás-Cabacés, T., & Purroy-Aritzeta, I. (2013). El doble estigma de la mujer consumidora de drogas: Estudio cualitativo sobre un Grupo de Auto Apoyo de mujeres con problemas de abuso de sustancias. *Alternativas, 20*, 9–22.

Natera, G., Tiburcio, M., García, E., Valeriano, Y., & Bernal, P. (2007). Desafíos para la implementación de un programa de intervención relacionado con el consumo de alcohol en comunidades indígenas. In S. L. Echeverria & V.C. Carrascoza (Compiladoras), L. E. San Vicente (Ed.), *Prevención y Tratamiento de Conductas Adictivas* (pp. 183–202). Editorial: Grupo ayr. ISBN: 978-970-32-4954-1.

Navarrete, F. (2008). Los pueblos indígenas de México: CDI, 2008. 141. Pueblos Indígenas del México Contemporáneo.

Oficina de las Naciones Unidas contra las Drogas y el Delito (UNODC). (2020). World health report 2020. Booklets, United Nations.

Pozas, A., & Ricardo. (1957). *El alcoholismo y la organización social. La Palabra y el Hombre, núm. 2, pp. 19–26.* Universidad Veracruzana.

Romer, M. (2003). Mujeres indígenas migrantes y sus experiencias urbanas. *Antropología. Revista Interdisciplinaria Del INAH, 70*, 65–74. Recuperado a partir de https://revistas.inah.gob.mx/index.php/antropologia/article/view/3037

Setién-García, C. (2020). El uso del término στίγμα (stigma) y su tradición latina en la literatura cristiana primitiva. *Revista de estudios Latinos, 20*, 71–90.

Sweetnam, D., & Morrissette, P. (2018). Alcohol abuse recovery through the lens of Manitoban First Nations and Aboriginal women: A qualitative study. *Journal of Ethnicity in Substance Abuse, 17*(3), 237–254.

Tiburcio Sainz, M. (2009). *Adaptación de un modelo de intervención para familiares de usuarios de alcohol en una comunidad indígena.* Tesis doctoral, Universidad Nacional Autónoma de México.

Vázquez, F., Camacho, J., & Díaz, E. (2022). Estrés y alcoholismo en un pueblo indígena del municipio de Jalpa de Méndez, Tabasco. https://www.researchgate.net/profile/Jose-Lopez-Cocotle/publication/362318059_Consumo_de_alcohol_en_adolescentes_de_una_secundaria_del_Estado_de_Tabasco_Mexico/links/62f1271288b83e7320bb443c/Consumo-de-alcohol-en-adolescentes-de-una-secundaria-del-Estado-de-Tabasco-Mexico.pdf#page=39

Vega, L., Rendón, A., Gutiérrez, R., Villatoro, J., Vargas, A., Juárez, A., & Trejo, S. (2015). *Estudio sobre patrones de consumo de sustancias psicoactivas en población indígena residente y originaria de la ciudad de México.* INP-IAPA.

Villatoro Velázquez, J. A., Reséndiz-Escobar, E., Mujica Salazar, A., Breton Cirett, M., Cañas-Martínez, V., Soto-Hernández, I., Fregoso-Itto, E., Fleis-Bautista, C., Medina-Mora, M. E., Gutiérrez-Reyes, J., Franco-Nuñez, A., Romero-Martínez, M., & Mendoza-Alvarado, L. (2017). Encuesta Nacional de Consumo de Drogas, Alcohol y Tabaco 2016-2017. Instituto Nacional de Psiquiatría Ramón de la Fuente Muñiz, INPRFM, Instituto de Salud Pública, Comisión Nacional contra las Adicciones,

Weisner, C., & Schmidt, L. (1992). Disparidades de género en el tratamiento de los problemas relacionados con el alcohol. *JAMA, 268*(14), 1872–1876. https://doi.org/10.1001/jama.1992.03490140080039

Wilsnack, R. W., Vogeltanz, N. D., Wilsnack, S. C., Harris, T. R., Ahlström, S., Bondy, S., Csémy, L., Ferrence, R., Ferris, J., Fleming, J., Graham, K., Greenfield, T., Guyon, L., Haavio-Mannila, E., Kellner, F., Knibbe, R., Kubicka, L., Loukomskaia, M., Mustonen, H., Nadeau, L., Narusk, A., Neve, R., Rahav, G., Spak, F., Teichman, M., Trocki, K., Webster, I., & Weiss, S. (2000). Gender differences in alcohol consumption and adverse drinking consequences: cross-cultural patterns. *Addiction, 95*(2), 251–265. https://doi.org/10.1046/j.1360-0443.2000.95225112.x

Chapter 17
Addictive Behaviors, Gender, and Stigma: Contributions to the Understanding of the Portuguese Case

Sandra Mendes, Sara Melo, and Idalina Machado

17.1 Introduction

Addictive behaviors and dependencies have been the subject of intense debate in social and human sciences, being analyzed by sociology, anthropology, and social work. The literature in these disciplinary areas, although it has focused on addictions and dependencies, has been scarce regarding the analysis of the impact of stigma associated with these conditions, especially when considering the gender dimension. Stigma, understood as an attribute that socially disqualifies an individual or group, affects not only how individuals with addictive behaviors are seen but also how they perceive and live their dependencies. The gender dimension, understood as intersectionality, adds a complex layer to this issue, as, on the one hand, men and women experience stigma differently, and on the other, they have distinct trajectories concerning their dependencies. This reflection aims to address these intersections and contribute to a broader view on the subject, based on the observation of the latest data published in the European Drug Report (EUDA, 2024), with results referring to the Portuguese reality in the years 2022 and 2023, in terms of use of psychoactive substances, as well as the data contained in the V National Survey on the Consumption of Psychoactive Substances in the General Population, Portugal 2022 Final Report, edited by ICAD (Balsa et al., 2023), the 2022 Annual Report—The Country's Situation in Terms of Alcohol (ICAD, 2023a), and the 2022 Annual Report—The Country's Situation in Terms of Drugs and Drug Addiction (ICAD, 2023b).

The authors intended to analyze how addictive behaviors and dependencies on legal and illegal psychoactive substances are influenced and shaped by stigma and gender and how the drug decriminalization policy in Portugal, dated 2001, can be

S. Mendes (✉) · S. Melo · I. Machado
Higher Institute of Social Work of Porto, Porto, Portugal
e-mail: sandra.mendes@isssp.pt; sara.melo@isssp.pt; idalina.machado@isssp.pt

T. Mota Ronzani (ed.), *Social Stigma and Drug Use*,
https://doi.org/10.1007/978-3-031-94813-8_17

interpreted considering these concepts. Anthroposociological theories were mobilized to explain the relationships between stigma, gender, and the use of psychoactive substances, proposing strategies for reducing stigma and incorporating the need for gender perspective in public policies.

17.2 Definition of Addictive Behaviors and Dependencies in a Liquid Modernity

17.2.1 Contributions from Classical Sociology

Addictive behaviors can be defined as repetitive and compulsive actions that, despite bringing negative consequences, are maintained by the individual due to a sensation of pleasure, relief, or necessity. Dependencies, in turn, can be translated as a relationship of psychological or physical subordination to a specific substance or behavior, which leads to a loss of internal control and persistence in use, regardless of its consequences.

Giddens (2002) and Bauman (2000) highlight the relationship between modernity (or post-modernity) and the intensification of addictive behaviors. In contemporary Western (or post-modern) society, marked by excessive consumption, resulting from the savagery of the capitalist market and by the incessant search for pleasure and quick gratifications, addictive behaviors can emerge from states of individual alienation, experiences of anomie, as well as responses to social pressures.

Bauman (2000) discusses the concept of *liquid modernity* marked by fluidity, uncertainty, and transience, typical of a constantly changing reality, contrasting it with the solid modernity of previous generations, where institutions, values, and social ties emerged with greater stability and predictability. In liquid modernity, the liquidity and volatility of relationships, identities, and commitments shape not only lifestyles but also consumption patterns, behaviors, and attitudes, marked by impulsivity in the pursuit of pleasure and immediate satisfaction, reflecting the eagerness to fill the sense of emptiness in the search for identity. It is in this logic of liquid modernity, marked by ephemeral consumption, centered on the speed of experience to the detriment of duration, that psychoactive substances can be understood, namely in the desire for relief, immediate satisfaction, pleasure, or alienation, in the experimentation of a transitory "self."

The concept of transience that Bauman (2000) proposes allows us to understand the consumption of legal and illegal psychoactive substances with different purposes and motivations: i) whether they are recreational motivations (instant pleasure and alienation), ii) whether they are motivations connected to the response of the fragmentation of the "self" and individualism, iii) whether they are motivations guided by the search for an identity that needs to be (re)signified or as a means of expression.

Dissatisfaction, as a product of this modernity, is reflected in individual compensations, both in the enjoyment of experiences and in material consumption, which function as palliative agents to deal with a reality perceived as chaotic and difficult to attribute meaning to.

Understanding the use of psychoactive substances (legal and illegal) requires an inter- and transdisciplinary approach, being certain that some contributions from classical sociology are a sine qua non condition, especially for understanding deviant behavior (from the norm established by a majority) as adaptive behavior.

To guide our lives with minimum security, our culture provides a system of values and norms that structure our ways of acting, thinking, feeling, and being in the world. This fact allows us to know how to act in a specific situation. This happens due to the internalization of our reference group's cultural norms and values, that is, through our socialization, the primary control mechanism that leads us to act under what is established.

However, no one consistently acts according to standardized norms and values. All of us, at some point or in a particular situation, deviate in some way from the cultural standard. Another aspect to consider is that not all behaviors that deviate from conventional norms translate into deviant behaviors. Thus, we can talk about non-conformity in the face of a behavior that, despite deviating from conventional norms, is, to some extent, tolerated by the population. This is the case, for example, of an individual who arrives late for a medical appointment. A behavior is considered deviant when it is perceived by the general (or majority) population as an intolerable behavior, such as the abusive consumption of psychoactive substances. The forces and processes that contribute to conformity constitute social control. As previously mentioned, socialization is the primary control mechanism.

Individuals develop self-control or internal control by internalizing norms and values, allowing them to act according to what is established. In addition to norms, individuals internalize the implied formal and informal sanctions, reinforcing conformity.

External social control constitutes the secondary control mechanism. This can be formal or informal. Both formal and informal control are associated with a system of sanctions. Sanctions can be positive or negative depending on the intended objective. If the goal is to reinforce a positive behavior, the sanction consists of a reward. If the goal is to dissuade the individual from a negative behavior, the sanction translates into a punishment. In the case of sanctions being applied by the general population, such as group distancing, we speak of informal social control. Sanctions can also be of various natures: physical, economic, social, and spiritual. Whether in the case of deviance or crime, social control derives from self-control and informal social control. A few formal instances can lead individuals to act according to norms, especially when these norms do not correspond to their reference group's values and norms.

It should be noted that acts cannot be considered deviant in themselves. Consuming alcohol at meals, for example, is an act that can be accepted at home, at a dinner with friends, or a family lunch in a restaurant. Whether or not it is a deviant behavior depends on the time, space, audience, and individual. Therefore, deviance is relative. The important thing is not the act but the audience. A behavior can be considered deviant in front of one audience and not in front of another. An act can be considered a crime in one place or society and not in another.

Durkheim was one of the first sociologists to focus on deviance and social control. His works, *The Rules of Sociological Method* (1995), *The Division of Labor in Society* (1989), and *Suicide* (1996), are a reference in this matter. For the author, deviance is a normal and necessary dimension in society. From his work, Durkheim (1966) argues that society directly influences individuals' behavior, especially in moments of anomie—states of social disorganization where norms and values lose their strength. The author demonstrates that social factors, different degrees of social integration of certain groups, and social regulation can influence deviant behaviors, such as the abusive consumption of psychoactive substances. Variables such as family situation, economic status, religion, sex, and age offer distinct conditions of social integration. In the context of dependencies, the lack of social ties and explicit norms can result in addictive behaviors as a form of adaptation or response to social crises. In settings where there is little social cohesion or confused normativity, addictive behaviors can emerge as forms of escape or compensation for the lack of a sense of belonging. This perspective is relevant to understanding the relationship between marginalized social environments and increased risk behaviors.

On the other hand, Becker (1963) presents the labeling theory, which postulates that deviance is not inherent to an act but rather a consequence of the application of social rules by others. Chemical dependency and other addictive behaviors are often the result of social labeling, where certain groups are stigmatized and marginalized due to their behaviors. Becker (1963) argues that the labeling process generates a cycle of stigmatization, where the individual begins to internalize the deviant role assigned by society, reinforcing behaviors that maintain dependency. This concept is important for analyzing how labels affect the identity of people who use drugs and alcohol, influencing their chances of recovery and social reintegration.

Thirdly, Bourdieu's (2010) concept of *habitus* provides a valuable lens for analyzing how the consumption of psychoactive substances is incorporated and normalized in specific social practices. From the author's perspective, *habitus* is a set of internalized dispositions that guide the practices and perceptions of individuals based on their social position and accumulated experiences. In the setting of addictive behaviors with substances (legal or illegal), the concept of *habitus* proves helpful in understanding how substance use is influenced by factors such as social class, culture, and social capital. For example, the use of alcohol or drugs can be seen as acceptable behavior or even valued in certain social circles. In contrast, in others, it is strongly condemned, which allows us to understand how consumption and dependency are shaped by social and cultural factors rather than being just a matter of individual choice.

17.2.2 The Concept of Stigma and Its Relevance in Understanding the Consumption of Psychoactive Substances

Stigma, widely discussed by Goffman (1963), refers to a devaluation process of individuals or groups possessing deviant characteristics or behaviors. In the analysis of addictive behaviors with the use of psychoactive substances, the *stigma* can be understood as a factor that exacerbates social marginalization and hinders access to treatments and support networks. This fact also serves to highlight why policies, services, and other community agents of the scientific community and civil society should abandon the concepts "drug user," "junkie," and "addicts" (when referring to People who use drugs), which can be considered archaic and deeply stigmatizing terms (recognizing the continuous use of these terms by the legal area). The language used to describe people who use drugs is far from neutral—it shapes public perception, reinforces institutional power, and influences the self-esteem of individuals.

In addition to Goffman (1963), Foucault (1987) contributes to this discussion by exploring how social norms and discursive practices shape what is considered "normal" and "pathological." Foucault (1987) questions the role of social and medical institutions in defining and controlling deviant behaviors, including dependencies. The author explores how social control and disciplining institutions shape the behavior of individuals. Addictive behaviors or dependency (or abusive consumption of Psychoactive Substances), seen through the Foucauldian lens, are understood not only as a medical pathology but as a social construction where norms are applied to regulate behaviors considered deviant. The author emphasizes the role of medical discourse and psychiatric institutions in defining what is normal or pathological, contributing to the stigmatization of dependents. Through Foucault (1987), we can analyze how power is manifested through control mechanisms, such as public health campaigns and rehabilitation programs, which often perpetuate unequal power relations and reinforce stigmas, especially when they do not consider gender differences and the cultural particularities of the individuals affected. Illich (1976) similarly warned that institutionalized language, especially in medicine, can dehumanize and disempower individuals, advocating instead for more humane forms of expression that foster autonomy and mutual care. Following this idea, we can understand the need to change how we talk about people who use drugs and drug use, for example, (i) through the use of a person-first language that recognizes the person as the person who uses drugs instead of "drug user" or "addict"; (ii) the use of respectful language that shows care and concern, rather than judgment; (iii) the use of linguistic codes that acknowledges and promotes the fact that harm reduction and recovery is a reality and can be seen different for everyone. As advocated by Bernstein (1971, 2001), language operates through social codes that either include or exclude, depending on one's class, cultural capital, and institutional alignment.

17.2.3 The Gender Perspective in Dependencies

Gender is currently recognized as an empirical variable of extreme importance in understanding many aspects of human behavior. However, despite its current use in various scientific domains, it often lacks adequate awareness of its conceptual and social importance. The terms "sex" and "gender" are frequently used interchangeably (Gould & Kern-Daniels, 1977), contributing to the misunderstanding of the assumptions brought by Biology and Social Sciences in various topics that are supposedly addressed "from a gender perspective." If, on the one hand, common sense tends to conceive gender as a property of individuals, the fact is that the progressive abandonment of biological determinism by Social Sciences researchers has led to the understanding of it as a collective and socially constructed product, a structuring element of social relations (Amâncio, 1994; Nogueira, 2001).

Feminist theories are distinct from other theoretical perspectives in that they are centered on women, distinguished by their interdisciplinary approach, and actively promote ways to achieve social justice. Three fundamental questions shape feminist theory: (1) "What is so special about women?" (2) "Why is the social world as it is?" and (3) "How can we change and improve the social world to make it a fairer place for women and all people?" (Ritzer, 2008).

Feminist theorists have also begun to question the differences between women, including how race, class, ethnicity, and age intersect with gender. In short, feminist theory is essentially concerned with the issue of giving voice to women and highlighting the various ways in which women have contributed to society (Ritzer & Goodman, 2003).

Although not all gender studies are feminist by nature (Chafetz, 1999), it is imperative to recognize that these have provided the most excellent foundations and theoretical innovations for gender studies in general (Järviluoma et al., 2003) by determining the importance of gender as a central dimension of human life, alongside other variables such as class and race that are transversal to it.

Symbolic interactionism has influenced a series of feminist theories: role theory, socialization theory, sociolinguistics, psychosociology, and sociology, which root their explanations in language and communication. The body of work theorizes that gender inequality is sustained because men dominate conversations. At the same time, women use verbal and body language in a way that weakens their abilities to be assertive. Labeling theory is a descendant of symbolic interactionism and is also used by feminist theories. Gender is reproduced because social scripts for task performance are specifically associated with one gender. As people go about these tasks, they perform gender roles (e.g., domestic work).

In what is considered one of the benchmark statements on gender from a constructionist perspective, West and Zimmerman (1987) conceive it not as a property of individuals but as a property that emerges from social interaction and that varies according to the interaction context in question: men and women act in always specific contexts and perform gender systematically, at all times and in all contexts. The interpretive grids of this paradigm, as advocated, in addition to being currently the most common approaches to the study of gender, represent an important advance in recognizing the importance of personal meanings as an organizational structure of individuals' daily lives. Being interactive and social, gender can be better theorized as a verb than as a noun, as it does not exist as a set of fixed roles established by culture or society, nor as a set of stable personality traits, but rather as a dynamic repertoire of meanings that is activated by individuals interacting with their social environments.

The gender perspective is essential to understand how addictive behaviors and dependencies are experienced and perceived differently, for example, by men and women. The social construction of gender imposes norms on masculinity and femininity that directly influence the way we relate to substances and addictive behaviors.

Butler (2011) argues that gender is a performative construction that establishes individual expectations and behavioral norms. These expectations influence, for example, how men and women are stigmatized for their abusive consumption of psychoactive substances, legal or illegal. For example, women who display addictive behaviors face greater social stigma due to the violation of traditional femininity norms, while men may face stigmas related to virility and emotional control. Following this, Connell and Messerschmidt (2016), in their revisit to the concept of *hegemonic masculinity*, highlight how risk behaviors, including substance abuse, are often associated with an idealized construction of masculinity. For the authors, hegemonic masculinity represents a dominant social construction that associates "being a man" with attributes such as strength, self-sufficiency, and resistance to vulnerability. Although recognizing hegemonic masculinity as dynamic, with internal contradictions and possibilities of movement toward gender democracy, this construction results in risky behaviors, such as excessive use of alcohol and other psychoactive substances, often naturalized and/or reinforced as part of the construction of this masculinity. This may explain different consumption patterns between men and women and how both genders seek treatment or deal with their consumption. Literature has shown that men tend to face more difficulties in seeking social or medical help, just as trans women tend to face greater difficulties in accessing treatment.

Authors such as Campbell (2000) and Ettorre (1992) also explore the intersectionality of gender, addiction, and stigma, showing how women, especially those from marginalized social groups, face significant barriers in treatment contexts due to gender biases. Rosenbaum (1981) showed that women who used heroin as a substance of consumption, unlike men, ended up using heroin in relational contexts and responded to emotional factors related to histories of trauma or abusive relationships. The experience of stigma is also apparently more intense, encompassing additional challenges. For example, in seeking treatment, women, especially when they were mothers, experienced difficulties/resistance due to fear of losing custody of their children.

The author presents as social and institutional barriers, particularly for women using heroin: (i) stigmatization and exacerbated moral judgment, as cultural expectations that associate the female role with care and protection, drug use appears in an antagonistic and fracturing position of these norms, resulting in a double stigmatization, that is, on the one hand, drug users and, on the other, women who inadequately perform their role as mothers ("bad mothers"); (ii) challenges related to motherhood, namely the fear of losing their children because, as studied by the author, child protection services considered drug use as a sign of neglect and a risky and dangerous environment for minors, leading to their institutionalization and the rupture of family ties; (iii) financial and relational dependence on partners, enhancing cycles of dependence or co-dependence and abusive relationships; (iv) limited access to treatment services aimed at women, since responses to substance use were, according to the author, historically thought for a male audience, disregarding specific needs of women, among which support related to reproductive health issues, traumas related to sexual violence and childcare; (v) vulnerability to violence and exploitation, as women who use substances such as heroin are often associated with situations of high vulnerability and physical, psychological, and sexual violence, resulting from abusive relationships or in exchange for food or substance for consumption (by partners or traffickers) (Rosenbaum, 1981).

17.3 The Portuguese Reality Regarding Drugs Today

17.3.1 Contextualization of Drug Policies in Portugal

In 2001, Portugal became a pioneer by decriminalizing the personal consumption of all drugs. Decriminalization does not mean legalization but a change in approach to drugs, shifting consumption from a criminal problem to a public health issue. Instead of prison, people who use drugs, when identified by law enforcement agents, are referred to dissuasion commissions, composed of psychologists, jurists, and social workers, for evaluation and guidance. This policy is based on the idea that addiction is a condition to be treated, not punished. The Decree-Laws no. 30/2000, 130-A/2001, and 183/2001 came to decriminalize the consumption of psychoactive substances and complement Portugal's National Drug Strategy 1999, reinforcing the principle of pragmatism and humanism by allowing the creation of Risk and Harm Reduction programs. As Borges et al. (2023) recall, this National Strategy for the Fight against Drugs saw its emergence in 1998 on the initiative of the Deputy Prime Minister when creating the Commission for the National Strategy to Combat Drugs, "with the aim of supporting the government in creating a public policy for the area of addictive behaviors and dependencies, at the time designated as 'fight against drugs,' due to the eternal bellicosity associated with the fight against drugs" (p. 291).

This model, focusing on prevention, reintegration, training, research, harm reduction, and combating trafficking, significantly reduced HIV infection rates and deaths related to overdoses and advocates for reducing the stigma associated with addictive behavior and dependencies. However, social reactions, the role of stigma, and cultural norms continue to influence how the general population applies and perceives this policy.

As we have seen previously with Durkheim (1989, 1995, 1996), social integration and regulation are fundamental for societal cohesion. The decriminalization of drug use in Portugal can be seen as an effort to reinforce social integration, offering people who use drugs an alternative to incarceration, which would further marginalize them. Instead, Portuguese policies seek to reintegrate people who use drugs into society through treatment programs, social support, and harm reduction and minimization programs.

Portugal's approach also reflects an attempt to improve social regulation, providing clear guidelines for treating and handling substance use replacing criminal punishment with public health strategies. This can be seen as an attempt to reduce social anomie, which, according to Durkheim (1989, 1996) and revisited by Merton (1957), is one of the factors leading to deviance and, potentially, substance abuse, as it posits that participation in behaviors such as drug use represents an individual-level response to successive failures in the conventional world (in education, employment, and material gains) and the subsequent rejection of this world.

Becker's (1963) *labeling theory* allows us to understand how the change in drug policies in Portugal can reduce the effects of labeling. Before decriminalization, drug use was strongly labeled as criminal behavior, associated with marginalization and social stigmatization. With this policy, Portugal tried to deconstruct this label, addressing people who use drugs as people who need medical and social care, not crime and punishment.

The shift from the label of "criminal" to "people who use" represents a conscious strategy to reduce stigma and facilitate rehabilitation. However, labeling persists in some sectors of society, and decriminalization faces challenges to be entirely accepted, especially when it comes to deeply ingrained social stigmas about drug use. This fact contributes to the difficulty of making well-structured, more humanistically pragmatic policies.

Decriminalization and treatment programs and harm reduction aim, theoretically, to treat all people who use drugs equally. However, as we saw through Bourdieu (2010), available resources, access to treatment, and rehabilitation opportunities can vary according to the social position of individuals and the volume of capital (economic, social, cultural, and symbolic) they possess. For example, individuals from favored social classes may have greater access to quality treatments. In contrast, those from more vulnerable social classes face additional challenges due to a lack of economic and cultural capital. The *habitus*, the acquired dispositions, can influence how different groups perceive and engage with the social and health services offered by the public system.

Even with decriminalization, stigma, as discussed by Goffman (1963), still plays a crucial role in drug policies in Portugal. Decriminalization tried to change public perception about drug use. However, stigma persists, especially against people who use drugs, such as heroin, cocaine, or crack, and oppressed groups, such as women and nonbinary people. These substances continue to be associated with contexts of poverty and marginalization, which affect how policies are implemented. Canêdo

(2023) and Pires (2025) have already pointed out that Portugal still lacks a gender perspective in drug policy.

People who use drugs (essentially those whose social position is, from the outset, more disadvantaged) and who accept treatment still face stigmatization processes, both in social and health systems. Discrimination can occur, for example, in work environments and interactions with health professionals and social workers, making the change process difficult. Despite the policy change that occurred more than twenty years ago in Portugal, stigma is a persistent barrier that limits the effectiveness of reforms and persists beyond legislative change.

Douglas's (1992) analysis of the cultural construction of risk is relevant to understanding how different substances are viewed in Portugal, even after the decriminalization. The distinction between "acceptable" and "unacceptable" substances reflects cultural values that are still strong in Portuguese society. For example, alcohol, which is culturally integrated and accepted, is often seen less negatively than illicit drugs. These cultural distinctions affect how risk behaviors are assessed and how prevention policies are formulated. The social acceptance of certain addictive behaviors (such as alcohol consumption) versus the condemnation of others reflects how risk is culturally constructed and negotiated in different social groups.

Decriminalization does not eliminate control but shifts it from a penal sphere to a medical, social, and public health sphere. The "dissuasion commissions" are an example of how the State continues to exercise power and control over drug users, albeit in a less punitive way. Foucault (1987) suggests that power is present in all forms of social regulation, and the discourse on public health can be a way to normalize deviant behaviors. Portuguese policies attempt to "normalize" people who use drugs by encouraging them to seek treatment and adopt behaviors considered healthier and less harmful. However, this normalization still occurs within a context of surveillance and monitoring, where people are observed and evaluated in terms of compliance with social norms regardless of their setting or background.

The gender perspective, discussed by authors such as Butler (2011) and Connell (2008), is also essential to understand that decriminalization offers a gender-neutral framework. However, in practice, women who use drugs face specific stigmas. They are often judged more harshly than men due to traditional norms of femininity, which include responsibility for the family and childcare. Specific policies that address the needs of women, such as treatment services aimed at mothers or victims of gender violence, are still insufficient in Portugal. This reality reveals the need for a more intersectional approach, which considers that gender, social class, and other variables influence how addictions are treated and socially viewed.

Pires (2025) has highlighted this concern in her research about the structural conditions of harm reduction services in Portugal, finding that most of the services that participate in the study seem not to be prepared to answer the specific needs of vulnerable groups, such as women, migrants, and the LGBTQIA+ community. Pires (2025) refers to the existence of institutional barriers and bureaucracy and the lack of an effective articulation with other fundamental dimensions of the human being, such as mental health, housing, or social protection. More financial investments to develop services adapted to these vulnerable groups must be a priority, with professionals trained in intersectionality, diversity, and human rights appointed to the study.

The Portuguese decriminalization policy is an attempt to reformulate stigma and address addiction from a public health perspective, but it also reveals the limits and challenges of implementing these policies.

17.3.2 Empirical Illustration of the Portuguese Reality from a Gender Perspective

In 2024, the Institute for Addictive Behaviors and Dependencies (ICAD) released relevant data on addictive behaviors in Portugal in its *2022 Annual Report—The Country's Situation Regarding Alcohol* (ICAD, 2023a) and *2022 Annual Report—The Country's Situation Regarding Drugs and Drug Addiction* (ICAD, 2023b) and through the *V National Survey on the Consumption of Psychoactive Substances in the General Population, Portugal 2022; Final Report,*[1] (Balsa et al., 2023) which reveal distinct trends in consumption and treatment. Men continue to represent the majority of illicit drug users. In 2022, over 80% of drug users seeking treatment in Portugal were men, especially in the age group between 40 and 59 years. These data indicate that men are more prone to regular and problematic use of illicit substances, such as cocaine and heroin.

One of the main results observed is the increase in alcohol consumption, especially among women, with a growth that almost quadrupled in cases of *binge drinking* (excessive consumption in a short period) between 2012 and 2022, corresponding, respectively, to 1 glass and 4 glasses. The increase in consumption among women in Portugal reveals changes in cultural norms about alcohol use, which were traditionally more tolerated among men. Accompanying the increase in consumption among women in Portugal is the increase in the evaluation of abusive consumption and alcohol dependence through the *Alcohol Use Disorders Identification Test.* We found that in 2012, the high-risk/harmful and dependence evaluation was at 0.1% and 0.8%, respectively. In 2022, although the level of dependence is at 0.3%, the high risk/harmful evaluated in women that same year increased to 2.5%. This pattern reflects the cultural construction of risk, as proposed by Douglas (1992), where the perception of consumption by women is still laden with stigma, which may hinder their access to appropriate treatments. The persistence of stigma shows that social policies need to continue to deconstruct gender prejudices. Indeed, for Douglas (1992), the notion of risk is social, cultural, and symbolically constructed

[1]According to the V National Survey on the Use of Psychoactive Substances in the General Population, Portugal 2022, Final Report, "the universe considered in the study is the population residing in Portugal between the ages of 15 and 74. The sample design follows a multi-stage, stratified design by clusters, with the selection of primary units (municipalities) and secondary units (statistical subsections) randomly proportional. The selection of the final observation units—the individuals—is carried out by systematic random sampling in the selection of households and using random number tables for the selection process of individuals within the household. The fieldwork resulted in 12,038 valid interviews. The results are weighted by sex, age group, and NUT II to ensure the representativeness defined in the theoretical sample for these three parameters. The calculations were made for a confidence level of 95%" (Balsa et al., 2023, p. 13).

by mechanisms that serve to differentiate the pure from danger and, more relevantly, to distinguish the "self" from the "others" (who have risk behaviors). For the author, risk is described as a moral and political construction that provides the basis for an appropriate cultural code in which risk is associated with guilt. Being a person at risk means daring to transgress cultural and symbolic boundaries and becoming a person in danger, or as referred to by Parkin (2013, p. 17), "a body to be feared."

Although data by gender or sex are not public regarding the primary motivations of the Portuguese population to drink alcohol, it is still relevant to indicate that, with 40.6% of responses, the population agrees that they drink "because it tastes good" (pleasure). As for the motivations for abstinence, lack of interest in drinking (50.2%) and health concerns (44.5%) stand out. We highlight the 21.9% of respondents who considered pregnancy or breastfeeding very important as a motivation for abstinence, while 58.7% considered this variable as not important at all. This result deserves some attention regarding the high risk of stigma toward pregnant women and the barrier to accessing treatment and support because of the internalized and social stigma.

Regarding the search for treatment for problems related to alcohol consumption, in 2022, this has been shown to have increased. The data show 4867 admissions for the start of treatment, with 1546 readmissions and 3321 new patients. As referred to in the *2022 Annual Report—The Country's Situation Regarding Alcohol* (ICAD, 2023), "outpatient users (+4%) increased for the second consecutive year" (p. 13), which may represent a greater recognition of the need for specialized support.

Also, the European Drug Report 2024,[2] published by the *European Union Drug Agency (EUDA)*, highlights distinct consumption patterns between men and women in Portugal, with significant implications for formulating social policies and interventions with gender sensitivity.

The analysis of Portuguese data reveals that drug consumption and the associated consequences vary according to gender, influencing both usage patterns and impacts on health and social behavior.[3]

[2] According to the EUDA (2024), the data collection sources are multiple and varied and have different territorial origins, depending on the provision of information from national partners and specific projects at the city territorial level. National surveys are carried out "based on representative and probabilistic samples. The surveys consist of self-reported data on current and past drug use, personal characteristics, and knowledge and attitudes towards drugs or other related topics (for example, health topics)." [authors' translation] In https://www.euda.europa.eu/data/stats2024/methods/gps_en.

[3] Both the European Drug Report (EUDA, 2024) and the ICAD Report (ICAD, 2023) assume the difficulty in obtaining representative data of the different profiles of substance users, as well as, in the case of the European report, legal and political constraints related to different countries, which may contribute to an underrepresentation of the results, hence the caution in reading. The authors of this chapter analyzed data from both reports, finding inconsistencies explained by the methodologies used and the target audience affected by the data collection instruments. However, they still believe that the results presented expose the trends of the situation regarding the behaviors of legal and illegal psychoactive substances in Portugal, making their analysis valid in this work.

In the Portuguese context, and according to the *V National Survey on Consumption of Psychoactive Substances in the General Population, Portugal 2022, Final Report* (Balsa et al., 2023), men continue to be the primary consumers of drugs, especially among those aged between 40 and 59 years, who represent the majority of overdose fatalities. Women, on the other hand, have shown a significant increase in alcohol consumption (as we have seen) and polydrug use (use of multiple substances simultaneously), a phenomenon that may be related to changes in social norms and use contexts, including their increasing visibility in social and professional environments previously dominated by men.

According to the same survey, tobacco consumption has shown a progressive increase in its lifetime prevalence record. In 2022, the data pointed out that 48% of the total population surveyed reported this consumption throughout their life, 36% in the consumption patterns of female individuals, with prominence in the age group of 35 to 44 years, and 61% in male individuals, with prominence in the age group from 45 to 54 years old. The average age of starting tobacco use in 2022 was 16 years for males and 17 years for females.

Regarding the use of sedatives, tranquilizers, or hypnotics, in 2022, this behavior was more prevalent among females, 16.9%, compared to 9% of males. The data shows a trend toward a decrease in this consumption from 2012 to 2022. The profile of people who consume sedatives at any time (throughout life, last 12 months, and last 30 days) differs from other substances consumed, as consumption among women prevails, except in situations of non-medically prescribed sedative use. In this situation, the differences are almost negligible between the sexes (3% throughout life in males and 4.7% throughout life in females). The underlying motivations for consumption highlight the search for a way to relax, being sick, and being depressed. Trying to forget problems or seeking states of higher spirits are also pointed out as relevant motivations by people who consume this type of substance.

Regarding the consumption of opioid analgesics, the consumption profile does not differ much from that of sedatives. The prevalence of consumption of these analgesics is higher in females (8.4%) compared to males (6.5%). The same reality remains in the type of consumption of opioid analgesics with non-medical use. 2.5% of females use this type throughout life, contrasting with 2.2% of males. The primary motivations pointed out for the consumption of this substance are related to states of illness (52%), relaxation (5.8%), and obtaining physical energy for work (4.2%), followed by depression (4%) and obtaining physical energy for leisure activities (2.8%).

The lifetime prevalence for any illicit substance, in the last twenty years, for women went from 7% in 2001 to 9.6% in 2022, while consumption in men went from 18.2% to 21.9%.

In 2022, according to the *2024 European Drug Report*, the prevalence of cannabis use is lower for women (1.2%) than for men (4.5%). Considering the data from 2016 (5.1%) collected by EUDA and the data from 2022 (2.8%), there is a decrease in people who have reported consuming this substance in the last 12 months. According to the final report of the *V National Survey on the Consumption of Psychoactive Substances in the General Population, Portugal 2022* (Balsa et al.,

2023), 51% of the consumers surveyed reported preferring to consume cannabis in herb form, 47.9% in resin, and less than 1% in oil. Regarding the most frequent places of consumption, the data provided does not categorize the answers by gender or sex. The general population surveyed refers to consuming frequently on a street, square, or garden (13.6%), 7.2% refers to consuming frequently at home, and 4.8% in bars and nightclubs. The non-categorization by gender does not allow us to show that women seek less visible or public places to carry out their consumption. This reality is transversal for all substances analyzed. Similarly, 10.7% refer to consuming frequently on vacation, 8.4% alone, and 7.4% when unemployed or without work. The data indicates that cannabis is a substance consumed in a recreational context (10.3% refers to consuming frequently on New Year's Eve, 7.9% at concerts/music festivals, and 5.3% to celebrate the end of classes). The motivations most frequently associated with this consumption are related to curiosity (35%), the need to feel an altered state of consciousness/feeling *high* (33%), and relaxation (20%). The same report (Balsa et al., 2023) states that the three main reasons for the consumption of this substance have remained unchanged since 2001. Risky consumption is always higher in men than in women. The symptoms of dependence on cannabis consumption in the population residing in Portugal decreased in women from 2017 to 2022 (0.4% to 0.2%, respectively).

Regarding cocaine use, according to the *2024 European Drug Report*, the prevalence of this consumption is lower for women (0.1%) than for men (0.3%). Considering the data from 2016 (1.2%) collected by EUDA and the data from 2022 (1.1%), this substance's consumption rate is almost maintained throughout life. The prevalence of lifetime consumption is higher in those aged 15 to 34. Portugal ranks 27th in a comparison of European countries (out of a total of 28), with a prevalence of cocaine use in the last 12 months. According to the final report of the *V National Survey on the Consumption of Psychoactive Substances in the General Population, Portugal 2022* (Balsa et al., 2023), throughout life, 76% of females indicate having been exposed to a low level (one to five times), to the offer of cocaine compared to males corresponding to 73%. Also, at the medium level (6 to 19 times) of exposure to the offer of cocaine, 18% were females, and 16% were males. Regarding high levels (20 times or more) of exposure to the offer of cocaine, males are more representative than females, 11% and 6%, respectively. Regarding the perception of the availability of the substance, 58.5% of females stated they considered it easy or very easy to obtain cocaine within 24 hours.

Regarding heroin use, it is predominantly male and remains almost unchanged, although its prevalence has decreased by a tenth from 2017 (0.5%) to 2022 (0.4%). This decrease was observed in both male (0.8% in 2017 to 0.7% in 2022) and female individuals (0.3% in 2017 to 0.2% in 2022). This type of consumption is concentrated in the older population, compared to the population aged 15 to 34 years; its prevalence in 2022 was 0.1% overall. The contexts of substance use are predominantly the home (27.8% responded frequently), workplace (17.6%), and street, square, or garden (15.3%). Heroin use is more frequent when the user is alone (31.3%), unemployed (27.8%), and during a weekend away from home (23.6%).

Regarding substance intake, 54% of heroin users reported smoking, 29% referred to injection, and 17% to inhalation. In Portugal, with the data from 2021 published in the European Drug Report 2024, men, particularly in the age group of 40 to 59 years, are more affected by overdoses associated with the use of heroin and cocaine. These data suggest that they more frequently engage in risky consumption patterns, including the use of injectable substances, which have severe negative impacts on physical and mental health. An older consumer profile with a long-term consumption trajectory is added to these indicators. According to the same report, Portugal continues to be the country with the fewest overdose deaths, a fact that could be interpreted as being due to its pioneering drug policies. These patterns reinforce the idea that gender stereotypes continue to influence how men and women consume and face drug-related problems. Traditional masculinity is associated with risk behaviors and public consumption, while female consumption, although increasing, is still affected by social stigma, leading to more discreet or hidden consumption practices. Butler's (2011) analysis of gender as a performative construction helps to understand the social pressures that influence the addictive behaviors of men and women. For women, drug use still carries a stronger stigma, especially when it deviates from traditional caregiving roles. This differentiation is reinforced by Goffman's (1963) theory of stigma, which points to exacerbated social judgment in cases where women consume substances in visible contexts, such as parties and work environments. This differential stigmatization may explain why women tend to use more discreet health services and adopt less visible consumption practices. At the same time, men are more prone to visible and socially accepted consumption, such as drinking alcohol in bars. The increase in consumption may be related to social changes and crises (such as the pandemic or economic transformations) that affect social cohesion. Policies that promote psychological support and health services are crucial to strengthen social ties and reduce addictive behaviors. The increase in the number of people seeking treatment or resorting to a harm reduction program may indicate a reduction in the stigma associated with substance use, possibly because of awareness campaigns and policies that decriminalize consumption.

In Portugal, some specific approaches try to consider gender issues related to addictive behaviors and dependencies, but this sensitivity is still developing and faces significant challenges. Some notable initiatives include (a) Gender-Sensitive Prevention and Treatment Programs. The Portuguese National Health System and public and private institutions that have been working on prevention campaigns and treatment programs have begun to consider the specific needs of women, especially regarding alcohol consumption and the use of illicit drugs. The gender-sensitive approach includes—Specialized care for all pregnant women or mothers, aiming to ensure care for both the woman and the baby—Treatment focused on traumas and specific experiences that more often affect women, such as domestic violence or past abuses and other outbreaks of violence; (b) Interventions in Family Contexts, few treatment centers in Portugal offer specialized support that recognizes the family and social responsibilities that may weigh more on women, such as child-rearing. These policies aim to facilitate access to treatment with family support structures, including childcare during therapy sessions; (c) Awareness Campaigns and Stigma Reduction, the ICAD has been conducting campaigns that address the issue of stigma, particularly for women, who often face additional barriers due to social gender expectations. These campaigns aim to educate the public about the reality of female addiction and reduce the prejudice associated with drug use by women. (d) Proactive activism of NGOs and communities regarding gender sensitivity in drug services and social intervention. Despite these initiatives, the inclusion of a gender perspective in the policies on addictive behaviors and dependencies in Portugal is still limited. Many treatment and prevention programs are still developed without fully considering the specificities of women and nonbinary experiences and the different impacts that substance use can have regarding gender singularities. There is a lack of data and studies focused on gender, which hinders the formulation of policies based on specific evidence for women and gender minorities. While there are movements toward more gender-sensitive policies, there is a need for greater intersectionality in approaches, considering not only gender but also factors such as social class, ethnicity, and trauma history. Integrating more detailed data can help create interventions that recognize these complexities. Some authors, such as Pires (2025), pointed out the lack of funded services for addictive behaviors, such as drug and alcohol use, especially in harm reduction responses. Such a reality comes as a barrier to implementing and developing long-term programs according to territorial equity, innovation, and adaptation to the needs of people who use drugs. The recommendation is clear on the need to integrate harm reduction as a strategic approach in the national and local plans of health, use of substances, mental health, housing, and social inclusion. Some services that work with people who use drugs mainly on a harm reduction approach are financed by the State as projects, and where planning for the future and consistent work is limited. The need to change this management model is urgent to transform effective service into recognized programs with adequate budgets to develop innovative responses. Portugal's drug policies and services must be more participative, with active discussions between national entities, NGOs, and the communities. An intersectoral approach is needed to guarantee human and social rights. We should recognize the social determinants but primarily promote them in the everyday lives of people who use drugs. To reach such a reality, the Portuguese State must protect the labor conditions and promote dignity and a stable job to those who work within harm reduction services, social workers, nurses, psychologists, physicians, and other relevant actors acting in drug settings.

17.4 Conclusion

Despite decriminalization, the State maintains normative control through public health measures. Dissuasion commissions exemplify how Foucauldian control remains, albeit in a more humanized form. This control influences how addiction is managed, encouraging treatments that aim to "normalize" behavior.

Social policies have proven effective in reducing mortality and increasing access to treatment but face the challenge of adapting strategies to different groups, especially considering gender variables. The public health-based approach, as opposed to the penal one, has been a key factor in reducing stigma and promoting a culture of prevention, aligning with theoretical suggestions for social integration and the deconstruction of negative labels.

Data from 2024 referring to 2022 show significant progress in Portugal but also highlight the ongoing need for social policies that consider gender and the cultural construction of risk. The success of decriminalization policies and treatment strategies reveals the importance of a holistic and integrative approach, considering both individual factors and social and cultural contexts. However, the apparent lack of investment in this matter, both financially and in terms of human resources and specialized services, should not be overlooked.

The decriminalization policy adopted in Portugal seems to assist in reducing stigma and encouraging treatment, but the data suggest that social structure and gender stereotypes still influence consumption patterns. Public policies must adapt to these differences, offering specific programs for women, including support for family and professional contexts and awareness campaigns that combat stigma.

The focus on polydrug use and the increase in alcohol and other substance use by women underscores the importance of intersectional approaches, which also consider how class and age influence addictive behavior. Interventions must be culturally sensitive and attentive to differences in the trajectories of men and women in the context of consumption and treatment.

This scenario demonstrates the ongoing importance of adapting social policies to dynamic contexts, considering public health norms and the social and cultural constructions that shape addictive behaviors.

References

Amâncio, L. (1994). *Masculino e Feminino. A Construção Social da Diferença*. Edições Afrontamento.

Balsa, C., Vital, C., & Urbano, C. (2023). *Relatório Anual do V Inquérito Nacional ao Consumo de Substâncias Psicoativas na População Geral Portugal 2022. Relatório Final*. SICAD – Serviço de Intervenção nos Comportamentos Aditivos e nas Dependências. https://www.icad.pt/DocumentList/GetFile?id=569&languageId=1

Bauman, Z. (2000). *Liquid modernity*. Polity Press.

Becker, H. (1963). *Outsiders: Studies in the sociology of deviance*. Free Press.

Bernstein, B. (2001). *Volume I: Theoretical studies towards a sociology of language*. Routledge.

Borges, M., Bragança, C., Camilo, A., António, P., Francisco, S., & Oliveira, P. (2023). Planeamento e redução de danos. Um modelo de gestão de prazeres e riscos centrado nas pessoas. In I. Casquilho-Martins & J. Fialho (Eds.), *Planeamento da intervenção social: conceção, ação e avaliação* (pp. 289–308). Almedina.

Bourdieu, P. (2010). *A Distinção. Uma crítica social da faculdade do juízo* (p. 70). Edições.

Butler, J. (2011). *Bodies that matter: On the discursive limits of sex*. Routledge.

Campbell. (2000). *Using women: Gender, drug policy, and social justice*. Routledge.

Canêdo, J. (2023, September 29–30). *MANAS: Contributos bottom-up para a inovação da política de drogas através de respostas à violência de género lideradas por pares*. Comunicação apresentado no SIAP – Pessoas invisíveis ou invisibilizadas? Abrir os olhos ao sistema de saúde. Porto. Disponível em, https://equipocesca.org/wp-content/uploads/2023/11/siap-2023-Porto-ponencia-Joana-Canedo.pdf

Chafetz, J. S. (1999). *Handbook of the sociology of gender*. Kluwer Academic/Plenum Publishers.
Connell, R. W. (2008). *Masculinities*. Policy Press.
Connell, R. W., & Messerschmidt, J. W. (2016). Hegemonic masculinity: Rethinking the concept. *Gender and Society, 19*(6), 829–859.
Decreto-Lei n.° 130-A/2001, de 18 de abril. Diário da República, Série I-A de 2001-04-18. https://diariodarepublica.pt/dr/detalhe/decreto-lei/130-2001-163640
Decreto-Lei n.° 183/2001, de 21 de junho. Diário da República, Série I-A de 2001-06-21. https://diariodarepublica.pt/dr/detalhe/decreto-lei/183-2001-362322
Decreto-Lei n.° 30/2000, de 13 de março. Diário da República, Série I-A de 2000-03-13 https://diariodarepublica.pt/dr/detalhe/decreto-lei/30-2000-410915
Douglas, M. (1992). *Risk and blame: Essays in cultural theory*. Routledge.
Durkheim, E. (1989). *Da divisão do Trabalho Social*. Editorial Presença.
Durkheim, E. (1995). *As Regras do método sociológico*. Editorial Presença.
Durkheim, E. (1996). *O Suicídio*. Editorial Presença.
Ettorre, E. (1992). *Women and substance use*. Springer.
European Monitoring Centre for Drugs and Drug Addiction. (2024). *European drug report 2024: Trends and developments*. https://www.euda.europa.eu/publications/european-drug-report/2024_en
Foucault, M. (1987). *Surveiller et punir: Naissance de la prison*. Gallimard.
Giddens, A. (2002). Modernidade e Identidade..
Goffman, E. (1963). *Stigma. Notes on the Management of Spoiled Identity*. Penguin Books.
Gould, M., & Kern-Daniels, R. (1977). Toward a sociological theory of gender and sex. *The American Sociologist, 12*, 182–189.
Illich, I. (1976). *Medical nemesis: The expropriation of health*. Pantheon Books.
Järviluoma, H., Moisala, P., & Vikko, A. (2003). *Gender and qualitative methods*. Sage.
Merton, R. (1957). Social structure and anomie. *American Sociological Review, 3*(5), 672–682.
Nogueira, C. (2001). *Um novo olhar sobre as relações sociais de género*. Fundação Calouste Gulbenkian.
Parkin, S. (2013). *Habitus and drug using environments. Health, place and lived-experience*. Ashgate Publishing Limited.
Pires, J. (2025). *Reforçar a redução de riscos e minimização de danos em Portugal. Recomendações estratégicas para políticas públicas* [Policy Brief]. R3 Riscos Reduzidos em Rede. Disponível em, https://sites.google.com/view/r3-riscosreduzidosemrede/notícias?authuser=0
Ritzer, G. (2008). *Modern sociological theory*. McGraw-Hill.
Ritzer, G., & Goodman, D. (2003). *Sociological theory*. McGraw-Hill.
Rosenbaum, M. (1981). *Women on Heroin*. Rutgers University Press.
Serviço de Intervenção nos Comportamento Aditivos e nas Dependências: Direção de Serviços de Monitorização e Informação/Divisão de Estatística e Investigação. (2023a). *Relatório Anual 2022 – A Situação do País em Matéria de Álcool*. ICAD – Instituto para os Comportamentos Aditivos e as Dependências. https://www.icad.pt/DocumentList/GetFile?id=604&languageId=1
Serviço de Intervenção nos Comportamento Aditivos e nas Dependências: Direção de Serviços de Monitorização e Informação/Divisão de Estatística e Investigação. (2023b). *Relatório Anual 2022 – A Situação do País em Matéria de Drogas e Toxicodependências*. ICAD – Instituto para os Comportamentos Aditivos e as Dependências. https://www.icad.pt/DocumentList/GetFile?id=604&languageId=1
West, C., & Zimmerman, D. (1987). Doing Gender. *Gender & Society, 2*, 125–151.

Index

A

Accessibility barriers, 189–201
Addictions, 5, 19, 47, 61, 71, 85, 106, 113, 131, 155, 189, 206, 220
Alcohol, 37–39, 47, 49, 61, 75, 101, 129, 137–141, 143–147, 169–171, 173, 175, 189, 195, 199, 207, 219–228

B

Behavioral addictions, 71–80

D

Diagnosis, 6, 20, 62–65, 77–79, 86, 159, 170, 194, 205
Discrimination, 3–5, 8–10, 15, 18, 20–23, 29, 31, 33, 34, 37, 38, 40, 45–47, 50, 53, 59–62, 64, 77, 86, 87, 90, 92–94, 104, 113–120, 125, 126, 130, 138, 142, 145, 156–161, 175, 176, 179, 182, 190, 192, 195–197, 220, 222, 223
Drugs, 4, 16, 33, 45, 61, 97, 113, 126, 137, 154, 170, 220
Drug use, 5, 7, 9, 15–23, 29–41, 46, 47, 49–54, 61, 100, 118, 126–127, 130, 132, 143, 154, 155, 199

F

Families, 5, 10, 21, 22, 34, 35, 38–40, 47, 49–53, 73, 74, 76, 77, 85–87, 93, 98, 102–104, 108, 117–120, 128–132, 142, 143, 147, 156–158, 167–169, 171–174, 176–182, 189, 190, 198, 199, 206–208, 210–216, 221, 223, 224, 226, 227

G

Gender, 10, 16, 18–23, 29–41, 45, 46, 50–54, 65, 74, 86, 98, 99, 115–119, 127, 130–132, 137–139, 141, 143, 145–147, 158, 167–182, 189–201, 205, 215, 220–222

H

Health, 4, 16, 30, 45, 60, 71, 85, 98, 113, 126, 137, 153, 168, 190, 206, 220
HIV, 7, 16, 39, 102, 141, 145–147, 153–161, 205
Homeless people, 32, 34, 35, 191

I

Intersectionality, 10, 15–23, 30, 48, 113, 115–119, 132, 159
Intrafamily violence, 167–182

L

LGBTQIA+ population, 138, 140, 141, 143, 145–147

M

Media, 9, 17, 32, 54, 86, 93, 117, 125–132, 159, 160, 175, 181, 182

T. Mota Ronzani (ed.), *Social Stigma and Drug Use*,
https://doi.org/10.1007/978-3-031-94813-8

O
Online intervention, 85–94

P
Poverty, 19, 29–41, 62, 118, 127, 169, 180, 191, 221
Psychoactive substances, 21, 97, 99, 100, 107, 114, 138, 143, 144, 147, 169–173, 175, 179, 180, 182, 191

S
Social exclusion, 6, 38, 49, 52, 86, 97–110, 115, 119, 126, 129, 141
Social stigma, 9, 49, 50, 115–117, 138, 214, 219, 224
Stigma, 3, 15, 29, 45, 60, 71, 85, 97, 113, 125, 137, 154, 170, 190, 205, 219
Stigma reduction, 7, 158
Substance use, 4, 5, 8, 9, 11, 20, 31, 33, 36, 38–40, 45, 47–52, 54, 63–66, 74, 85, 93, 97–100, 102–110, 113–120, 126, 127, 129–131, 137, 139, 143, 157–159, 167–182, 197, 222, 227

V
Video game addiction, 71–75, 78, 80
Vulnerable groups, 30, 32, 53, 74, 75, 93, 119, 144, 174, 191–193, 206

W
Women, 16, 20–22, 29–41, 46, 48, 50–54, 74, 88–90, 94, 102, 107, 115, 117–119, 130, 131, 137, 141, 142, 144–147, 156, 168, 174–176, 179, 180, 182, 190, 192, 194–201, 215, 219–228

Y
Youth, 98, 99, 137–147, 173

The manufacturer's authorised representative in the EU is Springer Nature Customer Service Centre GmbH, Europaplatz 3, 69115 Heidelberg, Germany. If you have any concerns regarding our products, please contact ProductSafety@springernature.com

Printed and bound by CPI Group (UK) Ltd, Croydon, CR0 4YY
01/10/2026
02225971-0005